Nursing Practice and Healthcare

Nursing Practice and Healthcare

Edited by **Cynthia Wison**

Callisto Reference
New York

Published by Callisto Reference,
106 Park Avenue, Suite 200,
New York, NY 10016, USA
www.callistoreference.com

Nursing Practice and Healthcare
Edited by Cynthia Wison

International Standard Book Number: 978-1-63239-775-1 (Hardback)

Printed in China.

Contents

Preface

This book was inspired by the evolution of our times; to answer the curiosity of inquisitive minds. Many developments have occurred across the globe in the recent past which has transformed the progress in the field.

This book traces the progress of the field of nursing, its practice and associated healthcare. It highlights some of its key concepts and applications. Nursing falls under the branch of healthcare and is mainly referred to as a practice of taking care of families, individuals and communities, so that they maintain or recover to optimum health. The topics included in this book have been contributed by international experts and will provide incredible insights to readers. This book is a compilation of chapters that discuss the most vital aspects and emerging trends in the field of nursing and healthcare. It is appropriate for students seeking detailed information in this area as well as for experts. This text will prove beneficial to nurses, practitioners, students and anyone else interested in this field.

This book was developed from a mere concept to drafts to chapters and finally compiled together as a complete text to benefit the readers across all nations. To ensure the quality of the content we instilled two significant steps in our procedure. The first was to appoint an editorial team that would verify the data and statistics provided in the book and also select the most appropriate and valuable contributions from the plentiful contributions we received from authors worldwide. The next step was to appoint an expert of the topic as the Editor-in-Chief, who would head the project and finally make the necessary amendments and modifications to make the text reader-friendly. I was then commissioned to examine all the material to present the topics in the most comprehensible and productive format.

I would like to take this opportunity to thank all the contributing authors who were supportive enough to contribute their time and knowledge to this project. I also wish to convey my regards to my family who have been extremely supportive during the entire project.

Editor

1

Challenges of Nurse Tutor Utilization of the Teaching Aids

Noel D. Mbirimtengerenji[1], Oluyinka Adejumo[2]

[1]Kamuzu College of Nursing, University of Malawi, Lilongwe, Malawi
[2]University of Western Cape, Cape Town, South Africa
Email: ndmbiri@kcn.unima.mw, adejumo@uwc.ac.za

Abstract

Introduction: Nursing is the largest healthcare profession in Malawi with more than 11,000 registered nurses (RNs), nurse technicians and midwives (NTM) practicing in hospitals and other settings like nursing colleges nationwide. Student preparation is mostly done by nursing tutors in all the nursing colleges using numerous types of teaching aids. Methods: Descriptive exploratory design which utilized both qualitative and sequential quantitative methods was applied to Iterated Purposive Probability Sampling (IPPS) of 10 nursing colleges in Malawi. This was done to 129 students and 82 nurse tutors in two structured questionnaires, 40 nurse tutors in-depth interviews and 10 students focus groups. There were 32 variables for the teaching aids under five ranked Likert scale and the Cronbach's Alpha was found to be 0.932 without standardisation and it was 0.952 after standard-disation. Results: Although nurse tutors show that they use manikins to teach (0.011 < p = 0.05), students seem not to agree on the utilization of the manikins during teaching both in class and at the clinical area (0.05; p = 0.05). There is also increased discrepancy between students and nurse tutors on internet utilization as the teaching aid as the Beta Coefficient value was (B = 0.202) for the nurse tutors and (B = 1.061) for the students basing on their experience. Use of patient as a teaching aid is very common in Malawi and both the nurse tutors and students agree that it is the realistic and best way in teaching and has a strong binary logistic regression with a model outcome of (OR = 1.431; 95%CI (0.890 ± 2.304); p = 0.139). Conclusion: There is a need to develop the teaching strategies that would be conducive with the current scarcity of the teaching aids. Use of patients if ethically followed remains the most effective and efficient teaching aid in developing countries.

Keywords

Teaching Aids, Nurse Tutor Work Experience, Student Study Experience

1. Introduction

Nursing is the largest healthcare profession in Malawi with more than 11,000 registered nurses (RNs) and nurse technicians and midwives (NTM) practicing in hospitals and other settings nationwide [1]. By 2020, Ministry of Labor Statistics projects that more than 20,000 additional nurses will be needed to work in acute care hospitals, long-term care facilities, community health centers, nursing schools, and other areas [2]. This implies that despite this number, many more qualified nurses must be prepared in programs offered by nurse tutors in nursing colleges to meet the nation's growing demand for healthcare in Malawi.

To fulfill Malawi shared goal in the preparation of a robust nursing workforce, there is a need to acknowledge the nation's full support of academic progression for nursing students in all nursing colleges. Nursing tutors are aligned with the nation's nursing council and association leaders in the belief that every nursing student and qualified nurses deserve the opportunity to pursue qualitative academic career growth and development. This student preparation is mostly done by nursing tutors in all the nursing colleges using numerous types of teaching aids [3]. This suggests nursing tutors have a big challenge to produce competent graduates from nursing students in colleges using effective quality and functional teaching aids. Therefore, the main aim of this paper is to explore the challenges of the teaching aids utilisation among nurse tutors in Malawi nursing colleges.

Nursing education in Malawi dates back from the colonial era where the European Christians through Sisters opened nursing schools in the country and used patients as teaching aids. All the Nursing Colleges that were under the Faith based organization grouped together for proper management of their hospitals and health related colleges. By 1980 the organization was called the Christian Health Association of Malawi (CHAM) and currently a part from numerous hospitals has at least 12 functioning nursing colleges [4]. The teaching resources from these colleges come from government funding and other international donations. There are only 5 government funded colleges and there is only one private nursing college. However, for more than 30 years now, Government of Malawi supports missionaries in running CHAM nursing colleges. But due to limited funding and resources, some nursing colleges have been closed at times which cause tutors and students to be fragmented in their learning process due to luck of basic teaching needs. In these colleges they produce diploma technical nurses who are capable of performing independently at primary health care level in the health system of the country. This means that they are given the responsibility to manage independently teaching resources and clinical services in the health centres across the country.

Although 85% of the CHAM nursing schools were still open by July 2013, there is critical shortage of basic student learning needs that cause nurse tutors to resign and look for greener pastures elsewhere, particularly in the United Kingdom [5]. Even those nurse tutors that still remain in the system of nursing education in Malawi find it hard to teach effectively or use modern methods of teaching strategies due to too many students, limited internet, and insufficient teaching aids. In response to this situation, government of Malawi doubled nursing student college intake. But there has been a limited response on human and material resource improvement of nurse tutors in the nursing colleges for them to function effectively [6]. This means that quality of nursing education is compromised in Malawi. This does not necessarily occur as a result of nature of curriculum but a reduced number of nurse tutors who are overstretched to cover many modules and courses within a given time. Although some nursing schools were operating while others were closed due to shortage of staff, quality of teaching was highly compromised [7]. As a remedy nurses council allowed clinical instructors with two weeks training on teaching strategies to take some modules and courses and teach in classes. This action only compromised the teaching standards in the colleges. Therefore, the main objective of this paper is to articulate the challenges of the nurse tutor in the utilization of the teaching aids. This paper is significantly making nurse tutors to be consciously aware on the need to properly use the available teaching aids in the colleges.

2. Methodology

The study design for this research is descriptive exploratory and utilized both qualitative and sequential quantitative methods. This study was conducted in Malawi from eight CHAM nursing colleges. There are about 2072 students in all the eight nursing colleges. And by 2014 there were 158 tutors in all the 8 CHAM nursing colleges and 2075 students in these colleges. Iterated purposive, Sampling (IPPS) has been chosen as the recommended sampling frame for nurse tutor teaching strategy needs. In order to achieve a sample worthy generalization quantitatively, the sample were obtained from the colleges basing on approximated (random probability) number of tutors and students respectively. Drawing sample from the population was done until the desired sample will be achieved and it will use the following sample proportion formula: Sample Size = $n/\left[1+\left(n/\text{population}\right)\right]$ *but* $n = Z^2P\left(1-P\right)/E^2$ (*Lemeshow, Hosmer, Klar & Lwanga*, 1990). Where n is sample size of tutors and students in colleges, P is the proportion of number of tutors or students and E is the margin error. This formula allowed 5% for expected margin of error (E) with 95% confidence level as the denominator. Z^2 is a constant score with a value of 1.96^2 (at 95% confidence level and 5% precision) [8]. So, using the same formula of probability sampling described above, it means that 129 students and 82 nurse tutors iterated randomly selected participated in the questionnaires. The questionnaire had a five ranked Likert scale with 17 items under the teaching aids. Moreover, qualitatively, 42 nurse tutors, four from each college, were purposively selected for in-depth interviews. The main variables included use of poster, figurative model, manual/modules, internet, video conference, workbook, library and patients.

It has to be added that 10 students in one focus group discussion for each nursing college also participated qualitatively.

Only those tutors that had undergone teaching methodology training, participated for the two questionnaires for the nurse tutor and the students. Only those students that have been in class for more than one year as their study experience participated in the study. All tutors who were just recruited and those on transfer and others like foreign expatriates were not included on the basis of lacking contextual experience of teaching strategy needs in Malawi.

The collected quantitative data were analyzed on SPSS software version 21.0 and the qualitative data was stored in ATLAS-ti 7.0. The data sheets were locked in drawers and the data in computers were protected by passwords only known to the researcher. Descriptive and inferential statistics in the form of frequencies, bivariate analysis and binary logistic regression were computed for tutors' teaching aids against the predictor variables of nurse tutor work experience and student study experience in different nursing colleges.

There are five ways on how this study controlled confounding variables. The most important method that were used are randomization, restriction, matching, stratification and inferential analysis. This study had an approval from ethical review boards from, University of Western Cape (UWC) and from University of Malawi (UNIMA) through COMREC. All nursing tutors' and students' participants were assured that no form of human rights violations would be encountered in the due course of the nationwide nursing tutor teaching aids assessment following the 1964 Declaration of Helsinki, the1978 Belmont Report [9]; Baltimore Treaty on Ethical Codes (BTEC) and the Nuremburg Codes in medical education research.

3. Results

3.1. Distribution of Nurse Tutors and Students on Use of Teaching Aids

The response rate on the results from the two questionnaires were 91% for students and 88% for nurse tutors. The Cronbach alpha was 0.912 standardised for nurse tutor Likert scale items and 0.941 for the student Likert scale items.

In **Figure 1**, the use of teaching aids particularly use of posters was spread into a linear graph. It was clearly noted that most of the nurse tutors from St Johns Nursing College strongly agreed on the use of posters in the last semester during teaching. But Mulanje Nursing College was the highest among those who strongly disagreed on the use of posters as a teaching aids. St. Joseph Nursing College was the least in the use of the posters as a teaching strategy when teaching during the last semester in class. Most of the nurse tutors pointed out that the main challenge is how to get the best poster on time during class as posters tend to be expensive.

However, in all colleges when Spearman correlation co-efficient was used in a two tailed test of significance analysis, use of posters by nurse tutors was found to be not correlated to the type of nursing college as the p-value was $0.023 < p = 0.05$. This means that use of posters by nurse tutors depends on the type of the college where the nurse tutor is teaching in Malawi nursing colleges.

It has also to be noted that use of overhead projector is still very high in most of the nursing colleges in Malawi as students from all colleges strongly agreed that their nursing tutors use overhead projector during teaching. Even using Spearman correlation co-efficient in a two tailed test of significance analysis, it was found out that use of overhead projector is strongly correlated to the type of the nursing college, that the nurse tutor is teaching, as the p-value was $0.002 < p = 0.05$. This also entails that the use of overhead projector is very common in all nursing colleges in Malawi. Students pointed out that poor electrical power always cause the teaching aid not to work effectively during class.

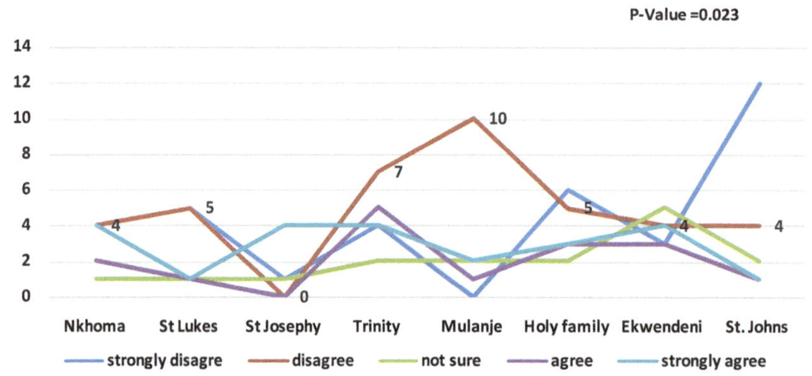

Figure 1. Distribution of tutors on the use of POSTERS in different college.

Furthermore, the use of LCD-power point presentation was compared with the type of the nursing college in a two tailed test of significance for Spearman correlation co-efficient, at 0.05 alpha level. Therefore, the null hypothesis that use of LCD was not correlated to type of nursing college was not rejected. Therefore, it was noted that student nurses strongly agreed that LCD is commonly used in their colleges during the last semester.

There was mixed feelings on the use of figurative models in different colleges in Malawi as students from Nkhoma Nursing College, Trinity Nursing College and Holy Family Nursing College strongly disagreed that their tutors used the models during clinical teaching in the last semester. However, when the Spearman correlation co-efficient was used to compare the use of the models and the type of the college for all the nursing colleges, there was no correlation as the p-value was $0.011 < p = 0.05$. This also suggest that although some colleges do not use the figurative models during teaching but generally in all colleges they models are used as statistically proven. Therefore, type of the college influence the utilization of the figurative models as teaching aid. Nurse tutors agreed that limited number and operation of the figurative model remain a challenge in their laboratories.

Although, students in all colleges indicated that they has computer laboratory, but there was mixed feeling towards the use of these computer laboratories due to poor maintenance of the old computers. Nkhoma Nursing College and Holy Family Nursing College are among the colleges where some students strongly disagreed that they use the computer laboratory. But when a two sided test of significance in bivariate analysis was used to compare the dependent variable use of computer and independent variable type of college in a Spearman correlation co-efficient, it was found out that use of computer is not correlated to type of nursing college as the p-value was $0.035 < p = 0.05$. This means that use of computer is not generally available in some colleges during the last semester although some nurse tutors complained that there is poor maintenance to the old computers that are available.

It has to be mentioned that use of internet is still a problem in some colleges of nursing in Malawi as nursing students had also mixed feelings towards the services. Trinity Nursing College, Holy Family Nursing College and St. Johns Nursing Colleges students strongly disagreed that they have used the services during the last semester both in class and at the clinical area. The main reason given was poor signal and limited distance coverage. However, most of the colleges' students also agreed that they have at times used the internet as a teaching aids during last semester. Moreover, when Spearman correlation co-efficient was used in a two tailed test of significance bivariate analysis, it was noted that use of internet was correlated with independent variable, the type of nursing college where students are learning as the p-value was $0.001 < p = 0.05$. This means that use of internet for students depends on the type of the nursing colleges that the student is learning.

In **Figure 2**, it was also noted that St. Johns Nursing College, Holy family nursing college and Trinity Nursing Colleges had the services of internet for their students as they strongly agreed on the use, although there was very slow signal both in class and at the clinical area.

The students had also a mixed feeling on the use of library as a teaching aid during teaching. All Nursing students from Nkhoma Nursing College strongly disagreed that they had used the library as a learning aid. While students from St. Lukes nursing College and St Joseph also disagreed that they use library often as a learning aid. However, when Spearman correlation co-efficient was done in a bivariate analysis with a two tailed test of significance, the null hypothesis that use of library is not correlated to type of nursing college was rejected as the

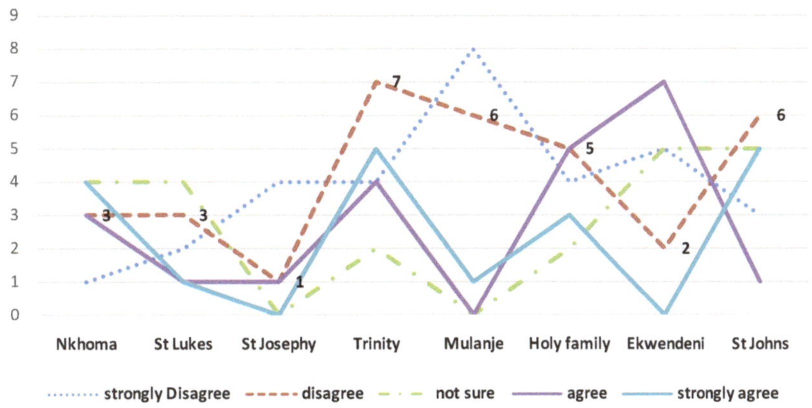

Figure 2. Distribution of use of internet by students in different colleges.

p-value was 0.003 < p = 0.05. This means that although some colleges do not use the library so often, but use of library is correlated to the type of the nursing college.

3.2. Distribution of Nurse Tutors Work Experience and Student Study Experience on Teaching Aids Utilization

When the nurse tutor work experience was compared with the teaching aids like use of poster in a bivariate analysis, It was noted that the p-value from Spearman correlation co-efficient was 0.046 < p = 0.05. This means that use of poster is correlated to tutors work experience during teaching both in class and at the clinical area. This is a true reflection of the tutor's perception as it was also noted that 63.2% of the tutors strong agree that they had used poster during teaching as a teaching aid during the last semester. However, this is different from student perspective as the p-value was not statistically significant at 0.101 > p = 0.05, thus when independent variable student study experience was compared with the use of the poster. This means that although use of poster depends on tutor work experience but the same use of poster does not depend on student study experience. This discrepancy lives much to be desired in teaching and learning process in Malawi nursing colleges (see **Table 1**).

It has also to be pointed out that use of manual or module was found to be highly correlated to the nurse tutors work experience. This was because the independent variable nurse tutor work experience is correlated to dependent variable use of module as the p-value was 0.040 < p = 0.05. This means that the Spearman correlation co-efficient favoured the alternative hypothesis that independent variable nurse tutor work experience is strongly correlated to dependent variable use of modules when teaching both in class and at the clinical area. But this was not the case with students as the p-value when we compared use of teaching module and student study experience was 0.887 > p = 0.05. This means that we fail to reject the null hypothesis that use of teaching modules is not correlated to student study experience. This means that use of teaching module does not depend on student study experience.

There was a board-line correlation between nurse tutors work experience and the use of internet as the p-value in the Spearman correlation co-efficient was 0.05 = p 0.05. This indicated that use of internet in nursing colleges depends on the work experience of the nurse tutors. This is a true reflection as the frequency statistics also revealed that 57.1% of more than 6 years nurse tutor experienced, strongly agreed that they had used the internet during the last semester both in class and at the clinical area during teaching. However, 70.8% of the students who have more than two year study experienced strongly disagreed on the use of the internet as a teaching aid in their colleges. Even the Spearman correlation co-efficient revealed that there is no statistical significant (p-value; 0.085 > p = 0.05) between student study experience and the use of internet in nursing colleges. This indicated that students do not highly use internet as a source of learning in Malawi.

67.7% of the more experience nurse tutors indicated that they strongly disagree on the use of video conference as a teaching aid both in class and at the clinical area. It was also found out that there was no statistical significance between use of video conference and nurse tutors work experience as the p-value was 0.197 > p = 0.05. This means that use of video conference does not depend on the nurse tutors experience. 70.3% of the students with more than two years student study experienced strongly disagreed that they had not used the video confer-

Table 1. Distribution of tutors' work experience & students study experience on and tutors' choice of teaching aids.

Choice of teaching aids variables	Work experience				Total	p-value	Students study experience N = 129				Total	p-value
	1 - 5 years		6 and more yrs		n (%)		Two year		More than two yrs		N (%)	
Use of posters							N	%	N	%		
Strongly disagree	1	12.5%	7	87.5%	8 (100)		7	30.4%	16	69.6%	23	
Disagree	7	77.8%	2	22.2%	9 (100)		6	37.5%	10	62.5%	16	
Not sure	2	66.7%	1	33.3%	3 (100)	**0.046**	10	62.5%	6	37.5%	16	**0.347**
Agree	10	37.0%	17	63.0%	27 (100)		14	35.9%	25	64.1%	39	
Strongly agree	12	34.3%	23	65.7%	35 (100)		17	48.6%	18	51.4%	35	
Use of figurative models from clinical laboratory												
Strongly disagree	0	.0%	7	100.0%	7 (100)		3	16.7%	15	83.3%	18	
Disagree	7	77.8%	2	22.2%	9 (100)		5	55.6%	4	44.4%	9	
Not sure	2	25.0%	6	75.0%	8 (100)	**0.009**	10	52.6%	9	47.4%	19	**0.101**
Agree	9	45.0%	11	55.0%	20 (100)		14	35.9%	25	64.1%	39	
Strongly agree	14	36.8%	24	63.2%	38 (100)		22	50.0%	22	50.0%	44	
Use of manual or module guides						**0.040**						
Strongly disagree	2	28.6%	5	71.4%	7 (100)		1	11.1%	8	88.9%	9	
Disagree	2	22.2%	7	77.8%	9 (100)		6	54.5%	5	45.5%	11	
Not sure	3	60.0%	2	40.0%	5 (100)		11	52.4%	10	47.6%	21	**0.887**
Agree	13	54.2%	11	45.8%	24 (100)		22	37.9%	36	62.1%	58	
Strongly agree	12	32.4%	25	67.6%	37 (100)		14	46.7%	16	53.3%	30	
Use of internet when teaching												
Strongly disagree	6	33.3%	12	66.7%	18 (100)		7	29.2%	17	70.8%	24	
Disagree	8	40.0%	12	60.0%	20 (100)		9	34.6%	17	65.4%	26	
Not sure	4	44.4%	5	55.6%	9 (100)	**−0.050**	11	47.8%	12	52.2%	23	**0.085**
Agree	8	38.1%	13	61.9%	21 (100)		14	46.7%	16	53.3%	30	
Strongly agree	6	42.9%	8	57.1%	14 (100)		13	50.0%	13	50.0%	26	
Use of video conference						0.197						
Strongly disagree	10	32.3%	21	67.7%	31		11	29.7%	26	70.3%	37	
Disagree	8	33.3%	16	66.7%	24		7	26.9%	19	73.1%	26	
Not sure	7	63.6%	4	36.4%	11		9	40.9%	13	59.1%	22	**0.004***
Agree	5	41.7%	7	58.3%	12		21	67.7%	10	32.3%	31	
Strongly agree	2	50.0%	2	50.0%	4		6	46.2%	7	53.8%	13	

This is an SPSS table in bivariate analysis comparing the nurse tutors work experience and students study experience against different teaching aids for nurse tutors in Malawi. The cut point of the bivariate analysis was 0.05 power value. The analysis was generated from Spearman correlation co-efficient in a two tailed test significance, excluding missing data.

ence as a teaching aid both in class and at the clinical area. But the Spearman correlation co-efficient in a bivariate analysis revealed $0.004 < p = 0.05$. This indicates that student study experience is strongly correlated to use of video conference. Therefore, utilization of the video conference depends on the student study experience. However, some students showed that video conference are rarely done in there colleges as they even do not have a working video screens.

When Spearman correlation co-efficient was used in a two tailed test of significance in a bivariate analysis, the null hypothesis that nurse tutors work experience is not correlated to use of research articles was rejected as the p-value was $0.021 < p = 0.05$. This means that nurse tutor work experience is highly correlated to use of research articles when teaching both in class and at the clinical area. This means that use of research articles by nurse tutors depends on the nurse tutors work experience.

3.3. Association of Nurse Tutors' Work Experience and Nursing Student Study Experience with Use of Teaching Aids

Binary Logistic regression was performed by selecting all dependent variables that showed statistical significance in the bivariate analysis and enter them into the model of logistic regression. This was done after dichotomising the five ranked Likert scale dependent variables to two covariates of "Agree" and "Disagree". "Disagree" was coded 0 to become constant value in our output but not presented in **Table 2**. "Agree" was coded 1 to become our interactive value in the output. With logistic regression analysis the findings reported in this study informed the importance of independent variables of their effect on the dependent variables` odds (see **Table 2**).

This suggest that the effect of the nurse tutors work experience and nursing student study experience influences the dependent variables on teaching aids. It has to be reminded that the main objective one was to explore the tutors teaching aids and how it affects learning with a focus on teaching aids utilization and the challenges. The independent variables or the predictor variables, like nurse tutor work experience and nursing student study experience were compared to different dependent variables on utilization of teaching aids.

The binary logistic regression analysis with the probability stepwise of 0.05 was used as the entry point and 0.1 as the removal point at 95% confidence level. The model also used 0.5 as the probability classification cut-off. In the outcome of the model Omnibus test of model coefficient was selected. It showed clear association of dependent variable use of poster and independent variable nurse tutor work experience as the Odds Ratio was OR = 1.192; 95%CI (0.767 ± 1.853); $p = 0.435$. This suggests that the more nurse tutor work experience that one has the more likely that she or he would use the posters when teaching both in class and at the clinical area. This was also the same when the logistic model was used on students. It was clear that the more student study experience that one has the more likely that she or he would use the posters both in class and at the clinical area as the Odds Ratio was OR = 1.226; 95%CI (0.539 ± 2.789); $p = 0.628$. This is a true reflection of the students as the p-value for Hosmer and Lemeshow test was strongly, statistically significant at $0.628 > p = 0.05$. Moreover, there was a positive direction of relationship between the dependent and predictor variables since the Beta Coefficient value for nurse tutors equation was B = 0.176 and Beta Coefficient value for student equation was B = 0.203. This means that the more the years of tutor work experience the more likely that she or he would use posters correctly in class and at the clinical area effectively.

It has been noted that there is no association between the use of the green board and the nurse tutor work experience during teaching in nursing colleges in Malawi. This was done after comparing the predictor variable nurse tutor work experience and the dependent variable use of the white or green board during teaching. A probability stepwise criteria of 0.05 was used for entry point and 0.1 was adopted for the removal point in the equation of the binary logistic regression. The classification cut-off point was set at 0.5. The results of the odds ratio was OR = 0.912; 95%CI (0.522 ± 1.594); $p = 0.747$.

It clearly illustrates that if there is an addition of one year as a constant value to the nurse tutor work experience there would be a likelihood chance of 0.912 times less for the nurse tutors to use whiteboard or green board during teaching. However, there has been a negative direction of the relationship between nurse tutor work experience and use of white or green board during teaching in class and at the clinical area. This is because the Logistic regression revealed a Beta Coefficient value of B = −0.092. This suggests that if there is an increase in the years for the nurse tutor during teaching there would be a likely decrease in the nurse tutors using the white or green board. But this is not the case with the Beta Coefficient value of the logistic regression equation

Table 2. Association of tutors work experience, students study experience and teaching aids.

Tutors who agree on teaching aids	Tutors work experience						Students study experience					
	B	WARD	sig	ODD	Confidence interval		B	WARD	sig	ODD	Confidence interval	
					Lower	Upper					Lower	Upper
Use of posters	0.176	0.610	0.435	1.192	0.767	1.853	0.203	0.235	0.628	**1.226**	0.539	2.789
Use of white/greenboard	**−0.092**	0.104	0.747	0.912	0.522	1.594	0.302	0.120	0.729	1.353	0.245	7.459
Use of projector	**−0.020**	0.010	0.922	0.981	0.663	1.451	-	-	-	-	-	-
Use of PowerPoint	**−0.230**	0.388	0.533	0.795	0.385	1.638	**1.688**	**3.558**	**0.059**	**5.407**	0.936	31.233
Use of training CD & DVD	**−0.367**	**2.524**	0.112	0.693	0.440	1.090	-	-	-	-	-	-
Use of figurative models	**−0.021**	0.007	0.932	0.979	0.596	1.607	0.235	0.222	0.638	**1.265**	0.475	3.370
Use of research articles	0.064	0.067	0.796	1.067	0.654	1.740	0.536	0.383	0.536	1.709	0.313	9.328
Use of work-book	0.370	**2.241**	0.134	1.447	0.892	2.349	1.112	0.857	0.355	3.040	0.289	32.011
Use of teaching manuals/modules	**−0.129**	0.213	0.644	0.879	0.509	1.518	0.104	0.021	0.884	1.110	0.272	4.535
Use of computer laboratory	0.369	**2.125**	0.145	1.447	0.881	2.378	**−0.819**	**4.332**	0.037	0.441	0.204	0.953
Use of internet	**−0.202**	0.662	0.416	0.817	0.503	1.328	0.060	0.019	0.891	**1.061**	0.452	2.490
Use of teaching CDs from books	**−0.388**	1.896	0.169	0.678	0.391	1.179	-	-	-	-	-	-
Use of chalk	0.342	**2.556**	0.110	10.408	0.926	2.143	-	-	-	-	-	-
Use of library	0.337	10.898	0.168	10.400	0.867	2.261	−1.121	5.723	0.017	0.326	0.130	0.817
Use of video conference	**−0.244**	0.520	0.471	0.783	0.404	1.521	**−1.447**	**9.129**	**0.003**	0.235	0.092	0.601
Small group discussions	−0.301	1.545	0.214	0.740	0.461	1.189	**−0.939**	**5.028**	**0.025**	0.391	0.172	0.888
Use of patients	0.359	**2.184**	0.139	1.431	0.890	2.304	**−0.630**	**2.113**	0.146	0.533	0.228	1.245

This is a logistic regression models with probability classification cut-off of 0.5 and the entry point of p-value of 0.05 in statistics of Hosmer-Lemeshow goodness of-fit. Basing on method of ENTER, the maximum iteration of 20, the equation had a probability of 95% confidence interval. The OR interpretation of above 1 was adopted for the predictor variables of nurse tutor experience and student study experience separately. All the categorical dependent variables under teaching aids and the predictor/independent variables were first tested in the bivariate analysis at p-value of 0.05. All constant values are not tabulated although the models produced. The degree of freedom was set at 1; all teaching strategy dependent and nurse tutor work experience and student study experience which are independent categorical variables were dichotomizedly coded correctly (with 0 = disagree or lack of the characteristic; 1 = agree, or the presence of the characteristic).

output (B = 0.303) from the student study experience and nurse tutors use of green and white board. The model output indicated that the more years the student study experience the more likely the student has on the use of the green or white board during learning in class. The only main challenge reflected by nurse tutors is dust and irritation from the chalk.

The Odds Ratio of the regression model in the Hosmer and Lemeshow test showed that OR = 5.407; 95%CI (0.936 ± 31.233); p = 0.059 when the predictor variable student study experience was associated with use of power point as learning aid in class. This clearly showed that for any extra added year, of nursing student study experience, there would be a likelihood more chance of 5.407 times that the students would use power point both in class and at the clinical area for learning.

But the similar model for the predictor variable nurse tutor work experience and dependent variable use of power point when teaching showed a negative Beta Coefficient value of −0.230. This definitely shows that any extra added year to nurse tutor work experience would cause a decrease in the utilisation of the power point as a teaching aid both in class and at the clinical area. Yes age has been found to have a strong effect on the utilization of the PowerPoint presentation through LCD. Older nurse tutors are not using the PowerPoint effectively.

It has also to be mentioned that there was strong association between independent variable nurse tutor work experience and the dependent variable, the use of computer laboratory as the odds ratio was OR = 1.447; 95%CI (0.881 ± 2.378); p = 0.145. This binary logistic regression results revealed that any addition of one year to the tutor work experience, it is expected to increase the chance of nurse tutors using the computer laboratory by 1.447 times. However, the students strongly disagreed that they use the computer lab in their school as the odds ratio was OR = 0.447; 95%CI (0.204 ± 0.953); p = 0.037. This means that for every one year of student study experience there would be a likelihood chance of 0.441 times less for nurse tutors to utilising the computer laboratory. Even the Beta Coefficient value from the binary logistic regression model showed (B = −0.819) a negative direction of the relationship between the student study experience and the nurse tutors utilization of the computer laboratory during teaching. This indicates that any increase to the years of the student study experience there would be a decrease to the nurse tutors utilization of the computer laboratory during teaching the students in Malawi nursing colleges. However, most of the computer Laboratories do not have enough equipment.

Use of the Internet was also found to be not associated to nurse tutor work experience. This was done after comparing the two variables in the binary logistic regression model. The model adopted the probability stepwise of 0.05 as the entry point in the equation and 0.1 as the removal point while the classification cut-off point was set at 0.5. The odds ratio results were OR = 0.817; 95%CI (0.506 ± 1.328); p = 0.416. This entails that if one year is added to the nurse tutor work experience there would be a likelihood chance of 0.817 times for the nurse tutors to use the internet during teaching in Malawi nursing colleges. Therefore, it is not common among the nurse tutors to use internet during teaching in the nursing colleges in Malawi. However, in the student data, there was a borderline association when independent variable student study experience was compared to dependent variable use of internet as the Odds Ratio was OR = 1.061; 95%CI (0.452 ± 2.490); p = 0.891. This indicates that for every one year of student study experience in the nursing college there would a likelihood chance of 1.061 times for the nurse tutors to use the internet. But in the same way, the nurse tutors totally disagree with the students as the Beta coefficient value in the logistic regression output showed −0.202. This means that the more years the nurse tutor has the less likely that she would use internet as a teaching aid when teaching both in class and at the clinical area.

There was also a strong association between independent variable nurse tutor work experience and dependent variable use of chalk in class when teaching as the Odds Ratio was OR = 1.408; 95%CI (0.926 ± 2.378); p = 0.145. The result are from the binary logistic regression model where 0.05 was an entry point in the probability stepwise criteria. The classification cut-off point was set at 0.5. This indicates that for every one year more of nurse tutor experience there would be a likelihood chance of 1.408 times more for the nurse tutor to use chalk during teaching both in class and at the clinical area. The Beta Coefficient value in the model also showed (B = 0.342) a positive direction of the relationship between the nurse tutor work experience and the use of the chalk during teaching in Nursing Colleges in Malawi. Therefore, Use of Chalk is still very common among the nurse tutors in Malawi nursing colleges.

There was also a discrepancy between students and nurse tutors on the use of library as a teaching aid. When students data was analysed in a binary logistic regression for the Hosmer and Lemeshow equation revealed that there is strong association between dependent variable use of library and the independent variable nurse tutors experience as the Odds ratio was OR = 1.400; 95%CI (0.867 ± 2.261); p = 0.168. This is very encouraging as the nurse tutors has shown that for every one year addition to their experience there is 1.400 times likelihood chance for them to use the library as a teaching and learning aid. However, the students did not agree on the use of the library as a teaching aid as the Beta Coefficient value was (B = −1.12). This indicated that the more years of student study experience the less likely that they would use the library as a learning aid during the class period and during the clinical period. But in these library most of the books are very old and very few. They are not enough for the growing number of the students.

It is clear that in all nursing colleges in Malawi, students and nurse tutors disagreed that they have used the video conference as teaching aid during teaching and learning. This was found after using the binary logistic regression model. In the model omnibus test of model coefficient was employed to compare the predictor variable nurse tutor work experience and the dependent variable use of video conference as the teaching aid during teaching. The results showed that the odds ratio was OR = 0.783; 95%CI (0.404 ± 1.521); p = 0.471. This indicates that there is no association between nurse tutor work experience and the utilization of the video conference among nurse tutors during teaching the students in Malawi. In the student data again there was no association between student study experience and the nurse tutors utilization of the video conference as a teaching aid during student teaching. Even the Beta Coefficient values of the binary logistic regression model clearly indicated the negative values of B = −0.244 for tutors and B = −1.447. This means that the negative direction of the relationship between the predictor variable nurse tutor work experience and the dependent variable utilization of video conference. In this case even the students are strongly disagreeing that they have ever used the video conference as a learning aid. Video conference tend to be expensive to have in these nursing colleges when limitation of budget influence nurse tutors not to use this teaching aid.

Use of patient as a teaching aid has also received mixed feelings from the students and the nurse tutors in this research. When nurse tutor work experience as an independent variable was compared to dependent variable, it was noticed that the odds ratio was OR = 1.431; 95%CI (0.890 ± 2.304); $p = 0.139$. This indicated that any one year increase in nurse tutor work experience would increase the likelihood chances of use patient as a teaching aid by 1.431 times. In this regard, when the independent variable student study experience was compared to dependent variable use of patient as a learning aid it was noted that the beta value of the regression model was negative direction of relationship (B = −0.630) This means that the if the nurse tutor gain more years of experience in the process of teaching she or he would less likely to be using the patient as a learning aid. This also entailed that nursing students disagreed that tutors use patients as the teaching aid during teaching both in class and the clinical area.

4. Discussion

Posters have long been recognized as an effective medium for disseminating information, particularly with respect to evidence-based practice in nursing. This research has revealed that posters are commonly used in nursing colleges in Malawi although they are expensive to get. But nurse tutors complain of the proper utilization which is a challenge in most of the nursing colleges. The main problem is the availability of the posters which lead nurse tutors not to frequently utilize during teaching. In Cincinnati, Ohio nursing colleges, posters are now also being used for staff education at the clinical level in the surgical, medical, cardiac, and open-heart intensive care units. The benefits are more widespread than originally imagined [10]. If the posters are in good condition they help quality improvement and needs assessment to students' posters can also help to identify and develop topics to present in class and at the clinical area. This process also helped overcome the rigidity in thinking that posters are only for academia. In addition, the opportunity fit well with the hospital's clinical ladder program, because the participating nurses could earn credit [10]. Today many posters are designed with Microsoft PowerPoint templates, but can also lay out the sections of the poster on a large piece of poster board before finalizing it.

Use of PowerPoint in Malawi nursing colleges has been very common among nurse tutors. PowerPoint utilization works with an LCD machine. The main challenge of the nurse tutors is on how to operate the LCD machine and the computer. While we do appreciate that Malawi nursing colleges have not more than 3 - 5 LCD machine against 15 - 20 nurse tutors to use in a class where not less than 150 students are learning, it becomes an administrative problem on not owing more of these teaching aids. This is because if they are many, more nurse tutors, can utilise and become acquainted to the operational system [11]. The primary roles that nurse tutors have is to perform as a teacher in class and at the clinical area. Teachers at every level prepare plans that aid in the organization and delivery of their daily lessons. These plans vary widely in the style and degree of specificity on use of the PowerPoint. Some instructors prefer to construct elaborate detailed and impeccably typed outlines in PowerPoint; others rely on the brief notes in the PowerPoint and present clearly. Therefore, mastering the use of LCD and computer would not be necessarily the only option but on how to create the PowerPoint in the computer. If the PowerPoint has been created properly in the computer and the words are not clouded, chances of clear presentation among many students is very possible.

Use of figurative models or manikins in Malawi nursing colleges is very challenging. Basically human simulation aims to imitate reality whilst offering a skills-based clinical experience in a safe and secure environment [12]. But this format of using the manikins is a very difficult process in Malawi. The challenge is not only the availability of the adequate manikins for a large student class but also on the technical utilization of the manikins by nurse tutors. It has to be noted that the availability of Manikins are donor related in Malawi nursing colleges as they are very expensive and only produced outside the country. Not many colleges have more than 5 working manikins and other anatomical figurative models. This gives tough time for nurse tutors to conduct a demonstration session to large class of students as one topic would consume more hours due to student group division.

Use of research articles when teaching is gaining ground in Malawi nursing colleges due to availability of the internet. But many nurse tutors and students disagreed that they use this type of teaching aid. This is because in most colleges the resource of research articles or journals are not up to the standard in most college libraries. In

Turkey, researchers conducted a study on how nurses perceive the barriers to and facilitators of research utilization [13]. However, this study lacked validity and reliability, and barriers and facilitators of research utilization were not reported in rank order. No further studies of the use of Evidence Based Practice in nursing have been attempted in Turkey. Therefore, in Malawi nursing colleges, there is even no proper orientation on how to use research article in getting latest literature on a particular subject.

It has been found that nurse tutor tutors mostly use workbook or teaching modules when teaching although students did not agree. The discrepancy is coming in because of the availability of the teaching modules where most students do finish learning the module without owing the single copy of the workbook. While the aim of the teaching module is to uplift the presence of self-directed learning among students in nursing but the availability of the teaching modules gives a big challenge. Another researcher pointed out that with the complexity and degree of change in practice today, nurses should be encouraged to take responsibility for their own learning [14]. Even in America Studies have been conducted to explore the amount of time nurses spend on self-directed learning using modules. When the students were asked to recall their learning experiences, and differences in memory, it was high. But in Malawi with few teaching modules it is very difficult to highly recall what they have learnt or covered in the module.

Use of the computer laboratory in Malawi nursing college is still to start in most colleges. Computer laboratory assist students to get current information concerning nursing globally, regionally and locally. Many colleges do not have computer laboratory where they can search information from the net or learn how to type assignments. This affects the computer skill and internet skills. There were no significant (0.145 $p < 0.05$) baseline between the computer and nursing lecture groups by education or computer skills [15]. Results also noted that showed significant differences between the two groups in cognitive gains and nursing student satisfaction ($p = 0.01$), with the computer group demonstrating higher student satisfaction and more cognitive gains than the lecture group. The groups were similar in their ability to demonstrate the skill correctly. But this is not the case with the third world developing country like Malawi as this study student odds ratio on computer utilization was 0.441. Although it is imperative to compare USA students and Malawi students but the availability of the computers reduce the quality performance of the nursing graduates at the same level with the USA student.

Although use of chalk could behave as the old fashion in some countries, but in Malawi it is still being used in class for student learning in the colleges. The challenge of the Chalk and nursing students is the availability of the dust to white uniform. White chalk could be easy to use but the coloured chalk tend to dent the nursing traditional white colour both to the students and the nurse tutors [16]. But what is amazing is that this is the common teaching aid for nurse tutors in Malawi. Therefore, a lot of the nurse tutors and students agreed that chalk cause discoloration of their uniform. With the complexity and degree of change in nursing practice today, nurses should be encouraged to take responsibility for their own learning [17]. However, even when adult nursing students are willing to assume responsibility for their own learning, they will have different aptitudes for certain kinds of learning like the use of chalk in class while putting on their traditional white uniform.

Use of patient has been statistically noted to be very common among nurse tutors and students in Malawi nursing colleges ($OR = 1.431$; 95%CI (0.890 ± 2.304); $p = 0.139$). This clear shows that nurse tutors use the patients when teaching as a teaching aid particularly in the clinical area. The reality teaching and hands on the patients create student confidence very early in the profession. In Malawi, students start touching the patient through care in year one by doing basing nursing care like bed bath and bed making. In this process students gain trust on procedures and master the skills very early [18]. It is very important to note that even nurse tutors when they are teaching in class they sometimes bring real patient like mild anaemic patient so as to show the signs and symptoms to students right away during teaching. This give credit to the learning process as it acts as a motivation to students and internalization of the information is very high. While simulation is becoming an option to modern nursing, but use of real patient as teaching aids cannot have a reality replacement.

5. Conclusion

Use of teaching aids is having a big challenge among nurse tutors because of shortage and poor funding. With adequate funding availability of the materials like manikins and LCD would cause remarkable nurse tutor improvement in teaching both in class and at the clinical area. Use of patient as a teaching aid if ethically followed remains the most realistic teaching in nursing for developing countries where simulation technology for Best Emergency Medical Education (BEME) is still limited. There is a need to develop the teaching strategies that would be conducive with the current scarcity of the teaching aids.

References

[1] Ministry of Health (2008) Annual Report; Nursing Section. Lilongwe.

[2] Ministry of Health (2012) Annual Report on Nurse's Performance: Capitol Hill. Lilongwe.

[3] Ministry of Health (2010) Biannual Conference, Karikuti Hotel. Lilongwe.

[4] Nurses Council of Malawi (2012) Annual Report on Nursing Education.

[5] Grigulis, A.L. (2010) Lives of Malawian Nurses: Stories behind the Statistics. PhD Thesis, Centre for International Health and Development, University College London.

[6] Nurse Council of Malawi (2006) Annual Report; Progress of Nurses in Development. Lilongwe.

[7] Chirwa, M. (2007) Performance of CHAM Nursing Schools. Lilongwe.

[8] Dennis, H. and Duncan, C. (2011) Introduction to Research Methods in Psychology. 3rd Edition, Loughborough University Press, Prentice Hall. www.pearsoned.co.uk/howitt

[9] Rivera, R. (2011) Research Ethics Training Curriculum. 2nd Edition, Family, Health International. www.fhi.org

[10] Gina, M. (2002) Posters Give Nursing Staff Consistent Information. *Critical Care Nurse*, **22**, 152. http://ccn.aacnjournals.org/

[11] Maunye, T.J., Meyer, S.M. and van, V.C.E. (2009) An Assessment of Teaching Strategies. Used by Lecturers at a Nursing College in Mpumalanga. *Curatiouis*, **32**, 30-37. http://dx.doi.org/10.4102/curationis.v32i3.1221

[12] Cant, R.P. and Cooper, S.J. (2010) Simulation-Based Learning in Nurse Education: Systematic Review. *Journal of Advanced Nursing*, **66**, 3-15. http://dx.doi.org/10.1111/j.1365-2648.2009.05240.x

[13] Yava, A., Tosun, N., Çiçek, H., Yavan, T., Terakye, G. and Hatipoğlu, S. (2009) Nurses' Perceptions of the Barriers to and the Facilitators of Research Utilization in Turkey. *Applied Nursing Research*, **22**, 166-175. http://dx.doi.org/10.1016/j.apnr.2007.11.003

[14] O'Shea, E. (2003) Self-Directed Learning in Nurse Education: A Review of the Literature. *Journal of Advanced Nursing*, **43**, 62-70. http://dx.doi.org/10.1046/j.1365-2648.2003.02673.x

[15] Jeffries, P.R. (2001) Computer versus Lecture: A Comparison of Two Methods of Teaching Oral Medication Administration in a Nursing Skills Laboratory. *The Journal of Nursing Education*, **40**, 323-329.

[16] Banning, M. (2005) Facilitation of Teaching Strategies in Nursing. *Nurse Education Today*, **25**, 502-508. http://dx.doi.org/10.1016/j.nedt.2005.03.007

[17] Polit, D. and Beck, C.T. (2003) Nursing Research: Principals and Methods. Williams Book Company, New York.

[18] Tomietto, M., Saiani, L., Palese, A., Cunico, L., Cicolini, G., Watson, P. and Saarikoski, M. (2012) Clinical Learning Environment and Supervision plus Nurse Teacher (CLES + T) Scale: Testing the Psychometric Characteristics of the Italian Version. *Giornale Italiano di Medicina del Lavoro ed Ergonomia*, **34**, B72-B80.

2

Concept Development and Implementation of Family Care/Caring Theory in Concentric Sphere Family Environment Theory

Naohiro Hohashi*, Junko Honda

Division of Family Health Care Nursing, Department of Nursing, Graduate School of Health Sciences, Kobe University, Kobe, Japan

Email: *naohiro@hohashi.org

Abstract

Caring is directed toward a variety of things. One of them is thought to be the concept of "family caring" aimed at families. This study attempts to clarify family caring and develop Family Care/Caring Theory (FCCT), with the aim of implementing it in conjunction with an existing family nursing theory, the Concentric Sphere Family Environment Theory (CSFET). In Japan and in Hong Kong, family ethnography (including formal interviews) was conducted. As a result, the item "family health care nurses and their colleagues" was added to the family external environment of the CSFET. In the family environment, evidence was obtained to the effect that the family system unit is cared for by the nursing professional, and conversely the family system unit cares for the nursing professional, in a circular transaction. Observing the two-dimensional plane formed by the structural distance and functional distance, family caring assumes a structure of concentric circles, and according to transactions, the structural distance and functional distance between the nursing professional and family system unit are gradually approached, and through deepening of mutual trust maintain an appropriate distance. Moreover observing the three-dimensional space-time continuum which is created through addition of the temporal distance, family caring forms a helical structure. As transactions are repeated along the temporal axis, the family system unit's self-actualization of other individuals and the self-actualization of the nursing professional are realized. Through these processes, a family care/caring relationship is reinforced and established. This is the concept of FCCT. Through future utilization in clinical settings this will be empirically substantiated, and it will be necessary to continue making creative corrections and revisions.

Keywords

Family Caring, Family Care/Caring Theory (FCCT), Concentric Sphere Family Environment Theory

*Corresponding author.

(CSFET), Family Health Care Nurses and Their Colleagues

1. Introduction

The objects of caring are not only human beings, but can be utilized in transdisciplinary domains so as to include animals, plants, things and ideas [1]. The objects of nursing, in addition to humans, also include families, groups, organizations, communities and so on [2]. In other words, caring that is directed at the family can also be considered within the concept of "family caring." While considerable research has been conducted regarding caring in the field of nursing, most of this involves from one individual to another, in other words, studies that are focused on caring from the nursing professional toward the patient. Consequently, caring assumes a one-way vector and interaction does not take place on a mutual basis [3]. Ray conducted research into caring in the organization of hospitals, from which the unique Theory of Bureaucratic Caring was developed [4]. In this theory, relational caring transcends the bounds of person to person, and occurs in professionals, hospitals and complex health care organizations that are affected by government policies or regulations. In the same manner, this includes hospitals, which are related to major centers of culture, such as cities or nations. However a caring theory does not exist that explains, by treating the family as a single system unit, the mutual caring between the family and nursing professional.

The family [5] that is the target of family nursing is defined as "a unit/organization as a system of the OR operation of individuals, *i.e.*, living people, having the cognition of belonging by other constituent member(s)." The family is a system unit, and family nursing, to realize the well-being of the family system unit, has been established as a specialized field of nursing studies [6]. In the frameworks of family assessment/intervention there are a number of family nursing theories, but none of them devote attention to family caring or focus on transactions between families and nursing professionals. In this study, as one family nursing theory, we propose to conduct concept development of family care/caring that focuses on transactions between the family and nursing professional.

The Concentric Sphere Family Environment Theory (CSFET) proposed by Hohashi [7] is a middle-range family nursing theory that focuses on the family environment that acts on the well-being of the family system unit. The family environment consists of "all entities (people, objects and matters) and phenomena that exist both within and outside the family system unit." The CSFET takes the form of a three-dimensional logical space-time continuum, consisting of three assessment axes (structural distance, functional distance, and temporal distance). Within these, the positioning of five systems (supra system, macro system, micro system, family internal environment system, and chrono system) enables the family system unit to be viewed in its entirety as a three-dimensional figure.

The supra system is "the external framework that encompasses the entire family environment, which produces the family environment and is directly or indirectly related to the family environment." This system includes religion, national and regional characteristics, language and so on. The macro system represents "family members' sphere of daily activities, which is situated relatively externally from the family system unit in terms of overall assessment of physical/objective and psychological/subjective aspects." It includes leisure environment, social resources, workplace environment, politics, economics and so on. The micro system represents "community in the nearby region, which is situated closer to the family system unit in terms of overall assessment of physical/objective and psychological/subjective aspects." It includes the local living sphere, neighbors, relatives and so on. The above three systems taken together are called the family external environment system. On the other hand, the family internal environment system refers to "the range within the family unit where mutual interactions between family members occur."

Changes in the family external environment system create changes in the family system unit, and changes in the family system unit cause changes in the external environment system. By means of these circular changes and reciprocal relations, the process of family growth and development [7] is created. The chrono system refers to "the time framework with a vector oriented from the present to the future."

The CSFET is characterized by structural distance and functional distance on its horizontal axes and temporal distance on its vertical axis as assessment axes. The structural distance indicates the level of physical/objective separation, and the functional distance, the level of psychological/subjective separation. Through these two distances, the relationship between systems can be assessed. The temporal distance refers to the amount of time between separate events, enabling assessment of growth and development of the respective systems.

Nevertheless in Version 2.4 of the CSFET, the position of the nursing professional who provides family care/caring is not clearly established in the family environment. Theoretically the nursing professional would be positioned in the family external environment system, with transactions occurring between the family and nursing professional, and it would be assumed that the relationship between the family and nursing professional could be assessed through the structural distance, functional distance and temporal distance. However, this has not been empirically substantiated. As the CSFET was developed and tested primarily utilizing family ethnography [8], utilizing this method to substantiate family care/caring and implementing it into the family environment of the CSFET will make it possible to update the version of the CSFET.

The aims of this study were 1) to empirically substantiate transactions between the family and nursing professional in order to construct a concept of family care/caring, and develop a Family Care/Caring Theory (FCCT); and 2) to improve the CSFET through qualitative and inductive implementation of family care/caring in the CSFET.

2. Methods

2.1. Hypothesizing the Construction of Family Care/Caring Theory

The basic hypotheses for development of CSFET/FCCT were as follows: The nursing professional is positioned within the family external environment system of the CSFET, and transacts with the family system unit, thereby influencing the family system unit. Conversely, it is provisionally postulated that the family system unit, influenced by the family external environment system, maintains family well-being through its transactions with the nursing professional. The above was structured, a model diagram drawn up, and the CSFET/FCCT draft produced.

2.2. Family Ethnography

In order to empirically substantiate the draft of the CSFET/FCCT and ensure its rigor, family ethnography [8] that focused on transactions between the family system unit and the nursing professional was implemented. According to growth and development segments for the family system unit [9], as it is possible for the structure and contents of the CSFET/FCCT to differ, in this study, it was directed at families with a variety of growth and development segments. Further, as the CSFET takes a holistic approach to the family and family environment, research proceeded with guidelines to study families having a variety of sociocultural backgrounds.

2.2.1. Field Work and Informal Interviews

In accordance with family ethnography, transactions between the family and nursing professional and notation from the perspective of mutual care were subjected to analysis. Field work was conducted in major urban areas and regional areas of Japan and in Hong Kong, with the informants including a variety of families and nursing professionals.

In the data-collection phase, participant observation, informal interviews and collection of existing materials were conducted. The participant observation was performed at visiting nurse stations, hospitals, private homes and so on. The subjects of informal interviews were individuals at the locations of the participant observations (nurses, public health nurses, midwives, physicians, etc.). Participant observations focused on transactions between families and nursing professionals, and notes were taken of observing and listening to family life and activities, impressions and thoughts by the observers and others. Visual data were collected through shooting of video movies, still photographs and sketches. These were all assembled and utilized to produce field notes.

The data obtained from participant observation and existing materials were confirmed in interviews, and while data obtained in the interviews were confirmed in participant observation and existing materials, multifaceted data collection was conducted, thereby increasing the rigor of the data. As for existing materials, necessary items were extracted from dissertations, books, statistical materials and various recordings.

Field work was conducted in regional areas in Japan by three people for 20 days in 2012 and three people for 16 days in 2013. In major urban areas in Japan, the field work was conducted by three people for 14 days in 2014. In Hong Kong, it was conducted by three people for 11 days in 2012 and by two people for 18 days in 2014.

2.2.2. Formal Interviews

In regional areas in Japan, in 2012 cooperation was obtained from social welfare corporations and high schools. The research plan was distributed and cooperation was requested for the research. Agreement to participate was obtained from 19 families. Then in 2013 cooperation was obtained from general hospitals, clinics, visiting nurse stations and a social welfare council, the research plan was distributed and cooperation requested. Twenty families agreed to participate.

In major urban areas of Japan, in 2014, cooperation was obtained from the community association in a public housing area whose residents were mainly elderly persons, the research plan was distributed and cooperation was requested. Fourteen families agreed to participate.

In Hong Kong, in 2012, cooperation was requested from a physical examination service organization, the middle school of the local Japanese school and a beauty salon operated by a Japanese man. The research plan was distributed to Japanese families residing in Hong Kong and cooperation was requested. Eight Japanese families residing in Hong Kong agreed to participate. Then in 2014 cooperation was once again requested from a physical examination service organization, the research plan was distributed to Japanese families residing in Hong Kong and cooperation was requested. Agreement to participate was obtained from seven families.

Utilizing the draft of the CSFET/FCCT, formal interviews were conducted with the families. The interview guide was focused on transactions between the family and nursing professional, with references to the Family Environment Assessment Index (FEAI) [10] and the Family Environment Map (FEM) [11], tools to assess the transactions between the family environment and family system unit based on the CSFET. A two-hour semi-structured interview was conducted with each participant family, which was recorded with the family's permission, and afterwards it was transcribed and made into part of the ethnography data.

At the end of each interview, with references to Graneheim's model of content analysis [12], the transcription was interpreted and analyzed from the perspective of the relationship between the family and nursing professional. Then after making revisions to the CSFET/FCCT the next interview was conducted. To ensure rigor, any questions were clarified and discussed until agreement was obtained among six nursing professionals. Also, in order to clarify the concept of caring, comparisons were made with previously conducted research [13]-[16], and arbitrariness was eliminated with the aim of consistency.

2.2.3. Construction of CSFET/FCCT

Based on the ethnographic data obtained as per the above, from categorizing the transactions between the family and nursing professional, the CSFET/FCCT was qualitatively and inductively reconstructed. To ensure rigor, data analysis was repeatedly discussed by two researchers and six practitioners with expert knowledge of family nursing, and their consensus obtained. Through the above process, the development of FCCT and an updated version of the CSFET were completed.

2.3. Ethical Considerations

In this study, field work was conducted at each location after gaining approval of the university's Institutional Review Board. When the field work was conducted, the responsible person at the site was given verbal explanation of the purpose of the research and confidential treatment, and permission was obtained for participant observation. The participants at the formal interviews received verbal and written explanations of the purpose of the study, confidential treatment and so on, and agreement to participate was given in writing.

3. Results

3.1. Concept Development of Family Care/Caring and the Construction of Family Care/Caring Theory

It has been empirically substantiated that from participant observations in the field and formal interviews, a mutually caring relationship exists between the nursing professional and the family system unit. For example, in one case where a family continued caring for a family member at home, until the very end, and a visiting nurse called on the dying person, it can be gleaned from remarks by members of target families such as "She entered into the feelings of family sufferings"; "She was there for us"; and "She watched over us," that the nursing professional had engaged in the practice of family caring while maintaining the appropriate structural distance and functional distance. Conversely from the practice of that family caring, it is also clear that the nursing professional is the recipient of caring by the target family. In other words, in this study, the transaction of caring between the family and nursing professional has been empirically substantiated. While it can be supposed that these factors are incorporated into the concept of caring as it currently exists, this study has constructed a new concept of "family care/caring" in transactions between the family and the nursing professional, which had not been clearly demonstrated up to now. Through this study, the concept of family care/caring was constructed and moreover deployed toward Family Care/Caring Theory. That theory is explained below (**Figure 1**).

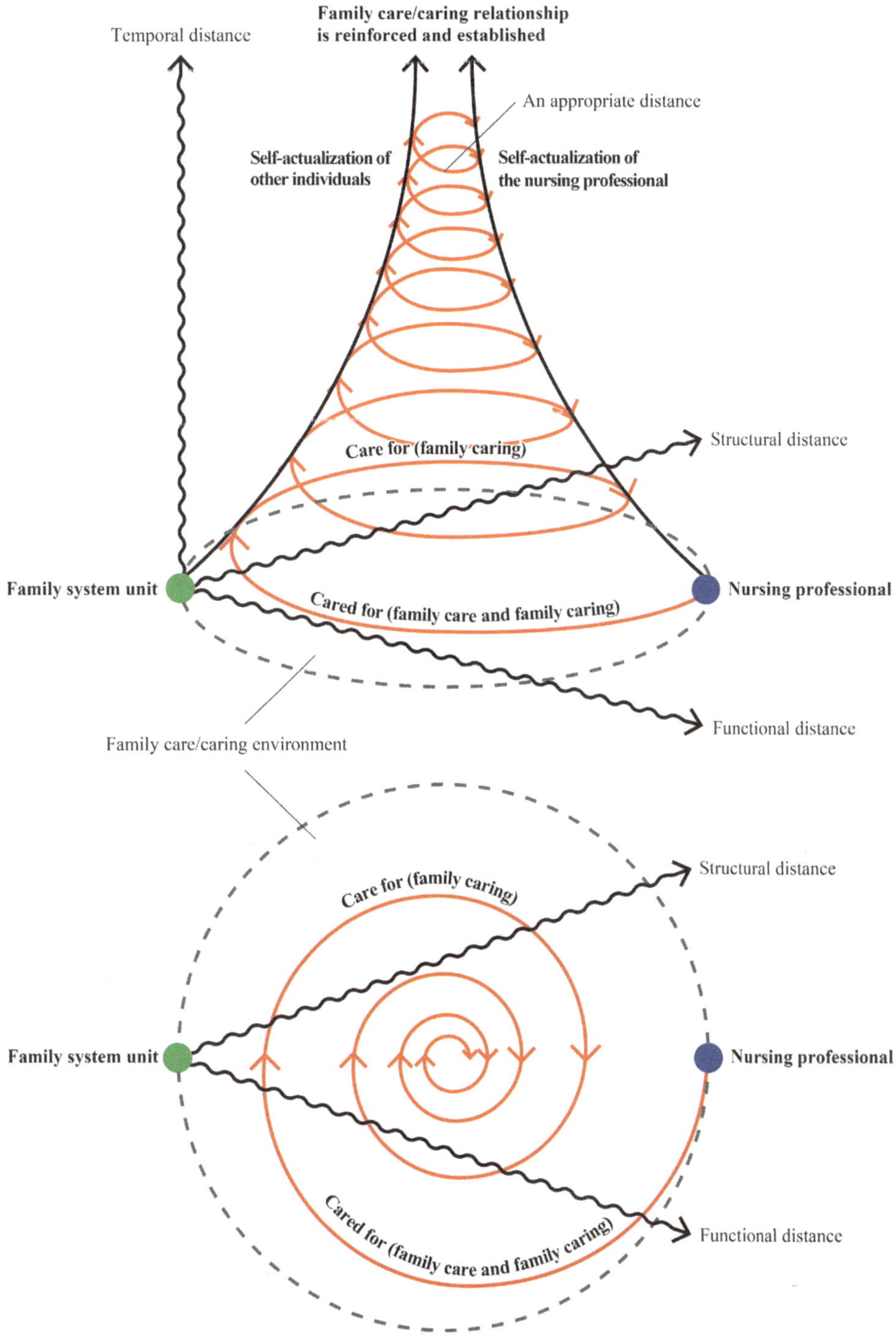

Figure 1. Model diagram of the Family Care/Caring Theory (FCCT) (Ver. 1.0).

Family care/caring forms the basic principle of family nursing, and is essential for the family system unit to maintain and improve family functioning independently and autonomously. In the family care/caring environment, which is within the family environment, the family system unit is cared for by the nursing professional, and conversely the family system unit cares for the nursing professional. The respective actions are deployed in a circular transaction (mutual act). Looking at the two-dimensional plane formed by the structural distance and functional distance, family caring forms a concentric circular structure and through these transactions, the structural distance and functional distance between the nursing professional and family system unit gradually move closer, maintaining an appropriate distance through deepening of mutual trust. Moreover observing the three-dimensional space-time continuum which is created through addition of the temporal distance, family caring forms a helical structure. As transactions are repeated along the temporal axis, the family system unit's self-actualization of other individuals, and the self-actualization of the nursing professional, are realized. Through these processes, a family care/caring relationship is reinforced and established.

In FCCT, family care, a compound noun, is defined as "acts of intervention aimed at maintaining and improving family functioning." Within the phenomena viewed as family care, family caring, a gerund, is defined as "knowing a family's beliefs, intentions and aspirations, to create an attitude of care for that family." Here, beliefs refer to "the way they conduct matters"; intentions refer to "thoughts concerning how they desire matters to be"; and aspirations refer to "things they wish to do." Family caring is guided by a manner of thought that is based on the family system unit in its entirety, and it is necessary for family intervention to focus on non-invasive methods of treatment.

3.2. Updating the Version of the Concentric Sphere Family Environment Theory

The CSFET implements the FCCT, and has been updated to Version 2.5 (**Figure 2**). In other words, "family health care nurses and their colleagues" have been added as an item in the family external environment system, and placed in the macro system of the CSFET. The nursing professional, while engaging in acts with the awareness that he or she is positioned in the family environment, is able to effect transformation of the family and family environment.

The relationship of trust between the family and nursing professional can be clarified by means of the structural distance, functional distance and temporal distance of the CSFET. At that time and place, how the relationship between family and nursing professional is formed, and moreover, the concept of time, that is, how the relationship between family and nursing professional is formed over the passage of time, in other words, it is necessary to give attention to the temporal distance of the CSFET. In the practice of family caring, an understanding of the FCCT and CSFET will be necessary.

4. Discussion

In this study, first, a conceptual meaning for family care/caring was created. The creation of a conceptual meaning is an approach to theory-building [17]. In other words, it undergoes a process of construction of FCCT from the creation of conceptual meaning. FCCT is a middle-range family nursing theory to explain a nursing phenomenon in which a relationship is created between the family receiving family care and the nursing professional who provides such care. This focuses on the process of establishing a family care/caring relationship between the family and the nursing professional. The mapping out of this theory is the Family Care/Caring Model (FCCM) as shown by the three-dimensional structural diagram (**Figure 1**) provided to facilitate visual comprehension. The degree of perception of distance in interpersonal relationships is represented by the concept of functional distance, but the relationship between the family system unit and family environment is not only the functional distance; it is also necessary to consider the structural distance, which refers to the degree of physical separation [7]. In the FCCT, which is based on the CSFET, the relationship of trust between the family and nursing professional can be clarified by the structural distance and functional distance. Through future use in clinical settings its effectiveness will be empirically substantiated, and it will be necessary to continuously engage in creative revisions.

The FCCT is constructed by layers of research by means of family ethnography. The family environment was reviewed over a wide scope, and it went through the process of development based on a diverse data that were obtained through permeation of family life and ways of thinking. Consequently it is believed that the objective, of a holistic approach to transactions between the family and nursing professional, was achieved.

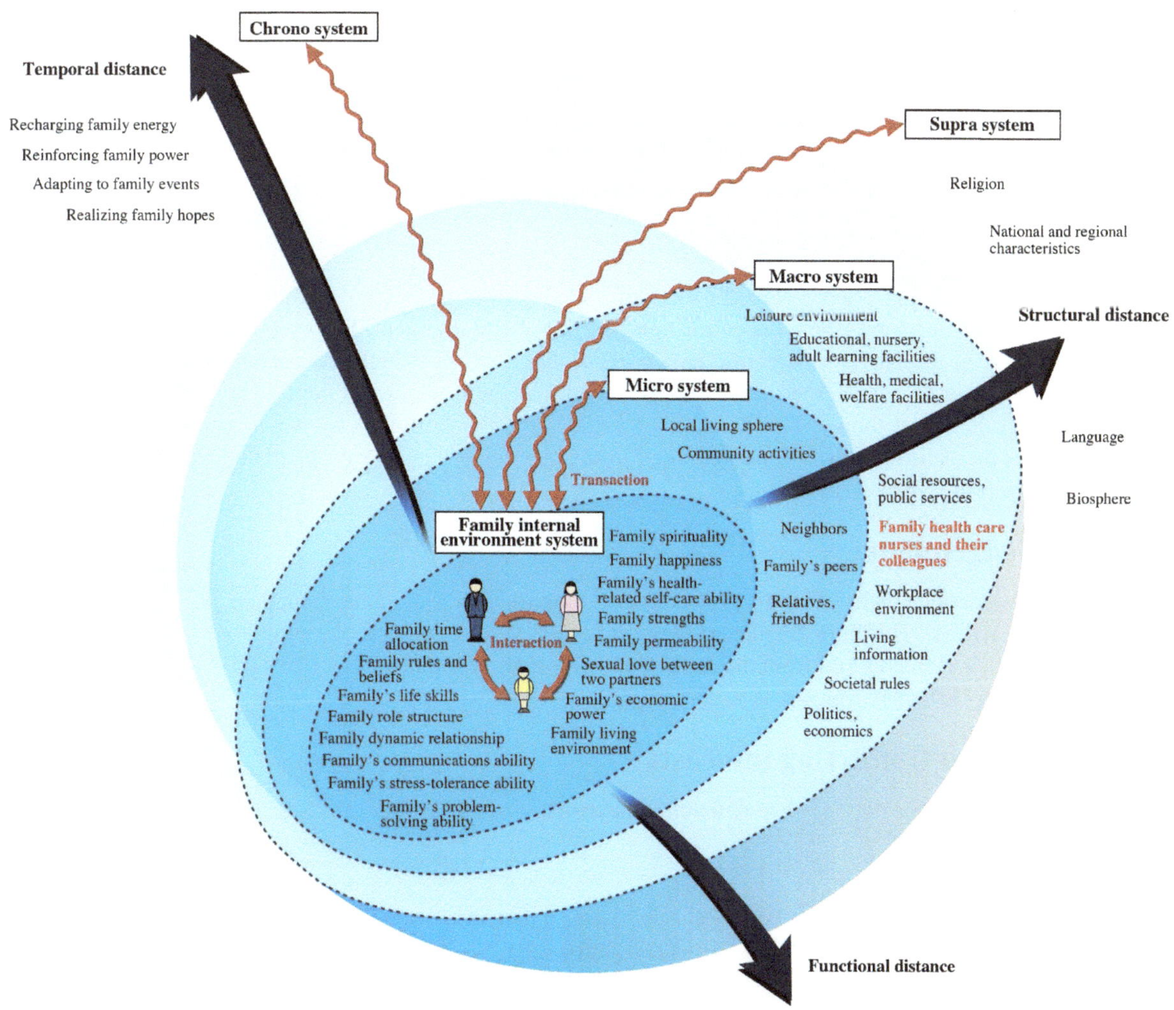

Figure 2. Model diagram of Concentric Sphere Family Environment Theory (CSFET) (Ver. 2.5).

Family nursing carries the connotation of family care and family caring, and it is believed that the quality of family nursing is determined by what sort of relationship built between the nursing professional and the family. In the CSFET/FCCT, through readiness to become close to the family, in other words, through empathy in understanding of the family and its world, it is important that a situation be constructed of "being together with the family." Moreover, the nursing professional, by self-knowledge, can achieve self-elevation, which is where the practice of family caring comes to be.

From the standpoint of the nursing professional, family caring promotes the growth and development of the family system unit, and improves family functioning (*i.e.*, the self-actualization of other individuals). The nursing professional, on the other hand, realizes self-healing and self-fulfillment is promoted (*i.e.*, the self-actualization). In this manner, the phenomena that develop between the family and nursing professional are the phenomena of family caring. The outcome of family care/caring is 1) self-actualization of other individuals; 2) self-actualization; and 3) establishment of a family caring relationship. In order to make for an effective and high quality moments of family intervention, which never recur twice in the same setting, establishment of a family caring relationship is a prerequisite.

The nursing professional feels "concern" toward the target family in his or her care, and must possess a clear desire for the family to realize its hopes to the greatest degree possible. The family care/caring environment is the family environment, the shared venue in which the family and nursing professional engage in family care/caring. It is necessary to also decide the direction of the functional distance between the family and nursing professional. In other words, in terms of functional distance as seen by the nursing professional, there is the functional distance by which the nursing professional cares for the family, and the functional distance by which the nursing professional is cared for by the family. The former is defined as the "active functional distance," while the latter is defined as the "passive functional distance," and the two are not necessarily of the same length. For example, in the case of family intervention that does not affect family beliefs [18], intentions and aspirations, active functional distance becomes overly shorter irrespective of the passive functional distance. In this case, it is necessary for the nursing professional to endeavor to build a relationship of trust.

5. Conclusion

The Family Care/Caring Theory (FCCT) was developed for the purpose of caring for the family system unit. This was implemented into the Concentric Sphere Family Environment Theory (CSFET), an existing family nursing theory. In the family care/caring environment, the "act" by which the nursing professional engages in family intervention on a concerned family with which he or she is dealing is family care. Then in the context of the culture of the target family, family care is provided, and the "attitude" by which intervention can enable a family to live on its own terms is family caring. For the practice of family caring, an understanding of FCCT and the CSFET will be indispensable.

Acknowledgements

The authors sincerely appreciate analytical assistance provided by Ms. Saina Taniguchi, Ms. Saori Komiya, Ms. Ai Washizu, and Mr. Hirofumi Mizukami, Kobe University. This project was supported in part by a Grant-in-Aid for Scientific Research (B) from the Japan Society for the Promotion of Science (JSPS) in Japan (Grant Nos. 24390498 and 15H05084).

Declaration of Conflicting Interests

The authors declare that they have no competing interests.

References

[1] Noddings, N. (2013) Caring: A Relational Approach to Ethics and Moral Education. 2nd Edition, University of California Press, Berkeley.

[2] Hohashi, N. and Honda, J. (2010) Family Functioning. In: Hohashi, N., Ed., *New Family Health Care Nursing: Theory, Practice and Research*, Medical Friend Sha, Tokyo, 38-45.

[3] Honda, J. and Hohashi, N. (2015) The Trend of Research Concerning "Caring" in Japan. *International Journal for Human Caring*, **19**, In Press.

[4] Ray, M.A. (1989) The Theory of Bureaucratic Caring for Nursing Practice in the Organizational Culture. *Nursing Administration Quarterly*, **13**, 31-42. http://dx.doi.org/10.1097/00006216-198901320-00007

[5] Hohashi, N. and Honda, J. (2014) "Unreciprocated Family Members" Issue (Hohashi). In: Hohashi, N., Ed., *Assessment Guide for Japanese Version of the Family Environment Map (FEM-J)*, Editex, Tokyo, 27-29.

[6] Hohashi, N. and Kobayashi, K. (2010) Methods of Treatment of the Family System Unit. In: Hohashi, N., Ed., *New Family Health Care Nursing: Theory, Practice and Research*, Medical Friend Sha, Tokyo, 16-25.

[7] Hohashi, N. and Honda, J. (2011) Development of the Concentric Sphere Family Environment Model and Companion Tools for Culturally Congruent Family Assessment. *Journal of Transcultural Nursing*, **22**, 350-361. http://dx.doi.org/10.1177/1043659611414200

[8] Honda, J. and Hohashi, N. (2010) Ethnography. In: Hohashi, N., Ed., *New Family Health Care Nursing: Theory, Practice and Research*, Medical Friend Sha, Tokyo, 399-404.

[9] Honda, J. and Hohashi, N. (2014) Development of a New Growth and Development Sectors for the Family System Unit. *Proceedings of the Sigma Theta Tau International's 25th International Nursing Research Congress*, Hong Kong, 25 July 2014, 822-823.

[10] Hohashi, N. and Honda, J. (2013) Japanese Version of the Family Environment Assessment Index (FEAI-J). Editex, Tokyo.

[11] Hohashi, N. and Honda, J. (2015) Assessment Guide for the English Version of the Family Environment Map (FEM-E). Editex, Tokyo.

[12] Graneheim, U.H. and Lundman, B. (2004) Qualitative Content Analysis in Nursing Research: Concepts, Procedures

and Measures to Achieve Trustworthiness. *Nurse Education Today*, **24**, 105-112. http://dx.doi.org/10.1016/j.nedt.2003.10.001

[13] Purnell, M.J. (2006) Development of a Model of Nursing Education Grounded in Caring and Application to Online Nursing Education. *International Journal for Human Caring*, **10**, 8-16.

[14] Emoto, R., Tsutsui, M. and Kawana, R. (2015) A Model to Create a Caring and Healing Environment for Nurses in Child and Family Nursing. *International Journal for Human Caring*, **19**, 8-12.

[15] Ray, M.A. (2009) Transcultural Caring Dynamics in Nursing and Health Care: The Dynamics of Contemporary Nursing. F.A. Davis Company, Philadelphia.

[16] Smith, M.C., Turkel, M.C. and Wolf, Z.R. (Eds.) (2012) Caring in Nursing Classics: An Essential Resource, Springer Publishing Company, New York.

[17] Chinn, P.L. and Kramer, M.K. (2011) Integrated Theory and Knowledge Development in Nursing. 8th Edition, Mosby, St. Louis.

[18] Wright, L.M. and Bell, J.M. (2009) Beliefs and Illness: A Model for Healing. 4th Floor Press, Calgary.

3

Cognitive-Behavioral Group Treatment for Men Voluntarily Seeking Help for Violence towards Their Intimate Partners: The Impact of Treatment Components 4 - 7 Years after Therapy

Stig Jarwson*, Merete Berg Nesset, Tom Palmstierna, Jim Aage Nottestad, Erik Søndenaa

St. Olavs Hospital, Forensic Department Brøset, Norwegian University of Science and Technology, Norway
Email: *stig.jarwson@stolav.no

Abstract

Background: Even though domestic violence is a major problem, only a few studies have examined the long term sustainability of treatment for men who voluntarily seek help to stop their violent behavior towards intimate partners. Women are exposed to a much greater degree of serious violence and sexual abuse compared to men. Objective: The aim of this study was to identify which elements of the treatment program batterers found most useful four to seven years after program completion. Design: The participants consisted of a sample of men who had gone through anger management therapy four to seven years previously. Data on violence were collected through self-report before and four to seven years after treatment, using a modified version of the Conflict Tactics Scales. Results: The decrease in physical violence was statistically significant: $t(36) = 8.43$, $p < 0.001$ with a large effect size (eta squared = 0.66). Psychological violence also decreased significantly: $t(36) = 9.21$, $p < 0.001$ with a large effect size (eta squared = 0.7). The results indicate that the most important anger management techniques were extensively applied in former patients of the anger management treatment program. In total, about two out of three patients still used the techniques after ending treatment four to seven years earlier.

Keywords

Intimate Domestic Violence, Cognitive Behavioral Treatment, Cognitive Techniques

*Corresponding author.

1. Introduction

Research on the effectiveness of treatment programs for partner-violent men has yielded mixed findings. In their evaluation of meta-analyses and experimental designs, Gondolf and Jones (2001) found little or no treatment effect. The studies included three, well-established batterer programs using a gender-based, cognitive-behavioral approach (n = 640). Completing a batterer program reduced the men's likelihood of re-assaulting by a percentage ranging from 44% to 64%, depending on the specifications used. Completing a 3-month program appeared to be as effective as completing a 5.5- or 9-month program [1]. In a recent Cochrane report [2], it was stated that in spite of many studies on the treatment of domestically violent men, the evidence of controlled studies is insufficient to draw conclusions on the effects. He also noted that most studies focused on the treatment of court-ordered clients and that many studies lacked a description of the actual content of the therapy.

A meta-analysis of 50 studies with a total of 1640 clients was conducted to determine whether cognitive therapy was an effective treatment of aggression and hostile power dominance [3].

Patient groups studied included abusive parents and abusive spouses, school children, clinical adolescents, juvenile delinquents, inmates, and college students. Effect sizes were calculated from self-reports of anger, dependent measures of anger and aggression, and behavioral ratings of aggression, and they were averaged across variables to produce one effect size per study. The effect sizes for the 50 studies ranged from −0.32 to 1.57 (SD 0.43) with all effect sizes but one being positive in value. The grand mean weighted effect size was 0.70 ($p < 0.001$), which means that the average patient who received CBT fared better than 76% of the patients who did not receive CBT. This corresponds to a treatment success rate of 67% for CBT compared with 33% for patients who received control treatments.

A study of the Brøset Model [4] showed that a 15-week manual, group-based CBT program significantly and substantially reduced self-reported violent behavior. After the initial assessment but before group therapy sessions, 26 men were randomly selected for immediate treatment or put on a waiting list.

In the treatment group, all kinds of self-reported partner-related violence were significantly reduced, while those on the waiting list did not reduce their partner-related violence. The results indicate that the group treatment had an effect in itself beyond the wishes and intentions of the men to reduce their partner violence.

Aim

The aim of this study was to identify which elements of the treatment program batterers found most useful four to seven years after program completion.

2. Methods

2.1. Subjects

Over a period of four years, 269 men completed the Cognitive behavioral group-treatment "Brøsetmodellen" (see below). A randomized sample of 85 men were selected and asked by mail to respond to a questionnaire as part of a follow-up study, concerning their current use of violence and use of the techniques from their treatment sessions. Ten of the eighty-five men were not traceable. Of the remaining seventy-five, four were unwilling to participate. From this sample (n = 71) 37 (52.1%) participated and 34 (47.9%) did not. A demographic comparison between the responders and the non-responders did not confirm any differences in age, education, income or violence before treatment.

The mean age of the responders was 41.8 (27 to 63). Most of them (67.6%) had the equivalent of a college education of 12 to 13 years , 27% had an academic education, 5.4% had no education after primary school (10 years), 91.9% lived in a spousal partnership, and 78.3% were fathers with one to three children (Mean = 1.9). At the follow-up, 62.9% lived in the same relationship as before treatment.

2.2. Treatment Description (Brøsetmodellen)

The treatment was based on the principles of Aaron Beck's cognitive therapy [5], with a treatment manual constructed by the first author (Jarwson) and colleagues [6] [7] In the first session, anger was described in terms of emotional, psychological, cognitive, and behavioral components.

The first aspect concerned the client-therapist relationship where the therapists reassures the clients that they were meeting with respect, warmth, and as "equal human beings". The second aspect of the individual sessions concerned the mutual assessment of the violence problem, creating a shared picture of the problem. Here the CTS assessments were part of the sessions. A third aspect of these individual sessions was reflections on the client's readiness to change, with emphasis on the client's acknowledgement of personal responsibility for his own behavior. If the client and his partner wished, a fourth session with them together reflecting on these themes was offered.

The cognitive group treatment approach combines a variety of techniques such as identifying core beliefs and assumptions that lead to misinterpretation of potentially violent situations. Also important is awareness of situational triggers leading to anger arousal. This may be followed by the patient learning to reframe the anger-arousing situation by rehearsing self-instructions. Self-instructions means that the person, when identifying negative thoughts in a situation, tells himself: "Stop! I am overreacting. This is my core belief and vulnerability talking" or "I can handle it. It is not his/her intention to hurt me." By identifying situational triggers and negative thoughts and feelings, the person may learn to react in a manner appropriate to the situation and avoid using violence.

The group therapy consisted of two equal parts (**Table 1**).

All sessions are guided by a manual, delivered by qualified therapists to a group of six to eight clients. Each session is of approximately 2 hours in duration.

Table 1. Preparatory and treatment phase of Brøsetmodellen.

Phase	Session focus
Individual therapy 3 - 4 hours	Recognizing motivation/readiness for change. In the individual sessions, the client learns the rationale of the method and the tools used in the group session. Measures schemas.
	Group therapy
Session 1. psycho-educative	Overview of the group and group rules Each participant's goal, expectations of the group What makes people angry into context with other emotions
Session 2 psycho-educative	Anger is an emotion and aggression is a behavior Event > distressed > "wronged" > anger > mobilized to attack Learn to gain control over anger through anger circle Reactions to triggers, thoughts, feelings, arousal, and behavior
Session 3 psycho-educative	The vulnerable self-image and self-esteem. Awareness of the vulnerability of negative thoughts, how the body reacts. Alternative coping strategies, time-out, yellow cards. Alternative thinking errors (Mindfulness shift focus)
Session 4 psycho-educative	Anger and violence in the family perspective, compassion, respect and cooperation in relationships Children perspective
Session 5 psycho-educative	Understanding automatic thoughts and learning about core beliefs and underlying beliefs Identifying the meaning of the event and our perceptions.
Session 6 - 12 Group therapy	Each client describes how the week has passed with regard to his violent behavior. Each client has to analyze his violent episode through the cognitive tools. Event > negative thoughts > interpretation > feeling > arousal > action. Using Socratic questions, the therapists encourage the clients to come up with constructive alternatives of behavior. The rest of the group participates by helping the client to define an acceptable alternative behavior.
Session 13 - 14 Group therapy	Understand their own core beliefs in order to recognize them, question them, and acquire techniques for challenging them. Cognitive distortions forming core beliefs and ways of addressing them are identified by using rehearsal and homework
Session 15 Group therapy	Group members evaluate each other and identify areas where they need to be cautious in the future.

2.3. Measures

Data on violence were collected before and four to seven years after treatment using a modified version of the Conflict Tactic Scale, CTS [8]. The CTS has been the principal method of measuring physical aggression among community samples of married couples or individuals dating. The CTS consists of a list of actions that a family member might use when in conflict with another family member, a friend or a stranger. The original CTS is intended to measure three constructs: Reasoning, Verbal Aggression, and Physical Aggression or Violence. In this study, the "reasoning" items from the CTS were dropped, and a section on material and sexual violence was added.

Clients who participated in the follow-up study answered the same CTS schema, and they registered the anger and violence throughout the previous year.

In this study, domestic violence is defined as the use of physical, psychological, or material violence by one adult towards a member of the household to cause harm, injury, or fear. Physical violence items involve throwing something, pushing, grabbing, shoving, slapping, spanking, kicking, biting, punching, hitting, or trying to hit with an object, beating, choking, threatening with weapons like a knife or a gun, and using weapons like a knife or a gun.

Psychological violence involves interrogating a partner when she has been out, calling her obscene names, or frightening her with threatening body language in intense jealousy. "Verbal Aggression" also means shouting at her, using verbal and symbolic means of hurting, such as insults or threats. Material violence was defined as behaviors such as pounding the wall or table as well as destroying property.

The violent acts were registered on a response scale with the options one, two, three times or more during the year.

The follow up questionnaire also focused on the target content of the intervention and asked ten questions concerning the use of crucial cognitive techniques in "the Brøset model" of anger management treatment [9]. The items were scored on a five-point ordinal rating scale reporting the frequency of utilization: 1 ("never"), 2 ("once"), 3 ("two to five times"), 4 ("six to ten times") and 5 ("more than ten times"). In the further analysis, categories 2 and 3 were combined into the new category "sometimes", and categories 4 and 5 were combined into the new category "frequently".

2.4. Ethics

The study was approved by the Regional Committee for Research Ethics (REK) and the Norwegian Data Inspectorate (NSD).

3. Results

The overall results showed that there was a decrease in physical and psychological violence at the follow up, four to seven years after treatment.

Physical violence and psychological violence were described in 70.3% and in 89.2% of the responders (N = 37) before treatment. Most participant (83.8%) reported a termination of physical violence at the follow-up, 10.8% were still physically violent and 5.4% were more physically violent four to seven years after treatment completion. A majority of the participants (59.4%) reported a termination of their use of psychological violence at follow-up, 32.4% were still psychologically violent, and 8.1% reported more psychologically violent behavior (see **Figure 1**).

The decrease in physical violence was statistically significant: $t(36) = 8.43$, $p < 0.001$ with a large effect size (eta squared = 0.66). Psychological violence also decreased significantly: $t(36) = 9.21$, $p < 0.001$ with a large effect size (eta squared = 0.7).

The results indicated that the most important anger management techniques were extensively applied in patients of the previous anger management treatment program. In total, about two out of three patients still used the techniques after ending treatment four to seven years earlier. The anger management circle was less used compared to the "time-out" techniques, recognizing body signals and anger management openness (Q9), but all techniques significantly approached in the patients repertoire (see **Table 2**).

A Friedman's Two-Way analysis of Variance by Ranks was conducted to evaluate the differences in frequency of using anger management techniques. A statistically significant difference between reports of "never

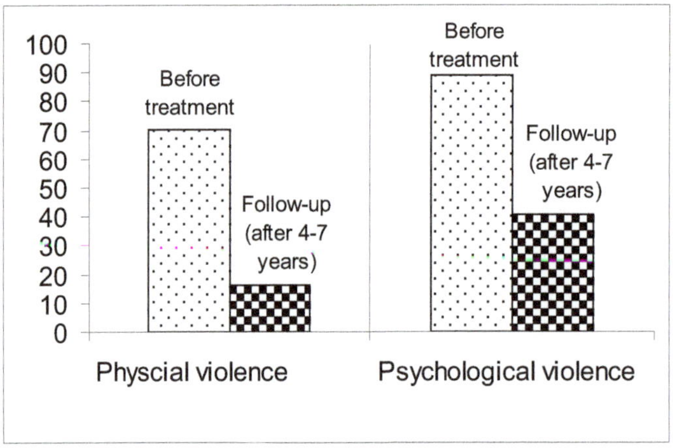

Figure 1. Self-reported violence before and at follow-up treatment.

Table 2. The frequency of using anger management techniques in all the patients (n = 37) and in patients with a self-reported positive treatment outcome.

Anger management technique	Frequently used in all patients (n = 37)	Frequently used in non-physical violent patients (n = 31)	Frequently used in non-psychological violent patients (n = 22)
Q1: circle of anger	15	13	10
Q2: "time-out" techniques	26	23	13
Q3: Recognizing body signals	25	23	14
Q4: Recognizing negative thoughts	23	21	15
Q5: Stop, making thought controlled	24	20	16
Q6: Evaluating missing interpretation	23	21	13
Q7: Evaluating the situation based on life-rules (expectations)	21	20	12
Q8: Take the responsibility of acting calm when humiliated	21	19	13
Q9: Discussing your anger problem	26	23	16
Q10: Focusing the self-confidence of acting without violence	26	22	15
Q11: Self-confidence avoiding violence	19	18	12
Mean number of techniques used	6.7 (sd = 3.4)	7.2 (sd = 3.3)	6.8 (sd = 3.8)

use" (Median = 14.1), "sometimes use" (Median = 19.8) and reports of "frequently use" [Median = 66.2, $p < 0.001$] arose.

4. Discussion

The results of the study of 37 former patients showed that a 15-week group-based anger management CBT program significantly reduced self-reported violent behavior. Further analysis showed that a number of anger management techniques that were emphasized in the program were substantially applied four to seven years after the treatment. Most participants reported applying several anger management techniques on a frequent basis. This result may be associated with the general decrease in self-reported spousal violence compared to the frequency of violent actions before the program. Timeout, recognizing body signals and negative thoughts, and discussing one's anger problem seemed most prominent among the tools they used. A balance of implicit and explicit techniques was emphasized in the group treatment, and the report was promising since in more than two out of three participants four to seven years after treatment, the former clients still frequently used these techniques. The relatively less frequent use of the "anger management circle" may indicate that an integrated comprehension of anger management belongs to an advanced level, but it is not necessarily useful to all patients. Few or no long-term follow-up studies exist on the effects of this type of treatment [2].

Additionally, few or no studies exist that investigate what motivates abusive men to stay in treatment. This fact makes interesting that all the men who started in the group sessions in our study also completed the program. The high completion rate among our subjects may seem out of the ordinary in view of other studies finding that non-court ordered men attend fewer sessions than court-ordered [10] [11].

These findings indicate that the treatment as a whole, including the initial individual sessions, was effective by itself, and also that it had effects over a long time span after treatment. Since 1960, Cognitive Therapy (CT) and Cognitive Behavioral Therapy (CBT), and programs with elements of CBT, such as the Duluth Model (Domestic Abuse Intervention Project DAIP, 1981), have frequently been used as treatment for men who abuse their female partners. The Duluth Model reflects the underlying feminist philosophy that violence is used by men to exert "power and control" over the behavior of their female partners. In recent years, the Duluth Model has been criticized for its lack of scientific research and for being impeded by the feminist ideological structure inherent in the patriarchal view of "power and control" [12]. Dutton and Corvo stated that men in treatment groups were more often characterized by powerlessness than by power and that the concept of power was misused by feminists.

The "Brøset Model" has a conventional Cognitive Therapy for anger as conceptualized by Beck [5] [13], working with automatic thoughts, logical errors, cognitive distortions, and core beliefs [14]. In the CBT group, self-disclosure is necessary for the group to gain access to covert cognitive processes that represent potential treatment targets. Feedback from the group, as well as the therapists, plays a role in helping to shift patients' distorted cognition and to reinforce more realistic appraisals.

Another important aspect is a therapeutic relationship built on warmth, empathy, and Socratic dialogue. This is in contrast to the moralistic attitude in CBT programs that has components from the Duluth Model [2]. The previous report [4] showed that a 15-week manual, group-based CBT program significantly and substantially reduced self-reported violent behavior at the end of treatment.

This follow up study on the Brøset Model four to seven years after treatment has some limitations, based on the small sample size and the lack of a control group.

Despite the methodological limitations of the response rate bias that self-reports represent, and the social desirability bias, the findings reported are interesting and important in their own right. Even four to seven years after treatment, when these men felt angry, many used the techniques they had learned to calm themselves down and consequently avoided violent situations. The skill-based training that was emphasized in the anger management program described above seemed to be an important and feasible element of the treatment many years after. This may indicate that being aware of bodily signs and negative thoughts when one is angry and—maybe most importantly—learning alternative ways to handle these situations, are potential moderating factors in the treatment of domestic perpetrators. The results in this study indicate that despite experiencing anger arousal, men can avoid acting out the anger if they receive the right tools to handle the angry feelings.

Controlled studies involving partner interviews and the separate techniques' impact may provide information on effective components of the improved treatment model.

References

[1] Gondolf, E.W. and Jones, A.S. (2001) The Program Effect of Batterer Programs in Three Cities. *Violence and Victims*, **16**, 693-704.

[2] Smedslund, G., *et al.* (2007) Cognitive Behavioral Therapy for Men Who Physically Abuse Their Female Partner. The Cochrane Library, JohnWiley & Sons, Ltd., Hoboken.

[3] Beck, R. and Fernandez, E. (1998) Cognitive-Behavioral Therapy in the Treatment of Anger: A Meta-Analysis. *Cognitive Therapy and Research*, **22**, 63-74. http://dx.doi.org/10.1023/A:1018763902991

[4] Palmstierna, T., *et al.* (2012) Cognitive-Behavior Group Therapy for Men Voluntary Seeking Help for Intimate Partner Violence. *Nordic Journal of Psychiatry*, **66**, 360-365. http://dx.doi.org/10.3109/08039488.2012.665080

[5] Beck, A.T. (1999) Prisoners of Hate: The Cognitive Basis of Anger, Hostility, and Violence. Harper Collins Publishers, New York.

[6] Haugan, G. and Jarwson, S. (2005) Kognitiv terapi ved vold og aggresjon [Cognitive Therapy of Violence and Aggression]. *Tidsskrift for kognitiv terapi*, **6**, 1-10.

[7] Jarwson, S. and Haugan, G. (2008) Violence and Anger: A Treatment Manual in Anger. In: Berge, T. and Repål, A., Eds., *Håndbok i kognitiv terapi*, Gyldendal Norsk forlag, Oslo, 349-378.

[8] Straus, M.A. (1979) Measuring Intrafamily Conflict and Violence: The Conflict Tactics (CT) Scales. *Journal of Marriage and the Family*, **41**, 75-88. http://dx.doi.org/10.2307/351733

[9] Jarwson, S. (2010) Effekten av manualisert kognitiv gruppeterapi for menn som frivillig søker hjelp mot vold i nære relasjoner: Effekten av kognitiv gruppeterapi etter deltakelse i Sinnemestring Brøsetmodellen 4-7 år etter avsluttet terapi.

[10] Daly, J.E., Power, T.G. and Gondolf, E.W. (2001) Predictors of Batterer Program Attendance. *Journal of Interpersonal Violence*, **16**, 971-991. http://dx.doi.org/10.1177/088626001016010001

[11] Gerlock, A.A. (2001) A Profile of Who Completes and Who Drops Out of Domestic Violence Rehabilitation. *Issues in Mental Health Nursing*, **22**, 379-400. http://dx.doi.org/10.1080/01612840116997

[12] Dutton, D.G. and Corvo, K. (2006) Transforming a Flawed Policy: A Call to Revive Psychology and Science in Domestic Violence Research and Practice. *Aggression and Violent Behavior*, **11**, 457-483. http://dx.doi.org/10.1016/j.avb.2006.01.007

[13] Beck, A.T. (1979) Cognitive Therapy and the Emotional Disorders. International Universities Press, New York.

[14] Young, J.E., Klosko, J.S. and Weishaar, M.E. (2003) Schema Therapy: A Practitioner's Guide. Guilford Press, New York.

4

Challenges of Nurse Tutors' Classroom and Clinical Performance When Teaching

Noel D. Mbirimtengerenji[1], Felicity Daniels[2], Penelope Martin[2]

[1]Kamuzu College of Nursing, University of Malawi, Lilongwe, Malawi
[2]University of Western Cape, Bellville, South Africa
Email: ndmbiri@kcn.unima.mw, fdaniels@uwc.ac.za, pmartin@uwc.ac.za

Abstract

Introduction: Nursing is a dual profession that involves teaching both in class and at the clinical area. Nurse tutors meet a lot of challenges in their profession through their cognitive, affective and psychomotor nursing performance. The aim of this paper is to determine the challenges of nurse tutor clinical affective, cognitive and psychomotor performance in Malawi. Methods: Mixed methods design was employed. Quantitatively, 129 students and 82 nurse tutors randomly selected were involved for the five ranked Likert Scale questionnaire, and 42 nurse tutors were involved in in-depth. While 8 focus group discussions were conducted in 8 nursing colleges. Descriptive and inferential statistics were used quantitatively for predictive variable of nurse tutor work experience and student study experience to compare with the dependent variables from the 39 cognitive, affective and psychomotor attributes. Results: Both nurse tutors and students are not impressed with nurse tutors cognitive, affective and psychomotor performance during teaching. There is inadequate clinical orientation to students [OR ≤ 0.302; 95%CI (0.096 ± 2.955); p ≥ 0.042] and inadequate funding from college administration [OR ≤ 1.013; 95%CI (0.271 ± 3.793); p ≥ 0.985] as a result it creates much pressure on teaching. Conclusion: There is a need to develop an effective teaching strategy that would be conducive and easy to use for the limited resource environments in Malawi.

Keywords

Nurse Tutor Challenges, Nurse Tutor Performance, Nurse Tutor Work Experience, Student Study Experience

1. Introduction

Clinical skills underpin nurses' professional practice and thus nurse tutors need effective opportunities to acquire, develop and master these skills [1]. Enabling practical skills development is a key dimension of nursing education [2]. It is stated that nurse tutors are charged with the responsibility of creating a learning environment and learning opportunities that are inviting, challenging and motivating, and that promote critical thinking and problem-solving skills to students. This is because nursing education must be both formal and informal that utilizes different teaching strategies both in class and at the clinical area.

Since nursing is a dual profession that involves teaching both in class and at the clinical area, Nurse tutors meet a lot of challenges in their profession through their cognitive, affective and psychomotor nursing performance. There must be much effort done by nurse tutors to let the students acquire these learning domains from different clinical settings as the tutors are perceived as role models in teaching. This challenges nurse tutors in ensuring that the integration of theory and clinical practice occurs basing on their cognitive, affective and psychomotor performance.

The integration of knowledge, skills, attitudes and values in a specified context is one of the cornerstones advocated by the outcomes-based approach to teaching nursing [3]. Such integration yields nurse tutor performance that must promote the professional care to patients. However, there have been increased challenges to the level of these performances of the nurse tutors in the clinical area in Malawi. Clinical performance of the nursing students depends upon the ward sisters and the nurse educator [4]. Clinical teaching is one of the core components of the role of the nurse tutors. Most of the clinical teaching of nursing students is done by nurse educators. However, there is no clear literature that has evaluated the clinical performance of the nurse tutors in Malawi basing on the cognitive, affective and psychomotor domains.

The philosophy of clinical instructions provides a framework for making curricular choices from among options and understanding the implications of alternate educational decisions, values and beliefs that provide structure and coherence for a curriculum [5]. Without structured instructions, the performance of the nurse tutor cannot be qualitative.

The way in which performance in nursing and midwifery is managed and measured is of concern to individual practitioners, managers, employing organizations, nursing educators and to patients. Most nurses and other health care practitioners in Malawi do not measure cognitive, affective and psychomotor nurse tutor performance correctly. By definition, performance is a reference to the nursing knowledge, skill or judgment possessed and applied by the nurse and/or midwife in the practice of the nursing and/or midwifery [6]. Cognitive performance focuses on the professional knowledge level of the nurse tutor when discharging duties in the clinical area. In this study, the professional cognitive performance of a nurse and/or midwife is unsatisfactory if it is below the standard reasonably expected of a nurse and/or midwife of an equivalent level of training or experience. The professional affective performance of the nurse tutor describes the professional attitudes that she or he discharges during teaching to nursing students in the clinical area while the professional psychomotor performance of the nurse tutor characterises the attributes of the nurse tutor that deals with the action oriented skills in the clinical area.

The fact that nurses spend more time with patients than do any other health care providers, patient outcomes are affected by nursing cognitive, affective and psychomotor quality care. This helps to give nurses much emphasis on determining the level of such performance during. Thus, improvements in patient safety can be achieved by improving nurse tutor performance attributes in clinical teaching to students. Another author [7] reviewed literature on nursing performance, which included cognitive, physical, and organizational factors that affected performance. It is noted that nurse's work system often does not accommodate human limits and capabilities and that nurses work under cognitive, perceptual, and physical overloads which in turn, impinge clinical performance. Specifically, nurses engage in multiple tasks under cognitive load.

Matching teaching and learning to students is often not possible hence the notion that educators have to adopt a variety of teaching styles to accommodate a variety of learning styles [8]. Diversity in the use of teaching styles is crucial for the attainment of cross-cutting core competencies and achieves better performance in nursing in the clinical area.

It is important for teachers to realize that learners in nursing are adult learners and, according to Knowles's theory. They possess the characteristics of self-concept with plenty of experience to connect new knowledge for meaningful understanding and interpretation of thoughts and feelings. Literature has also pointed out the concerns about the lack of skills and experience of some nurse tutors, and suggested that this can contribute to the poor performance of nursing students. They claim that some tutors are not specialized enough in their fields of knowledge, and that results in a drop in learners' motivational levels [5].

The quality of some nurse tutors performance is equal to that of the ward sisters who are not specialized in their field. On the other hand, tutor participants voice their needs to management to specialize in different fields, but there is limited support from management [9]. Nurse tutors complain that they do not get any study leave or long leave and cannot even attend developmental professional course which mostly demotivates them.

Moreover, several recent high profile cases of poor nurse tutor practice in nursing have been documented in Malawi [10]. Individual and institutional have highlighted the importance of managing and learning from poor performance. Scholars have recently defined poor performance as: "any aspects of a practitioner's conduct which: pose a threat or potential threat to patient safety; expose services to financial or other substantial risk; undermine the reputation or efficiency of services in some significant way; and are outside acceptable practice guidelines and standards". However, this definition has yet to be evaluated against practice and the extent to which it proves to be a robust and shared definition of poor performance among nurse tutors, necessary to assess, best manage and improve practice is yet unknown in Malawi. Whilst current global guidelines define poor performance primarily in relation to patient safety and risk, in nursing practice, more than 20% of nurses are suspended for professional incompetency reasons in nursing education [11].

Tutors have access to a mix of courses to improve teaching psychomotor skills and knowledge. Registered nurses with generic nursing degrees have access to scholarships to upgrade their qualifications in Malawi. For example, Kamuzu College of Nursing (KCN) has been training nurse tutors at degree level mature entry for more than 15 years. In this programme, experience registered nurses are selected from different hospitals and attend to a two year Bachelor of Science degree in nursing education. Some courses that they learn are the teaching strategies in nursing; curriculum development, curriculum administration and teaching practicum as the skill acquisition process in readiness to their tutorship deployment in the country' nursing colleges. KCN also developed a short course in teaching methodology for assistant tutors and clinical instructors from CHAM institutions [12]. Therefore, a reasonable number of the qualified nurse tutors with a degree are deployed into the nursing schools [13]. There has not been any study that evaluates the cognitive, affective and psychomotor clinical performance of these nurse tutors. To this effect, the aim of this paper is to determine the challenges of nurse tutor clinical cognitive, affective, and psychomotor performance in Malawi. This study is an eye opener to both nursing administrators and nurse educators on the improvement of the classroom and clinical cognitive, affective and psychomotor performance during teaching.

2. Methodology

The study design for this research was descriptive exploratory mixed methods which utilized both qualitative and sequential quantitative methods. This research was conducted in Malawi from CHAM nursing Colleges. There were 158 tutors and 2075 students in all the CHAM nursing colleges by 2013.

Iterated purposive, Sampling (IPPS) frame for nurse tutor performance was used. In order to achieve a sample worthy generalization quantitatively, the sample were drawn from the colleges basing on approximated (random probability) number of tutors and students respectively. Drawing sample from the population was initiated until the desired sample was achieved and used the following sample proportion formula: *Sample Size* = $n/\left[1+\left(n/population\right)\right]$ *BUT* $n = Z^2 P(1-P)/E^2$ Where n is sample size of tutors and students in colleges, P is the proportion of number of tutors or students and E is the margin error [14]. This formula allowed 5% for expected margin of error (E) with 95% confidence level as the denominator. Z^2 was a constant score with a value of 1.96^2 (at 95% confidence level and 5% precision [14]. So, this suggest that 129 students and 82 nurse tutors iterated randomly selected, participated in the performance study. Moreover, 42 nurse tutor squalitatively, four from each college, were purposively selected for in-depth interviews on the cognitive and psychomotor performance attributes. Furthermore, 10 students in one focus group discussion for each nursing college were also involved qualitatively.

As inclusion criteria, only two or more years of work experienced nurse tutors participated particularly on cognitive and affective performance attributes in Focus Group and In-Depth Interviews. Only those tutors that had undergone the teaching methodology training participated for the two questionnaires of nurse tutor questionnaire and student questionnaire. Only those students that have been in class for more than one year as their study experience participated in the study.

There were three main instruments used for this study; two **structured** questionnaires; the In-depth interview (**IDI**) and Focus Group Discussion (**FGD**) that articulated the affective and cognitive performance of the nurse tutors. The three instruments were administered concurrently to intensify the construct and face validity and reduce recall bias. 39 cognitive, affective and psychomotor performance attributes were classified and levelled in a five ranked Likert scale questionnaire.

The collected quantitative data were entered on SPSS software version 20.0 and the qualitative data was stored in ATLAS-ti 7.0. Descriptive statistics in the form of frequencies, bivariate analysis and binary logistic regression basing on the cognitive, affective and psychomotor performance attributes were computed for tutors' for all the 38 performance attributes against the predictor variables of nurse tutor work experience and student study experience in different nursing colleges.

The research used bivariate spearman correlation coefficient and binary logistic regression. Nurse tutor work experience and student study experience were used as independent and predictor variables against different nurse tutor performance variables as dependent variables. This was done to generate relationship tables, correlation tables from bivariate analysis and binary logistic regression tables. Only variables that showed correlation in the bivariate analysis were used in the binary logistic regression models to deduce the odds ratio, confidence interval and the beta coefficient results

This research used four criteria for establishing the trustworthiness of qualitative data from the tutors, students and administrators: These were credibility, dependability, confirmability, and transferability. Bias was reduced by doing face to face interview during data collection to iterated randomized nurse tutors and students [15]. Categorizing the participants into three different strata of tutors, student and administrators also helped to reduce bias. Use of limited time on data collection also assisted to reduce bias in the study. The inferential data analysis that focused on bivariate and binary logistic regression helped to reduce bias and control confounding [14]. The content validity for the instruments in the study was maintained by requesting opinions of the experts from two international universities; thus, University of Malawi, and University of Western Cape.

The internal consistency was measured with Cronbach's alpha as the performance attributes were more than 30 in the five ranked Likert scale [16] and variation of alpha values was determined in each item. This was so as Cronbach's alpha is an index of reliability associated with the variation accounted by the true score of the "underlying variables [17].

There were five ways on how this study controlled confounding variables. The most important methods that were used were randomization, restriction, matching, stratification and inferential analysis [14]. This study had an approval from ethical review boards from, University of Western Cape (UWC) and from University of Malawi (UNIMA) through COMREC. All nursing tutors' and students' participants were assured that no form of human rights violation would be encountered in the due course of the nationwide nursing tutor-student clinical performance following the 1964 Declaration of Helsinki; [14] [18] the 1978 Belmont Report; Baltimore Treaty on Ethical Codes (BTEC) and the Nuremburg Codes in medical education research.

3. Results

Nurse tutor performance when teaching in the clinical area were analysed using the tutors' perspective and the students' perspective in a five ranked Likert scale. There were 39 different cognitive, affective and psychomotor performance items that focus on nurse tutors. The Cronbach's alpha which is the reliability statistics was measured and the outcome from the SPSS was 0.954. Generally both nurse tutors and students are not impressed with nurse tutors performance during teaching. This is also the same to nurse tutors and students who clearly indicated dissatisfaction with the nurse tutors' cognitive, affective and psychomotor performance at the clinical area.

In **Figure 1**, the affective performance of nurse tutors on care of **student social support** at the clinical area was analysed. 21% (27) n = 129 of the students from Trinity Nursing College and St. Johns Nursing College agreed that nurse tutors have sense of care during teaching nursing procedures to students. While 19% (24) n = 129 of the students from Ekwendeni Nursing College agreed that their nurse tutors have sense of support and care during teaching both in class and at the clinical area. It was Mulanje nursing College that had the least of the number of students that agreed that their nurse tutors have sense of support and care during teaching both in class and at the clinical area.

Figure 2 illustrates the distribution of students on how they perceive their tutors **show interest in clinical learning**. 65% (13) n = 20 of the students from St. Johns Nursing College strongly agreed that their nurse tutors effectively show interest in clinical learning of the students when teaching. This was followed by Trinity Nursing College where the data illustrates that 54.5% (12) n = 22 of the students agreed that their nurse tutors show

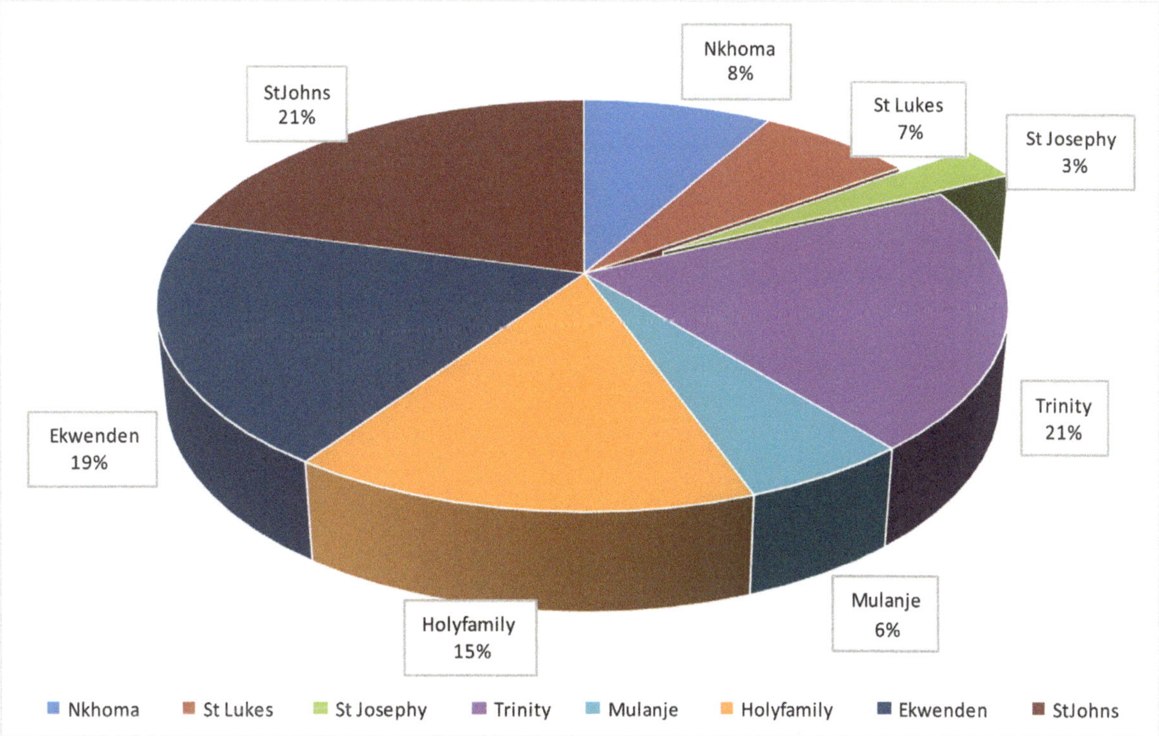

Figure 1. Distribution of students on those that agreed that tutors have sense of care and social support.

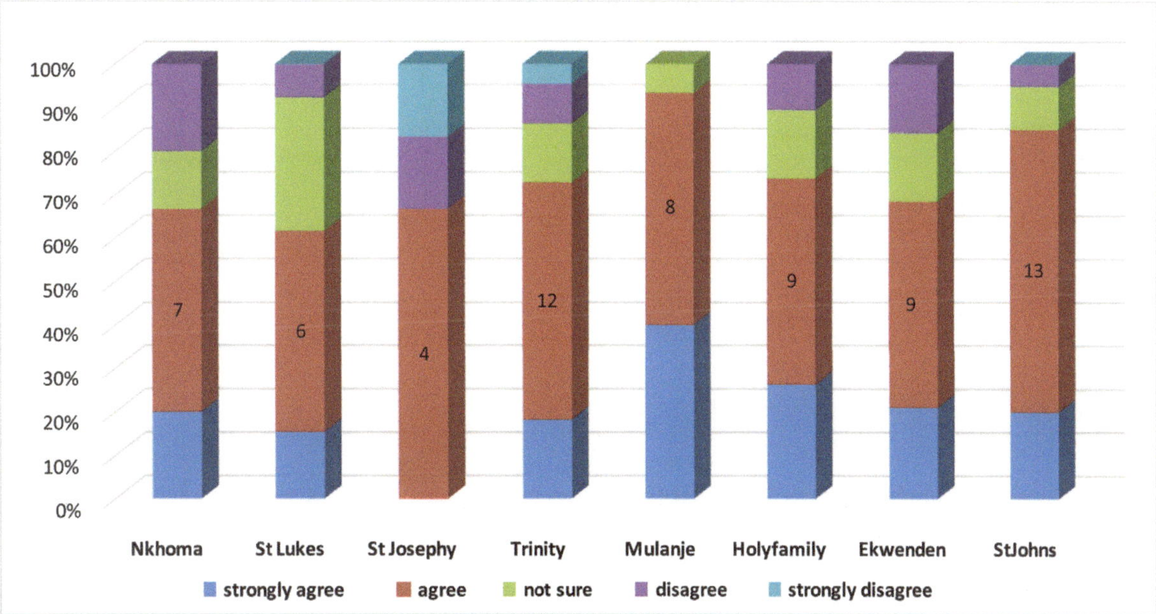

Figure 2. Students distribution on how their tutors show interest in clinical learning.

interest in clinical learning of the students. Holy Family nursing College and Ekwendeni Nursing College also showed high number of students who agreed that their nurse tutors show interest in clinical learning of the students. However, 48.4% (6) n = 13 of the students from St. Lukes nursing College were not sure whether their nurse tutors show interest in clinical learning of the students. This is very pathetic as it shows that students were afraid to say the truth about their nurse tutors affective performance on clinical learning of the students. But in general, 52.7% (68) n = 129 of the students from all nursing colleges agreed that they show interest on clinical student learning. This entails that affective performance of students on student clinical learning is very low. This is because clinical learning of the students is paramount to quality nurses in the country. However, some nurse tutors were very defensive on the affective and psychomotor Performance in class. For example a nurse tutor in St. Lukes Nursing College pointed that:

Am found where am supposed to be found, if am supposed to be in class am in class unless there are very tentative reasons, if am supposed to be at the clinical area, am at the clinical area unless there are very uncontrollable reasons and when am in class am supposed to teach I go there to teach and when am in the clinical area I go there to supervise, demonstrate and I also make sure I do what am supposed to do.

In **Figure 3**, the psychomotor performance of **nurse tutors on demonstration of clinical procedures** were also assessed to the students. In Trinity nursing college 68.1% (15) $n = 22$ of the students agreed that their tutors effectively demonstrates on clinical procedures during teaching. Almost all students from Mulanje Nursing College agreed that their nurse tutors demonstrate effectively on clinical procedures during teaching particularly in the clinical area. However, 73% (14) $n = 19$ of the students from Ekwendeni Nursing College also agreed that their nurse tutors perform effectively during demonstration of clinical procedures particularly at the clinical area. Generally, only 54.3% (70) $n = 129$ of the students from all the nursing colleges agreed that their nurse tutors effectively demonstrates clinical procedures both in class and art the clinical area. However, most of the nurse tutors complained that due to critical scarcity of the equipment, improvisation has remained a remedy during demonstration that reduces quality of the procedures during teaching.

The teaching cognitive and affective performance of the nursing tutors on gender sensitivity during teaching in the clinical area was also analysed in both the students and nurse tutors. 68% (15) $n = 22$ of the students from Trinity Nursing College agreed that nurse tutors are gender sensitive during teaching (see **Figure 4**). But some students explained that the main challenge of the nurse tutors is limited availability in the clinical area as a result they do not discharge their clinical skills frequently to students.

52.6% (10) $n = 19$ of the students from Holy Family nursing college also agreed that their nurse tutors are gender sensitive when teaching both in class and at the clinical area. However, 58.1% (75) $n = 129$ of the students agreed that **nurse tutors are gender sensitive** and understand the gender roles and sexual differences of the students. But one of the male nurse tutors pointed out that the main challenge is that nursing profession is female dominated, therefore, male nurses feel inferior at times to too many female faculty staff in the colleges.

In **Table 1**, the psychomotor performance of the nurse tutors in clinical area was also assessed particularly on the ability to act as a guide as opposed to dominating the group during teaching. 43.7% (7) $n = 16$ of the nurse tutors in Nkhoma Nursing school agreed that they have ability to act as a guide as opposed to dominating the

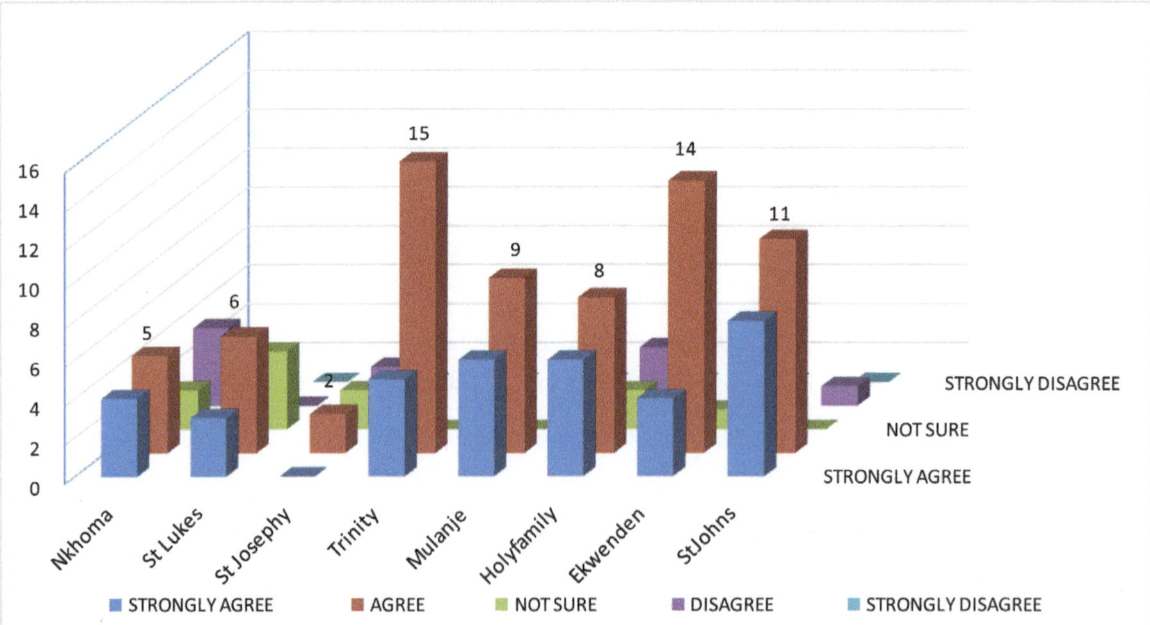

Figure 3. Students distribution on how their tutors effectively demonstrate on clinical procedures.

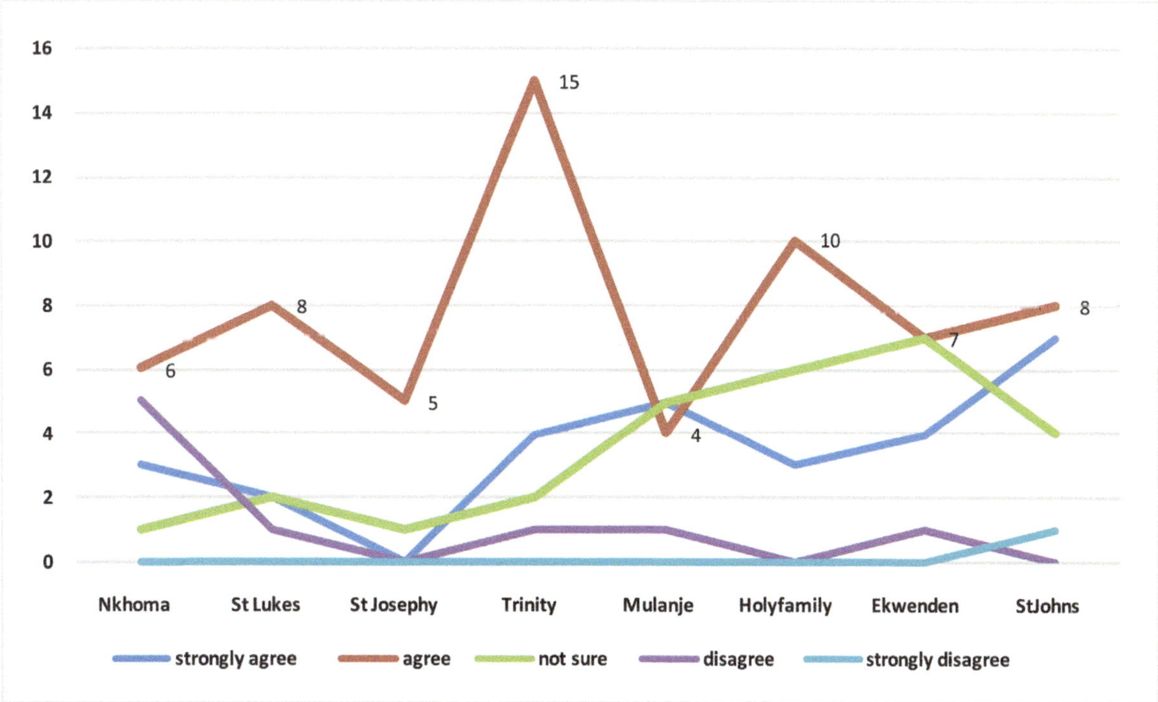

Figure 4. Distribution of students on how their nursing program is gender sensitive.

group in both the class and at the clinical area =. But in the same college 46.7% (7) $n = 15$ of the students agreed that indeed the nurse tutors have the ability to act as a guide as opposed to dominating the group of the students. While 40% (6) $n = 15$ of the nurse tutors in Ekwendeni nursing college agreed that they act as a guide to students rather than dominating in the group. But 42.1% (8) $n = 19$ of the students in Ekwendeni Nursing College agreed that nurse tutors act as guide rather than dominating the group. Generally 48.8% (40) $n = 82$ 0f the nurse tutors from different colleges agreed that they act as a guide to students rather than dominating the group. Moreover, 47.8% (61) $n = 129$ of the students from different nursing colleges agreed that their nurse tutors act as a guide rather than dominating during teaching both in the class and at the clinical area. However, a lot of nurse tutors explained that the increased dominance during teaching comes in on topics that students have limited experience like anatomy and physiology. Student do not participate actively during teaching, thereby causing cognitive dominance of the nurse tutors during teaching.

The teaching psychomotor performance of nurse tutors on **guiding clinical students on resource mobilisation** was also looked into during analysis. 53.3% of the nurse tutors in Ekwendeni Nursing College agreed that they guide nursing students on clinical resource mobilisation during teaching at the clinical area. Moreover, 63.1% of the students from Ekwendeni Nursing College also agreed that the nurse tutors guide the students on clinical resource mobilisation. And there were 50% of the students from St. Joseph who agreed that the nurse tutors guide students on clinical resource mobilisation during teaching in the clinical area. However, 56% (46) $n = 82$ of the nurse tutors from all the nursing colleges in Malawi agreed that they guide the nursing students on resource mobilisation both in the classroom during procedure demonstration and at the clinical area. in addition 56.5% (73) $n = 129$ of the students from different colleges of nursing agreed that nurse tutors guide nursing students on resource mobilisation during teaching particularly in the clinical area. This means that both students and nurse tutors are agreeing that the psychomotor performance of the nurse tutor on resource mobilisation is generally met during teaching both in class and at the clinical area. But a lot of nurse tutors pointed out that they struggle to mobilise resources due to limited funding. Many procedures are demonstrated to students under equipment improvisations (see **Table 2**).

Furthermore, in **Table 1**, the nurse tutors psychomotor performance of discharging **skills in accordance to ward policy** was also assessed. 43.8% of the nurse tutors in Nkhoma Nursing College agreed that they help the students to perform skills in accordance to ward policy during clinical teaching. But 73.3% of the students in the same Nkhoma nursing College agreed that nurse tutors in this college help them perform skills in accordance to

Table 1. Distribution of the nurse tutors and students on tutor performance in different colleges.

VARIABLE		In which college do you teach or learn																	
Cognitive/affective/ psychomotor	**Co-variates**	**Nkhoma**		**St. Lukes**		**St Joseph**		**Trinity**		**Mulanje**		**Holly family**		**Ekwendeni**		**St Johns**		**TOTAL**	
		tut	stud	tut	stud	tut	stud	tut	stud	tut	stud	tut	stud	tut	stud	tut	stude	tutor	stude
Ability to act as a guide as opposed to dominating the group	Strongly agree	7	3	2	2	0	1	2	5	4	5	8	2	1	2	2	4	**26**	**24**
	Agree	7	7	3	6	3	2	2	10	4	4	5	13	6	8	10	11	**40**	**61**
	Not sure	2	4	0	4	1	2	1	4	2	4	0	3	5	7	1	3	**12**	**31**
	Disagree	0	1	0	0	0	1	0	3	0	2	1	1	2	2	0	1	**3**	**11**
	Strongly disagree	0	0	0	1	0	0	0	0	0	0	0	0	1	0	0	1	**1**	**2**
	TOTAL	**16**	**15**	**5**	**13**	**4**	**6**	**5**	**22**	**10**	**15**	**14**	**19**	**15**	**19**	**13**	**20**	**82**	**129**
Inadequate attention to related strategies that maximise success	Strongly agree	6	2	1	1	0	1	3	0	3	4	3	3	5	3	4	4	**27**	**18**
	Agree	2	3	3	4	0	2	0	4	3	5	6	8	4	2	6	5	**24**	**33**
	Not sure	7	7	1	5	2	1	0	8	3	5	2	6	3	10	3	7	**21**	**49**
	Disagree	1	3	0	2	0	2	1	8	1	1	3	2	3	4	0	3	**9**	**25**
	Strongly disagree	0	0	0	1	0	0	1	2	0	0	0	0	0	0	0	1	**1**	**4**
	TOTAL	**16**	**15**	**5**	**13**	**4**	**6**	**5**	**22**	**10**	**15**	**14**	**19**	**15**	**19**	**13**	**20**	**82**	**129**
Appropriate personal and professional attitudes and practices	Strongly agree	5	2	2	1	2	1	1	4	3	3	5	4	4	3	4	4	**26**	**22**
	Agree	8	10	3	8	2	3	2	13	5	8	8	13	8	8	8	10	**44**	**73**
	Not sure	3	2	0	3	0	1	0	5	1	4	1	1	1	5	1	5	**7**	**26**
	Disagree	0	0	0	0	0	1	2	0	1	0	0	1	2	3	0	0	**5**	**5**
	Strongly disagree	0	1	0	1	0	0	0	0	0	0	0	0	0	0	0	1	**0**	**3**
	TOTAL	**16**	**15**	**5**	**13**	**4**	**6**	**5**	**22**	**10**	**15**	**14**	**19**	**15**	**19**	**13**	**20**	**82**	**129**
Willingness to take responsibility for their own behaviour	Strongly agree	3	2	0	3	0	1	2	3	3	4	4	3	5	4	2	6	**19**	**26**
	Agree	10	4	4	3	3	3	3	13	5	5	9	13	3	11	8	9	**45**	**61**
	Not sure	2	6	1	4	1	1	0	4	2	4	1	2	2	3	2	2	**11**	**26**
	Disagree	1	2	0	2	0	1	0	2	0	2	0	1	4	1	1	0	**6**	**11**
	Strongly disagree	0	1	0	1	0	0	0	0	0	0	0	0	1	0	0	3	**1**	**5**
	TOTAL	**16**	**15**	**5**	**13**	**4**	**6**	**5**	**22**	**10**	**15**	**14**	**19**	**15**	**19**	**13**	**20**	**82**	**129**

ward policy. At Holy Family Nursing College, 35.7% of the nurse tutors agreed that they help students to perform in accordance to ward policy. However, 73.6% of the students agreed that their nurse tutors help them during teaching in the clinical area in accordance to the ward policy. Generally, 45.1% (37) $n = 82$ of the nurse tutors from different nursing colleges in Malawi agreed that they help nursing students to perform at the clinical area in accordance to the ward nursing policy. It was very encouraging to note that 60.5% (78) $n = 129$ of the nursing students agreed that the nurse tutors help the nurse students in different colleges to perform at the clinical area in accordance to the ward policy. Some nurse tutors pointed out that the critical challenge is limited availability and exposure to ward policies by the nurse tutors.

Provision of ongoing feedback to students for growth during teaching both in class and at the clinical area was also assessed as a psychomotor performance to nurse tutors (see **Table 2**). 80% of the nurse tutors in St. Lukes Nursing College agreed that they provide ongoing feedback to nursing students during teaching for growth both in class and at the clinical area. While only 38.5% of the nursing students from the same St. Lukes Nursing College agreed that their nurse tutors provide ongoing feedback to the students during teaching both in class and at the clinical area. Furthermore 50% of the nurse tutors in Mulanje Nursing College agreed that they provide nursing students with ongoing feedback during teaching. But 53.3% of the nursing students agreed that their tutors provide ongoing feedback to students for growth during teaching both in class and at the clinical area. 46.3% (38) $n = 82$ of the nurse tutors from different nursing colleges agreed that they provide ongoing feedback to nursing students during teaching both in class and at the clinical area. However, most nurse tutors noted that provision of feedback is mainly compromised when the nurse tutors have limited interaction with the students.

60.5% (78) $n = 129$ of the nursing students from different nursing colleges agreed that the nurse tutors provide ongoing feedback to nursing students during teaching both in class and at the clinical area. This entails that many nurse tutors disagree that they provide ongoing feedback to nursing students during teaching. Therefore, the psychomotor performance of nurse tutors on provision of ongoing feedback to students during teaching is very limited both in class and at the clinical area.

Table 2. Distribution of the nurse tutors and students on performance in different nursing colleges.

VARIABLE		In which college do you teach or learn																	
Cognitive/affective/ psychomotor	Co-variates	Nkhoma		St. Lukes		St Joseph		Trinity		Mulanje		Holly family		Ekwendeni		St Johns		TOTAL	
		tut	stud	tut	stud	tut	stud	tut	stud	tut	stud	tut	stud	tut	stud	tut	stude	tutor	stude
	Strongly agree	9	3	1	2	3	1	3	3	4	8	9	3	7	3	7	6	43	**29**
Help student perform skills in accordance with ward policy	Agree	7	11	4	8	1	3	2	16	5	5	5	14	7	10	6	11	37	**78**
	Not sure	0	0	0	0	0	2	0	1	0	2	0	0	1	5	0	3	1	**13**
	Disagree	0	1	0	0	0	0	0	2	1	0	0	0	0	1	0	0	1	**4**
0.006 t/0.005st	Strongly disagree	0	0	0	3	0	0	0	0	0	0	0	2	0	0	0	0	0	**5**
	TOTAL	16	**15**	**5**	**13**	**4**	**6**	**5**	**22**	**10**	**15**	**14**	**19**	**15**	**19**	**13**	**20**	**82**	**129**
	Strongly agree	6	3	1	2	1	1	2	3	4	4	6	3	6	2	7	4	7	**22**
Provide ongoing feedback to the student for growth	Agree	7	8	4	5	3	3	3	18	5	8	7	11	5	12	4	13	4	**78**
	Not sure	2	1	0	1	0	2	0	0	0	3	0	2	4	4	2	2	2	**15**
	Disagree	1	2	0	3	0	0	0	1	0	0	1	2	0	1	0	1	0	**10**
0.07 t/0.069st	Strongly disagree	0	1	0	2	0	0	0	0	1	0	0	1	0	0	0	0	0	**4**
	TOTAL	16	**15**	5	**13**	4	**6**	5	**22**	10	**15**	14	**19**	15	**19**	13	**20**	13	**129**
	Strongly agree	7	2	0	1	1	1	2	3	5	4	7	2	3	2	3	3	28	**18**
Moved group actively in positive direction	Agree	5	9	5	6	2	2	3	15	3	9	7	14	9	11	6	16	40	**82**
	Not sure	4	2	0	4	1	1	0	2	1	2	0	1	3	3	3	1	12	**16**
	Disagree	0	2	0	2	0	2	0	2	1	0	0	1	0	3	1	0	2	**12**
0.1 t/0.085st	Strongly disagree	0	0	0	0	0	0	0	0	0	0	0	1	0	0	0	0	0	**1**
	TOTAL	16	**15**	**5**	**13**	**4**	**6**	**5**	**22**	**10**	**15**	**14**	**19**	**15**	**19**	**13**	**20**	**82**	**129**
	Strongly agree	6	3	2	3	0	0	2	6	4	6	7	3	4	0	3	5	28	**26**
Formulated questions to stimulate further inquiry	Agree	7	6	3	6	3	2	3	12	5	5	6	14	6	14	10	12	43	**71**
	Not sure	3	5	0	3	1	3	0	0	0	3	1	1	4	5	0	2	9	**22**
	Disagree	0	1	0	0	0	0	0	4	1	1	0	1	1	0	0	1	2	**8**
0.05 st	Strongly disagree	0	0	0	1	0	1	0	0	0	0	0	0	0	0	0	0	0	**2**
	TOTAL	16	**15**	**5**	**13**	**4**	**6**	**5**	**22**	**10**	**15**	**14**	**19**	**15**	**19**	**13**	**20**	**82**	**129**

When the nurse tutors were asked on how they improve their teaching psychomotor performance, a nurse tutor from Nkhoma Nursing College added that:

I make sure that I don't miss my classes, and I make sure that I follow the curriculum when am preparing my notes so that I don't go overboard, and I make sure that I take maybe content that is too little and then I consult other people, when there is need to, other tutors who have been in the profession longer than myself when I see that am not conversant with other things. And then I also continuously practice in the skills lab on my own just to remind myself or to keep up to date my skills on performing different sets of skill that I need.

Therefore, punctuality, curriculum abidance and consultations improve the nurse tutor teaching cognitive, affective and psychomotor performance in Malawi nursing colleges.

The concept of **formulating questions to stimulate students'** further inquiry during clinical teaching by nurse tutors was also analysed as a cognitive performance (see **Table 2**). 43.7% of the nurse tutors from Nkhoma Nursing College agreed that they formulate questions to stimulate further inquiry to students during teaching. While 40% of the students from Nkhoma Nursing College agreed that nurse tutors in their college formulate questions to stimulate further inquiry during teaching both in class and at the clinical area. 75% of nurse tutors in St. Joseph Nursing College agreed that they formulate questions to stimulate further inquiry to students during teaching. But only 33.3% of the students from St. Joseph Nursing College agreed that their nurse tutors formulate questions that stimulate students' further inquiry. The main challenge is that most nurse tutors are not having high qualification like master's degree that help them to articulate properly during teaching. However, 52.4 (43) $n = 82$ of the nurse tutors from different nursing colleges agreed that they formulate questions that stimulate further inquiry during teaching the nursing students in class and at the clinical area. 55% (71) $n = 129$ of the students from different nursing colleges agreed that their nurse tutors formulate questions that stimulate them for further inquiry. Therefore, it entails that the cognitive performance of nurse tutors on formulating questions is above average in all nursing colleges.

50% of the nurse tutors from Nkhoma Nursing College agreed that they **alleviate students stress in the clinical area** during teaching as an affective performance. But only 25% of the students from Nkhoma Nursing College agreed that their nurse tutors alleviate students stress in the clinical area during teaching. Moreover, 64.2% of the nurse tutors from Holy Family Nursing College agreed that they alleviate students stress in the clinical area during teaching. But, only 26.3% of the students from Holy Family Nursing College agreed that they alleviate students stress during teaching. Generally from different nursing colleges 48.8% (40) $n = 82$ of the nurse tutors agreed that they alleviate the students stress in the clinical area during teaching. However, only 45.7% (59) $n = 129$ of the nursing students from different nursing colleges in Malawi agreed that their nurse tutors alleviate students stress during teaching both in class and at the clinical area. This therefore, this study suggests that nurse tutors affective and psychomotor performance on student stress management during teaching in class and at the clinical area is very low. The main challenge, still focus on the availability of the nurse tutors, in the clinical area. Students are sent to different hospital for clinical practice, but follow up of the students to these hospital depend on funding from the college administration. Most nurse tutors pointed out that in a six weeks allocation students may be followed only three to five days by their clinical instructors.

Another important area where teaching psychomotor performance of the nurse tutors was checked is on **provision of student opportunities for personal practice** at the clinical area. 40% of the nurse tutors from St Luke Nursing College agreed that they provide students with opportunities for personal practice in the clinical area during teaching. 46.2% of the students from the same St. Luke Nursing College agreed that their nurse tutors provide them with opportunities for personal practice during teaching at the clinical area.

At St. Joseph 80% of the students disagreed that their nurse tutors provide them with an opportunities to practice in the clinical area during teaching. But 50% of the nurse tutors in the same St. Joseph Nursing College agreed that they provide their students with the opportunities to practice in the clinical area. However, in general, 47.5% (39) $n = 82$ of the nurse tutors from different nursing colleges strongly agreed that they provide the nursing students with opportunities to practice in the clinical area during teaching. 26.4% (34) $n = 129$ of the students from different nursing colleges strongly agreed that their nurse tutors provide them with opportunities to practice in the clinical area during teaching. Therefore, it is clearly that nurse tutors psychomotor performance on the provision of students an opportunity to practice in the clinical area is very low in Malawi nursing colleges. The major challenge on commonly on the number of hours that the students are exposed to their clinical instructors thus nurse tutors. Students are mostly found with the ward nurses who have limited skills on clinical instructions.

The **fitting of the training to the skills level** of the students was another teaching psychomotor performance that was assessed in the nurse tutors. 56.2% of the nurse tutors in Nkhoma Nursing College agreed that they fit the training material to the skills level of the students. But only 46.6% of the students from the same Nkhoma Nursing College agreed that their nurse tutors fit the training material to the skills level of the students during teaching both in class and at the clinical area. However, 40% of the students from Nkhoma Nursing College disagreed that nurse tutors fit their training material to the skills level of the students during teaching. At St. Johns Nursing College, 46.1% of the nurse tutors agree that they fit the training material to the skills level of the students during teaching. But 70% of the students agreed that their nurse tutors fit the training material to the skills level of the students during teaching. Generally after asking the question to all eight nursing colleges, 53.7% (44) $n = 82$ of the nurse tutors from all the colleges agreed that they always fit the training material to the skills level of the students during teaching both in class and at the clinical area. But 55% (71) $n = 129$ of the nursing students from all the nursing colleges in Malawi agreed that their nurse tutors fit the training material to the skills level of the students during teaching. Therefore, the cognitive and psychomotor performance of the nurse tutors in Malawi on fitting the training material to the skills level of the students during teaching has been very high as both the students and the nurse tutors agree that they do fit the training. However, nurse tutors complained that due to shortage of nursing staff in the hospital, first year students are seen performing procedures that they have not yet learnt in class.

But apart from fitting the training, some nurse tutors pointed out that they must also be goal oriented when teaching, for example a nurse tutor from St. Joseph Nursing College noted that:

Maybe I would say people say I am goal oriented and since I am goal oriented I don't allow people to do other things apart from the things I want them to do; if I am goal oriented then it means we have to meet the objectives you have set. And I make sure that students work in the limit to achieve those objectives; let's say maybe you have been assigned to do certain amount of work and you set limits. By such...such time I want this one to be complete and you have to make sure that at such time that job or that work is completed by students and me. And if students are not working accordingly then you have to make a proper follow up and make sure that you facilitate that process. When am talking to the student am audible enough the student are able to get what am saying!

So, if nurse tutors are goal oriented they can provide quality services to the student thereby promoting health in the clinical area.

25% of the nurse tutors in Trinity Nursing College agreed that they **pair the experienced skills based health education providers with the new students** at the clinical area.

But 54.5% of the nursing students agreed that their nurse tutors pair them with the experienced skill based health education providers. But 50% of the nurse tutors from St. Johns Nursing College disagreed that they pair the experienced skill based health education providers with their new students in the clinical area. While only 20% of the students from St. Johns Nursing College disagreed that their nurse tutors pair them to the experienced skill based health education providers in the clinical area. However, 46.3% (38) $n = 82$ of the nurse tutors from all the eight nursing colleges agreed that they pair the nursing students to the experienced skill based health education providers in the in clinical area. And 48% (62) $n = 129$ of the students from all the eight nursing colleges in Malawi agreed that their nurse tutors pair them to the experienced skill based health education providers during teaching in the clinical area. In this psychomotor performance item, it is clear that nurse tutors do pair nursing students to the qualified health education providers who would help in the clinical training for quality care and development of the students on clinical skills. However, pairing of student from different level of training is difficult due to different clinical student allocation. It might happen that first year students who are doing clinical fundamental nursing are paired with third year students who are doing maternal nursing. In such conditions the type of the wards might be different thereby denying the chance of pairing for mentoring.

The nurse tutor affective performance on the **students' encouragement on team work** was also assessed. 64.2% of the nurse tutors from Holy Family Nursing Colleges agreed that they encourage students on team work during teaching both in class and at the clinical area. And 63.2% of students from Holy Family Nursing College agreed that their nurse tutors encourage the students on team work during teaching both in class and at the clinical area. 75% of the nurse tutors from St. Joseph agreed that they encourage team work among students during teaching. Moreover, 66.6% of the nursing students from the same St. Joseph Nursing College agreed that their nurse tutors encourage them on team work during teaching both in class and at the clinical area. In addition, at St. Johns Nursing College 53.8% of the nurse tutors agreed that they encourage nursing students to team work during teaching. 50% of the nursing students from St. Johns Nursing College also agreed that their nurse tutors encourage them to team work during teaching both in class and at the clinical area. But generally after assessing in all the eight nursing colleges 52.4% (43) $n = 82$ of the nurse tutors agreed that they encourage nursing students in their respective colleges to team work during teaching. 51.9% (67) $n = 129$ of the students from all the eight nursing colleges agreed that their nurse tutors encourage them to team work during teaching both in class and at the clinical area. Therefore, nurse tutor teaching affective performance level on encouraging of the students to team work during teaching is very high in Malawi nursing colleges. However, when bivariate analysis was used to compare the independent variable type of the college where the nurse tutor is teaching and the dependent variable, nurse tutors encouragement of the team work. The null hypothesis that type of the nursing college is not correlated to nurse tutors encouragement to team work was rejected. This is because the p-value was $0.033 < p = 0.05$. This suggests that type of the college was highly correlated to nurse tutors encouragement of the students to team work during teaching. The result indicates that nurse tutors encouragement to team work of the students depends on the type of the college where the nurse tutor is working. Although some students said that the big challenge of team work is laziness of some students who do not participate fully in group discussions.

Another nurse tutor from Nkhoma Nursing College during in-depth interview also pointed out that they must be humble when approached by students:

My presentation I don't go there proposing like am too senior to the students. I really make sure that I humble myself before my students so that I am closer to their level, so that they understand what I am telling them because many students we teach they have a degree of low self-esteem. We are teaching nurse NMTs; nurse mid-wife technician, so you look at somebody and with a degree or masters and in my case to them they only look at your masters degree not what you are teaching so if you are not careful you don't deliver anything they just look at you as somebody with a lot of pride so by the end of the day they will only pick any comment you say they will rate, because she is much educated this is why she is saying so; they will rate you with academic status or your financial status if they know you. So, I really make sure that I just deliver the content without offending my students and if I happened that I offended them I say sorry so that by the end of the day they don't grasp that negative comment but they keep the main message.

Therefore, being humble to students during teaching, although you have high qualification, promotes team work thereby increasing the interest and performance of the nurse tutor.

The nurse tutors were also asked on how they generally perform with the students in the clinical area, particularly on the facilitation of the team work. And one of the nurse tutors from Ekwendeni Nursing College said:

Students usually have a duty roster and you have to make sure that everybody is following the duty allocation. Secondly these students are supposed to have objectives for the day so you make sure that you check whatever the student has planned to do from their objectives. And from your own plans, you also identify tasks that have to be done together with the students depending also on the ward that you are working. So you still have to work hand in hand to identify appropriate clients and patients with the students because sometimes they may not know clients or patients to choose. So, you have to facilitate that learning process by choosing the system to choose appropriately or with the actual teaching usually when I need to teach them according to the deadlines that they have. and also mainly when you have arrive in the ward, first of all you meet the students you have to discover before you start, if everybody and everything is ok then after you have gone through objectives then you also select some procedures that you want to do. Then after you have achieved whatever you had planned for the day before you close you also meet the group and discuss what they have learnt that day how best they could do those things and how they plan to improve so you work with them and give them the necessary feedback.

Therefore, facilitation of clinical student objectives and selection of appropriate clients for student learning enhance the teaching psychomotor performance of the nurse tutors in the clinical area.

The psychomotor performance of the nurse tutors working with students in **the laboratory** was also measured. 87.5% of the nurse tutors from Nkhoma Nursing College agreed that they work effectively in the laboratory with students to improve their skills. While 60% of the students from Nkhoma Nursing College agreed that their nurse tutors work effectively in the laboratory with students to improve their skills. 60% of the nurse tutors from Mulanje Nursing College also strongly agreed that they work effectively with their students in the laboratory to improve their nursing skills. But 33.3% of the students from Mulanje Nursing College agreed that their nurse tutors work effectively with them in the laboratory to improve their skills. 73.3% of the nurse tutors in Ekwendeni Nursing College agreed that they work effectively with the nursing students in the laboratory to improve their nursing skills. However, generally 52.4% (43) $n = 82$ of the nurse tutors from all the eight nursing colleges agreed that they work effectively with the students in the laboratory to improve their skills. But 55% (71) $n = 129$ of the nursing students from different nursing colleges in the country agreed that their nurse tutors work effectively with them in the laboratory to improve their skills. This suggests that nurse tutors psychomotor performance of working effectively with students in the laboratory is above average and it helps to improve the students' clinical skills. But when Spearman Correlation Coefficient was used to compare the type of the nursing college and the effective working with students in the laboratory by nurse tutors, the outcome of the p-value was $0.054 \leq p = 0.05$. This suggests that there is a board-line correlation between the type of the nursing college and the nurse tutors effectively working with students in the laboratory. This indicates that effective working of the nurse tutors in the laboratory with students is influenced by the type of the nursing college where the nurse tutor is working. But some lecturers pointed out that teaching students in the laboratory becomes a challenges due to large numbers and limited equipment.

4. Association of Nurse Tutor Work Experience and Student Study Experience on Tutors Performance

The variable of **inadequate clinical orientation to students** was measured as a nurse tutor psychomotor performance to see the statistical association using logistic regression in **Table 3**. The logistic model opted the

Table 3. Association of tutors work experience, students study experience and tutor clinical performance.

Tutor who AGREE on PERFORMANCE variables	Tutors work experience						Students study experience					
	B	WARD	sig	ODD	Confidenc interval		B	WARD	sig	ODD	Confidenc interval	
					Lower	Upper					Lower	Upper
Inadequate clinica orientation	**−1.196**	**4.152**	**0.042**	0.302	0.096	0.955	0.031	0.005	0.944	**1.032**	0.430	2.474
Too little-time to clinical practice	0.514	0.572	0.450	**1.672**	0.441	6.344	**1.844**	**5.165**	**0.023**	**6.324**	**1.289**	**31.030**
Infusion health without foundation	0.360	0.227	0.634	**1.433**	0.326	**6.295**	**−1.731**	**4.370**	**0.037**	0.177	0.035	0.898
Weak leadership	**−0.239**	0.121	0.728	0.787	0.204	3.039	**−1.080**	**4.735**	**0.030**	0.340	0.128	0.898
Lack of teaching material	**−0.024**	0.002	0.967	0.976	0.312	3.054	**−0.063**	0.022	0.882	0.939	0.407	**2.163**
Inadequate funding	0.013	0.000	0.985	**1.013**	0.271	3.793	**−0.989**	**6.688**	**0.010**	0.372	0.176	0.787
Recognition behaviour	0.523	0.450	0.502	**1.687**	0.366	7.771	0.612	**1.855**	0.173	**1.845**	0.764	4.452
Willingness to take responsibility	**−0.762**	0.732	0.392	0.467	0.081	2.675	**−0.161**	0.097	0.756	0.851	0.308	2.351
Concerned with Social student issues	0.447	0.270	0.603	**1.564**	0.290	8.449	0.105	0.033	0.856	**1.110**	0.358	3.446
Sense of student care	0.341	0.158	0.691	**1.406**	0.262	7.550	**−0.462**	0.679	0.410	0.630	0.210	1.889
Accurate teaching knowledge	**−1.119**	**2.513**	0.113	0.327	0.082	1.303	0.091	0.036	0.850	**1.095**	0.427	2.807

This is a logistic regression models with probability classification cut-off of 0.5 and the entry point of p-value of 0.05 in statistics of Hosmer-Leme show goodness of-fit. Basing on method of ENTER, the maximum iteration of more than 20 items were entered. Only those that show statistical significance were tabulated. The equation had a probability of 95% confidence interval. The OR interpretation of above 1 was adopted for the predictor variables of nurse tutor experience and student study experience separately. All the categorical or dependent variables and the predictor/independent variables were first tested in the bivariate analysis at p-value of 0.05. All constant values were not tabulated although the models produced due to table spacing. The degree of freedom was set at 1. All nurse tutor performance variables were regarded as dependent variables and nurse tutor work experience and student study experience which are independent or predicator variables. All categorical variables were dichotomizedly coded correctly (with 0 = disagree or lack of the characteristic (); 1 = agree, or the presence of the characteristics. The disagree was treated as a constant value.

probability for stepwise of the entry level of 0.05 and the removal level of 0.10. In this the model, which was omnibus test model of coefficient the outcome of the odds ratio was OR $\leq$ 0.302; 95% CI (0.096 $\pm$ 2.955); p $\geq$ 0.042. This was after predictor variable nurse tutor work experience was compared to dependent variable inadequate clinical orientation to students. In this outcome where the logistic method was ENTER, it clearly entails that the more years the nurse tutors have both in class and at the clinical area, the less likely that nurse tutors would have adequate clinical orientation to students during teaching in the clinical area. Even the Beta value of the analysis was showing a negative direction of relationship between the predictor variable and the dependent variable as it was B = −1.196. This means that for every increase in year of work for nurse tutors both in class and at the clinical area, there will be a decrease for the clinical orientation to students. Therefore, having more years of nurse tutor work experience in Malawi nursing colleges leads to nurse tutor limited or poor clinical orientation of students. Furthermore, this was the same in the students' perceptions as the omnibus test model of coefficient outcome of the odds ratio, Beta value, the Ward, correlations and the confidence interval were adopted. The results illustrated that OR $\leq$ 1.032; 95% CI (0.430 $\pm$ 2.474); p $\geq$ 0.944. In this outcome the probability was the main predictive values with standardisation as the specific residuals. This means that there was strong association between the predictor variable of student study experience and the dependent variable of inadequate clinical orientation to students by nurse tutors. Therefore, for every one year addition in the student study experience in all nursing colleges in Malawi, there would be 1.032 times of nurse tutors inadequate clinical orientation to students during teaching both in class and at the clinical area. Furthermore, students pointed out that the challenge of clinical orientation is the availability of the nurse tutors.

The psychomotor performance of the **nurse tutors on little concentrated time on the learning tasks** with student to clinical practice was also entered into the logistic model. This was done where the dependent variable was compared to the nurse tutor work experience as the predictor variable. This was done after dichotomising the predictor and dependent variables. In this logistic regression model the option of omnibus test of coefficient was used with probability for stepwise criteria of 0.05 in entry and 0.5 as the classification cut-off. Using the ENTER method the outcome of the odds ratio, Beta value, the Ward, correlations and the confidence interval were adopted. So, the results showed that OR $\leq$ 1.672; 95% CI (0.441 $\pm$ 6.344); p $\geq$ 0.450. This indicates that there is strong association between the predictor variable nurse tutor work experience and the dependent variable nurse tutors too little time to clinical practice during teaching. For every one year increase on the nurse tutor work experience there would be 1.672 times more likely that the nurse tutors have too little concentrated time on the student learning tasks to the clinical practice. Therefore, clearly entails that in Malawi nursing colleges, having more experience for nurse tutors would be resulting to poor nurse tutors performance on **too little concentrated time with the students learning tasks** in the clinical area for teaching.

Even the Beta Coefficient value of the Binary Logistic Regression equation showed a positive direction of relationship although in a decimal figure of $B = 0.514$. This illustrates that any increase in the nurse tutor work experience would result to slight increase of the performance of nurse tutor on concentrated time to students clinical practice for learning. Moreover, in another related omnibus test of coefficient model, it focused on the student study experience as the predictor variable in comparison with dependent variable of too little concentrated time with student clinical learning. The results of the model after using the ENTER method and probability for stepwise criteria of 0.05 in entry and 0.5 as the classification cut-off was $OR \leq 6.324$; 95% CI (1.289 ± 31.030); $p \geq 0.023$. This also means that there is a strong association between student study experience and nurse tutors' concentrated time on student learning tasks at the clinical area. For every one year extra in the student study experience there would be a likelihood of 6.324 times more for nurse tutors to have little concentrated time to clinical practice on student learning tasks.

Even the Beta Coefficient value of the results was $B = 1.844$. This showed that there is a positive direction of the relationship between student study experience and the nurse tutors little concentrates time with students learning tasks in the clinical area. For any increase in the student study experience in Malawi nursing colleges, there would be a likely increase of the nurse tutors to have too little concentrated time on student learning tasks in the clinical area.

Lack of teaching material is very devastating challenge among nurse tutors in Malawi and the variable was evaluated using the logistic regression analysis. In the omnibus test model coefficient, the probability for stepwise criteria was 0.05 at entry and 0.5 as the classification cut-off. This was done to compare the predictor variable nurse tutor work experience and the dependent variable nurse tutors lack of teaching material in the colleges and at the clinical area. The outcome of the model was an odds ratio of $OR \leq 0.976$; 95% CI (0.312 ± 3.054); $p \geq 0.967$ (see **Table 3**). This indicates that there is no association between the nurse tutor work experience and the nurse tutors **lack of teaching material** both in class and at the clinical area. For every one year increase in nurse tutor work experience there would be a probability likelihood of 0.976 times for the nurse tutors to lack teaching materials. Therefore, the nurse tutor work experience does not associate with lacking of teaching materials in Malawi nursing colleges. Even the Beta Coefficient value showed ($B = -0.239$) a negative direction of the relationship between the nurse tutors work experience and the nurse tutors lacking of teaching materials both in class and at the clinical area. This suggests that for any increase in nurse tutor work experience there would be a decrease in the nurse tutor lacking the teaching material in the nursing colleges during teaching both in class and at the clinical area. Moreover, in the student data when student study experience as a predictor variable was compared to the lack of teaching materials, there was no statistical association. This was done after omnibus test of model coefficient where the probability for stepwise criteria included 0.5 as the classification cut-off. The results of the equation revealed the odds ratio of $OR \leq 0.939$; 95% CI (0.407 ± 2.163); $p \geq 0.882$. This suggests that for every one year addition to the student study experience in all nursing colleges in Malawi there would be a probability likelihood of 0.939 times for nurse tutors to have lack of teaching materials. So, student study experience has very limited or no association with the lacking of materials for teaching in nursing colleges. For the Beta Coefficient value of the results (see **Table 3**), it clearly showed that ($B = -0.063$) there is a negative direction of the relationship between student study experience and the lacking of teaching materials in nursing colleges. For any increase in years for the student study experience there would a decrease in the nurse tutors lacking of teaching materials both in class and at the clinical area. Therefore, lacking of teaching material is not associated with student study experience.

It has to be mentioned again that **inadequate funding** by nursing administration for teaching is also a major challenge as it was found to be associated with nurse tutor experience. This was done after using the binary logistic regression with omnibus test of model coefficient. In the model the predictive value of probability stepwise criteria of 0.05 at entry and 0.1 at removal and 0.5 as the classification cut-off. The results of the equation clearly showed the odds ratio of $OR \leq 1.013$; 95% CI (0.271 ± 3.793); $p \geq 0.985$. The model indicates that there is a strong association between predictor variable nurse tutor work experience and the dependent variable inadequate nursing administrative funding for nurse tutor teaching in all the nursing colleges in the country. For every additional year of the nurse tutor work experience there would be a probability likelihood chance of 1.013 times more on the inadequate nursing administrative funding in the nursing colleges in Malawi. Therefore, more nurse tutor work experience has a probability likelihood chance of inadequate nursing administration funding in nursing colleges. Although the Beta Coefficient value was in a decimal point ($B = 0.013$) but it also illustrated the positive direction of the relationship between the nurse tutor work experience and the nursing administrations' inadequate funding to the teaching programs.

But the students had different perception towards the funding issue of their nursing colleges. Using the same logistic regression model, with omnibus test model of coefficient, the results of the odds ratio revealed $OR \leq 0.372$; 95% CI (0.176 ± 0.787); $p \geq 0.010$. This means that there was no association between the student study experience and inadequate nursing administrative funding. For any one year addition to the student study experience there would be a probability likelihood chance of 0.372 times of nursing administration having inadequate funding. This means that nursing administration do not have a big problem with funding the nurse tutors during teaching. Moreover, the Beta Coefficient value from the binary logistic regression equation showed $B = -0.989$. This is an illustration of negative direction of the relationship between the student study experience and the administrative inadequacy of funding the nurse tutors during teaching. So any increase in years to the student study experience would result to the decrease of the inadequacy of administrative funding in the nursing colleges. This entails that in nursing colleges the students feel that any increase in their study experience would not affect the funding structure of the nursing college.

The cognitive performance of the nurse tutors on **accurate teaching knowledge and adequate personal comfort** with teaching was also analysed using the logistic regression model. In the model the probability stepwise criteria of 0.05 was selected for entry level and 0.5 was also adopted as the classification cut-off point in the equation. This was done as predictor variable was compared with dependent variable accurate teaching knowledge and adequate personal comfort with teaching. The result of the equation included the odds ratio of $OR \leq 0.327$; 95% CI (0.082 ± 1.303); $p \geq 0.113$. This illustrate that there is no association between the predictor variable nurse tutor work experience and the accurate knowledge of teaching and adequate personal comfort with teaching. for every one year extra in the nurse tutor work experience there would be a likelihood chance of 0.327 times for the nurse tutors accurate teaching knowledge and adequate personal comfort with teaching students both in class and at the clinical area. Even in the Beta Coefficient results it clearly showed that ($B = -1.119$) there is a negative direction of the relationship between the predictor variable nurse tutor work experience and the dependent variable accurate teaching knowledge and the adequate personal comfort with teaching. If there is an increase in the student study experience in years there would also be a likely increase of the nurse tutors accuracy in teaching knowledge and adequacy in personal comfort with teaching. However, there were different perceptions from the students. Using the same logistic regression model where a probability stepwise criterion of 0.05 for entry was selected and the 0.5 as a classification cut-off point was also adopted. This was done to compare the student study experience as the predictor variable and the nurse tutors accurate knowledge in teaching and adequate personal comfort with teaching. The outcome which also included the odds ratio was $OR \leq 1.095$; CI (0.427 ± 2.807); $p \geq 0.850$. This clarifies that there is strong association between student study experience and the nurse tutors accurate teaching knowledge and adequate personal comfort with teaching. The results from the regression analysis shows that if one year is added to the student study experience there would be a likelihood of 1.095 times more for the nurse tutors to have accurate teaching knowledge and adequate personal comfort with teaching. Even the Beta Coefficient value from the results showed that ($B = 0.091$) there is a positive direction of relationship between the predictor variable student study experience and the dependent variable nurse tutor accuracy in teaching knowledge and adequacy in personal comfort with teaching. This implies that in Malawi if there is any increase in years of student study experience there would also be an increase in the nurse tutor accuracy in teaching knowledge and adequacy of personal comfort with teaching both in class and at the clinical area.

5. Discussion

Generally, in this study it has been found that both nurse tutors and students are not impressed with nurse tutors cognitive, affective and psychomotor performance during teaching. This is also the same to students who clearly indicated dissatisfaction with the nurse tutors' cognitive, affective and psychomotor performance both in class and at the clinical area. It has been noticed that different nursing colleges in Malawi have different sense of support to students in the clinical area.

The concept of nurse tutor psychomotor performance on **lecturing during the entire class** period has a big problem to students' process of learning. In this study students have clearly described nurse tutors to be teaching the entire class period despite level of experience. Student cannot cope up with pressure of such learning. When the students are tired there is always need to let them relax and get extra energy through fresh air, nutrition and reduced thinking capacity. But when the students are continuously learning without resting, the concentration span of their brain is severely reduced, that cause poor contribution and participation. Attention and concentration are the most powerful assets of human beings, and if correctly used, they can have numerous benefits in education [19]. At the same time it is very difficult to master content if the concentration span is reduced. A descriptive survey was conducted to assess the impact of teaching time that is classes for two hour, on attention and concentration of student nurses. The finding showed that 44% students had good attention and concentration in the first two hours of learning, 46% students had an average attention and concentration and 10% of students had poor attention and concentration score during the teaching and learning activities. It is clear that teaching beyond 2hours continuously reduces concentration span of the nursing students. Another author [20] did a study to assess the ability of the students to recall content taught during a lecture. Results show that most of the students were able to recall the initial content of the lecture soon after the class which indicates that they were more attentive during the beginning of class and gradually they become less attentive. This study reveals that to achieve full attention and concentration of the students, lengthy classes should have breaks or some learning activities, to make the class enjoyable. It is important for the students to pay attention and concentrate because it enhances their competency and skills to memorize the content for a longer period of time. There are many factors which can affect attention and concentration of nursing students in the classroom, such as duration and method of teaching, novelty and repetition of topic, surrounding environment, interest and including health and emotional status. If nursing students do not pay attention during teaching learning activities, they will be involved in other activities such as private conversations, dropping pen or pencils, excessive movement of body parts, passing notes to others. The environment of a professional college is very challenging. When an individual enters in a professional college as a student she/he has to prepare himself for higher education which demands attention and concentration during classes for future growth. Therefore, it is a big challenge for nursing students to learn during the entire class period.

The psychomotor performance of nurse tutors on **demonstration of clinical procedures** was also assessed to the students and to the nurse tutors themselves. Generally, it was noticed that only 54.3% (70) n = 129 of the students from all the nursing colleges agreed that their nurse tutors effectively demonstrates clinical procedures both in class and at the clinical area. Nurse tutor performance of demonstration needs to be appreciated by the students at the clinical area. If the nurse tutor performance on demonstration of clinical procedure is below standard some students can easily identify as they read widely in books about such procedures. The nurse tutors reputation on the students may reduce. Skill acquisition is viewed as complex due to the double demand of developing how to actually perform the skill in question as well as developing a professional understanding of theoretical and social aspects involved in such performance by the nurse tutor [21]. Social aspects are expressed through eye contact, voice, body language, and attention directed towards the "patient". Experiencing procedures from the perspective of the patient gives the students opportunity to reflect on whether their expressions are in accordance with distinctive features of a caring concern. But when the nurse tutor fails to these skills students tend to despise the performance of such nurse tutor.

Another concept under teaching affective performance of the nurse tutors were on the **willingness** to take responsibility for their own classroom and clinical behavior during teaching. Nurse tutor are supposed to take more responsibility on the clinical and classroom behavior that would lead to student quality learning process. But only 47.3% (61) n = 129 of the students throughout the nursing colleges in Malawi agreed that their nurse tutors have a willingness to take their own responsibility during teaching both in class and at the clinical area. This is a very awkward situation as nurse tutors dedication must be shown during teaching both in class and at the clinical area. In another study, results showed that the main factors leading to a lack of responsibility on clinical teaching by educational staff include lack of control and a sense of conflict, stress and anxiety in the ward-teaching situation, lack of peer support and an inability to plan ahead for such work. The most pervasive feature which emerged, however, was the felt lack of available time for clinical work in comparison to their other duties. This is discussed in terms of role strain. Differences in response between nurse tutors performance in the clinical area were studied and showed that all the problems found appear to be greater among the nurse tutor groups. This may be a consequence of a further finding that clinical nurse tutors are more likely to make finer and more frequent distinctions between the aims and problems of ward- and school-based teaching [22].

The teaching performance of nurse tutors on guiding clinical students on **resource mobilisation** was also looked into during analysis. 56.5% (73) $n = 129$ of the students from different colleges of nursing in Malawi agreed that nurse tutors guide nursing students on resource mobilisation during teaching particularly in the clinical area. This means that both students and nurse tutors are agreeing that the performance of the nurse tutor on resource mobilisation is generally met during teaching both in class and at the clinical area. Resource mobilization is a key in Malawi nursing colleges as nurse tutors teach under critical resource constraints [23]. Nurse educators in Malawi nursing colleges face several challenges. There are insufficient numbers of different resources, particularly in rural or under-served areas of the country. They face large work-loads in the face of increasing student numbers with limited resources. There is inadequate continuing professional development which influences the quality of teaching and clinical accompaniment and supervision of students; lack of orientation or induction programmes for nurse educators in many nursing colleges, insufficient up-skilling in new technologies, lack of a structured strategy for nursing educators to acquire new knowledge and skills; and an exodus of nurse educators due to occupation specific dispensation (OSD) and rural allowance. If nurse tutors are given adequate resources for teaching they cannot quit their prestigious employment and work in the non-governmental organizations.

6. Conclusion

This study has shown that an effective cognitive, affective and psychomotor nurse tutor performance requires an adequate funding in the nursing colleges in Malawi. There is a strong need to develop effective teaching strategies that can be conducive in developing countries where equipment is very scarce. Nurse tutor performance is not dependent on tutors alone but the type of students and the administrative accountability.

References

[1] WHO (2010) Statistical Year Book. Sub-Saharan Region, New York. www.who.int

[2] Carlisle, C., Calman, L. and Ibbotson, T. (2009) Practice-Based Learning: The Role of Practice Education Facilitators in Supporting Mentors. *Nurse Education Today*, **29**, 715-721. http://www.sciencedirect.com/science/article/pii

[3] Waterson, E., Harms, E., Qupe, L., Maritz, J. and Makobe, K. (2006) Strategies to Improve the Performance of Learners in a Nursing College; Part I: Issues Pertaining to Nursing Education. *Curationis*, **29**, 56-65. www.ncbi.nlm.nih.gov/pubmed/16910135

[4] Msiska, G., Smith, P., Fawcett, T. and Munkhondya, T.M. (2015) Where Is the Grade Coming from? Problems and Challenges in Evaluating the Clinical Performance of Nursing Students. *Open Journal of Nursing*, **5**, 470-481.

[5] Mbirimtengerenji, N.D. and Adejumo, O. (2015) Utilization of the Teaching Strategies among Nurse Tutors in Malawi Nursing Colleges. *Open Journal of Nursing*, **5**, 276-294. http://www.scirp.org/journal/ojnhttp://dx.doi.org/10.4236/ojn.2015.53031

[6] Nurses Council of Malawi (2009) Annual Report on Nursing Education. Lilongwe.

[7] DeLucia, P.R., Ott, T.E. and Palmieri, P.A. (2009) Performance in Nursing. *Reviews of Human Factors and Ergonomics*, **5**, 1-40. http://rev.sagepub.com/content/5/1/1.short

[8] Chilemba, E.B. and Bruce, J.C. (2014) Teaching Styles Used in Malawian BSN Programmes: A Survey of Nurse Educator Preferences. *Nurse Education Today*, **35**, e55-e60. www.elsevier.com/nedt http://dx.doi.org/10.1016/j.nedt.2014.12.015

[9] Grigulis, A.L. (2010) Lives of Malawian Nurses: Stories behind the Statistics. PhD Thesis, Centre for international Health and Development, University College London, London.

[10] Msiska, G., Munkhondya, T.M. and Chilemba, E. (2014) Undergraduate Students' Perceptions of the Role of the Nurse Educator during Clinical Placements in Malawian. *Open Journal of Nursing*, **4**, 836-847. http://dx.doi.org/10.4236/ojn.2014.412089

[11] Richman, S.B. (2010) A Process Model of the Link between Parenting Practices and Academic Behavior. Poster Presented at the Fifth Annual Institute of Education Sciences Research Conference, Washington DC. www.sesp.northwestern.edu/docs/cv/4790916114fa17c0b3b01a.pdf

[12] Mbirimtengerenji, N.D. and Adejumo, O. (2015) Challenges of Nurse Tutor Utilization of the Teaching Aids. *Open Journal of Nursing*, **5**, 516-527. http://dx.doi.org/10.4236/ojn.2015.55055

[13] Caffrey, M. and Graeme F. (2006) Health Workforce "Innovative Approachesand Promising Practices" Study: Attracting and Retaining Nurse Tutors in Malawi; Capacity; Project USAID Global Health/HIV/AIDS and the Africa Bureau Office of Sustainable. Development, Lilongwe. www.intrahealth.org/

[14] Mbirimtengerenji, N.D. and Adejumo, O. (2015) Challenges of Student and Nurse Tutor Interactions in Malawi Nursing Colleges. *IJSR-International Journal of Scientific Research*, **4**, 2277-8179. http://theglobaljournals.com/ijsr/articles.php?val=NTEwOQ==&b1=137&k=35#sthash.DPp234In.pdf

[15] Polit, D. and Beck, C.T. (2003) Nursing Research: Principals and Methods. Williams Book Company, New York. https://books.google.co.za/books?isbn=0781746256

[16] Tomietto, M., Saiani, L., Palese A., Cunico, L., Cicolini, G., Watson, P. and Saarikoski, M. (2012) Clinical Learning Environment and Supervision plus Nurse Teacher (CLES+T) Scale: Testing the Psychometric Characteristics of the Italian Version. *Giornale Italiano di Medicina del Lavoro ed Ergonomia*, **34**, B27-B80. www.ncbi.nlm.nih.gov/pubmed/23326942

[17] Ministry of Health-MoH (2012) Annual Report on Nurse'S Performance. Capitol Hill, Lilongwe.

[18] Roberto Rivera (2011) Research Ethics Training Curriculum. 2nd Edition, Family Health International, North Carolina. www.fhi360.org

[19] Lamba, S., Rawat, A., Jacob, J., Arya, M., Rawat, J., Chauhan, V. and Panchal, S. (2014) Impact of Teaching Time on Attention and Concentration. *IOSR Journal of Nursing and Health Science*, **3**, 1-4. www.iosrjournals.org

[20] Ministry of Health-MoH (2010) Biannual Conference, Karikuti Hotel, Lilongwe, Malawi Nurses Council of Malawi (NCM). 2007 Annual Report; Progress of Nurses in Development, Lilongwe.

[21] Bjørk, I.T. and Kirkevold, M. (2000) From Simplicity to Complexity: Developing a Model of Practical Skill Performance. *Journal of Clinical Nursing*, **9**, 620-631. http://dx.doi.org/10.1046/j.1365-2702.2000.00328.x

[22] Jones, J.A. (2005) A study of Nurse Tutors' Conceptualization of Their Ward Teaching Role. *Journal of Advanced Nursing*, **10**, 349-360.

[23] Barua, A. (2013) Methods for Decision-Making in Survey Questionnaires Based on Likert Scale. *Journal of Asian Scientific Research*, **3**, 35-38. http://www.aessweb.com/pdf-files/35-38.pdf

5

Registered Nurses' Experiences with Clinical Teaching Environment in Malawi

Thokozani Bvumbwe*, Atupele Malema, Mep Chipeta

Faculty of Health Sciences, Mzuzu University, Mzuzu, Malawi
Email: *bvumbwe.t@mzuni.ac.mw, atupelemalema@gmail.com, mepcoretta@gmail.com

Abstract

Clinical practice remains an integral part of nursing curriculum because clinical practice provides students with an opportunity to achieve professional competence. Creating a conducive learning environment for students is responsibility of academic staff, clinical nurses and students alike. However, studies in Malawi have reported poor clinical learning environment for students. This study therefore aimed at exploring nurses' experiences of clinical teaching environment in Malawi. The study used a qualitative research design utilizing a descriptive phenomenological approach. Participants were randomly identified from teaching hospitals across Malawi by nursing managers to attend a six week clinical preceptorship training at one University nursing college. Immediately before commencement of the training, participants were invited to voluntarily participate in a focus group discussion pertaining to their experiences with clinical environment. We conducted focus group discussions with 9 trainees in 2013 and 12 trainees in 2014 training cohorts. Findings reveal that nurses meet a number of challenges in teaching students in the clinical area. Four themes emerged from the study, namely, inadequate faculty support, poor clinical teaching environment, poor competence among nurses and unsupportive working conditions. Nurses require support from academic staff and their managers to ensure a conducive clinical teaching environment.

Keywords

Preceptors' Experiences, Clinical Learning Environment, Clinical Teaching

1. Introduction

Nursing is a practice based profession. Nursing education aims to develop professional clinical competencies

*Corresponding author.

and to enhance the quality of nursing care [1]. Clinical practice therefore remains an integral part of nursing curriculum. Clinical practice provides nursing students with an opportunity to work with patients where they develop higher level of thinking skills in order to achieve professional competence. Clinical practice setting allows students to put into practice what they have learnt during theory. A positive and supportive clinical practice setting influences integration of theory and practice [2].

Despite a debate on whether nursing educators are supposed to take up a clinical teaching role or an educationist orientation [3] [4], in Malawi nursing educators are expected to take students through blocks of theory and practice and clinical teaching is one of their core roles [5]. However, Malawi experiences shortage of nursing educators and clinical nurses have become the main players in students' clinical teaching [6]. This has resulted in a call for innovative approaches to clinical teaching and learning that will see clinical nurses effectively taking up the role of teaching students in the clinical area. Globally preceptorship model is extensively being used in nursing programs to facilitate clinical learning [7]. Students require adequate support, supervision, and teaching to facilitate achievement of learning during their clinical placement [8]. There is high evidence of effective learning when students are placed in clinical settings that encourage teaching and learning during care delivery [9].

Students have reported attainment of appropriate competency, confidence and skills that equip them to function within dynamic and complex settings when their learning involves a preceptor [10]. Clinical preceptors become experienced nurses working right in the practice setting foster independence and developing skills, competencies and confidence among students. Literature has consistently recognized preceptorship as a strategy to maximize the benefits of clinical practice in terms of promoting professional socialization [11]. However, little is known about the nurses' experiences with the clinical teaching environment. This study therefore aimed at exploring registered nurses' experiences of clinical teaching environment in Malawi. Findings of the study are relevant for nursing training colleges and hospital nursing managers so that they can work together to maximize students' clinical placements. Findings reveal gaps that exist for registered nurses to effectively support students' clinical learning. Findings give a baseline for transformative nursing education initiatives that aim at improving the clinical teaching environment.

2. Methodology

This study used a qualitative research design along the principles of the descriptive phenomenological approach. Phenomenological research aims "to capture as closely as possible the way in which the phenomena is experienced" [12]. The study aimed at exploring registered nurses' experiences of the clinical teaching environment in Malawi.

2.1. Participants

Thirty two registered nurses attended a six week clinical preceptorship training course in two cohorts at a public nursing University college in Malawi in 2013 and 2014. Participants for the study were drawn from 15 hospitals across the country where nursing students from various nursing colleges are allocated for clinical practice. The training participants were identified by their hospital nursing managers from various departments. Before commencement of the training participants were invited to voluntarily participate in a focus group discussion pertaining to their experiences of the clinical teaching environment in their respective clinical sites. A total of 21 nurses participated in the study. Nine out of 15 trainees participated during a 2013 cohort while 12 out of 17 participated during a 2014 cohort.

2.2. Data Collection

Two focus group discussions were separately conducted in 2013 and 2014. Focus group discussion was appropriate for the study because discussions provided preceptorship trainees with an opportunity to discuss their lived experiences of clinical teaching and clinical teaching environment. Researchers conducted the focus group discussions before participants commenced the training in order to have the preceptorship trainees' real experiences that are not influenced by what they would learn during the training. Participants were briefed on the purpose and procedure of the discussion. Both focus group sessions were audio recorded after getting informed consent from participants. The focus group discussions took 45 minutes and 60 minutes for the first and second session respectively. Two general questions were used for the discussions "how is the learning environment for students at your clinical sites" and "what is your experiences teaching students in the clinical area?" Active listening, paraphrasing, reflecting and probing were used to facilitate the discussions.

2.3. Data Analysis

Data collection and analysis were done concurrently. Content analysis, a systematic coding and categorizing approach was used. The researchers listened to audio recorded discussions carefully and data was transcribed verbatim. Transcribed data was read repeatedly to gain a deeper sense of the content. Careful and repeated reading of transcribed text helped researchers to identify patterns and trends of participants' responses. The researchers identified codes which were later categorized based on their similarities and differences. Finally the categories were grouped and four themes emerged.

2.4. Trustworthiness

The academic rigor of qualitative research is extremely significant. The trustworthiness of this study was ensured using two approaches. Firstly a "member checking" method was used. The researchers contacted five of the participants to verify and confirm the authenticity of the results. The researchers shared the summary of data analysis and results with five participants to check whether the developed concepts really reflected the insights and ideas that were discussed during the focus group discussions [13]. Secondly "peer checking" was used to check the credibility of the data analysis. Two academic members of staff were independently requested to identify concepts and codes from the data. These were compared with the researchers' developed codes, categories and themes. Differences were adjusted and harmonized through a discussion.

2.5. Ethical Issues

The study was done as part of a larger doctorate study titled "A critical analysis of strategies aimed at improving nursing education in Malawi" whose approval was granted by Humanities and Social Sciences Research Ethics Committee of the University of KwaZulu Natal (HSS/0986/012D) and the National Health Sciences Ethics committee of the Ministry of Health in Malawi (NHSRC # 1154). During the entire research process consideration was given to non-coercion, informed consent, participants' anonymity, freedom of participants to withdraw anytime they so wish to without being penalized. Participants were reassured that their responses would be kept confidential and their identities would not be revealed in research reports and publications.

3. Results

3.1. Demographics Characteristics of Participants

The sample consisted of 9 registered nurses in 2013 and 12 registered nurses in 2014. The study had a total of 6 males and 15 females. Majority of the participants were aged between 31 - 40 years. There were 8 registered nurses from central hospitals, 11 from district hospitals and 2 from health centres. All participants had more than 3 years of service except one who had less than 3 years of service. All participants were holders of a bachelor's degree in nursing except for one who had a diploma in nursing.

3.2. Emerging Themes

The study findings show that registered nurses experience various challenges in training students in the clinical setting. Findings reveal that registered nurses performance in training students is affected by various that include lack of resources, poor support from academic staff, overcrowding of student and general poor working conditions. The findings of the study have been presented under four major themes; inadequate faculty support, poor clinical teaching environment, poor competences among nurses and unsupportive working conditions.

3.2.1. Inadequate Faculty Support

The study reveals that there is poor support from academic staff. Majority of the participants expressed dissatisfaction with support they receive from faculty members. Participants reported that more often students come to the clinical area unaccompanied by their college teachers. This usually leaves students with little idea of what they are supposed to do during clinical placements. Participants noted that the college teachers' visits to the clinical area are usually infrequent. Participants said

"*Students come to the clinical area without any accompaniment from their colleges… sometimes with poor or no communication about their coming*"

"*academic staff may come only for assessments*".

It was observed that many students report for clinical allocation without clinical objectives or personal objectives and goals. The training colleges inadequately prepare clinical nurses to receive and manage students. The participants' excerpts include:

"*the way students come for clinical allocation is as if their teachers did not know that students will be leaving for clinical practice at that time. Whether students leave the objectives by their own making… but their teachers could have made sure that before students come to clinical area, they should bring clinical objectives*".

Another participant emphasized the need for faculty to put clinical allocation requirements in order before students report for clinical placement. The participant stated:

"*life becomes easy for clinical nurses if students bring their log books, clinical objectives, clinical diaries and possibly students clinical duty rosters. Personally when students come without clinical objectives I send them back to college to collect them from their teachers … am saying this because a nurse finds somewhere to start from when students know what they have come to do at that particular allocation … especially when they bring clinical objectives*".

Some participants indicated that they receive little guidance from faculty. They indicated that much as one might enjoy teaching students in the clinical area, little support and guidance frustrates them. One participant highlighted:

"*… with the experience I have working with students, I don't find it difficult to support students and facilitate their learning. The major problem is that the schools keep changing clinical plans without updating us or giving us adequate guidance … sometimes you look incompetent when you demand something from students and they tell you that that's not what we are supposed to do. Honestly speaking it could be very satisfying if the colleges could give us advance guidance before students report for clinical practice*".

Another added:

"*College staff should not just dump student at the clinical area. They should at least follow them up to check if they are doing what they are supposed to do. I need to say this because how do they expect them to evaluate students if the surely don't follow and teach them regularly?" … I have personally participated in students' evaluation with college staff who never followed the students. In such instances … they expect that you do all the students' evaluation. Usually because we also come to work in shifts, you might have not worked with the students adequately*".

However participant also reported that some colleges provide the required support and guidance. Participants said:

"*… some colleges give adequate attention to student's clinical allocation … There is always a teacher coming with students when they are coming for the first time*".

"*… colleges invite us for briefing before they send students to our clinical sites*".

These findings highlight the ineffective collaboration that exists between training institutions and clinical practice settings. Participants' responses clearly indicate that the responsibility of training students in the clinical setting was supposed to be coordinated between the colleges and clinical setting.

3.2.2. Poor Clinical Teaching Environment

Findings of the study show that the clinical learning environment in most cases has not been to the expectation of the students and nurses themselves. The majority of participants reported lack of resources as a big problem for nurses to effectively teach student. A participant said:

"*… our clinical area lacks appropriate resources for teaching students. Imagine even the mere gloves are an issue in the ward. How can students do some procedures without protecting themselves*".

Another participant agreed:

"*there is too much improvising in most hospitals including my own hospital. Now what happens is that no matter how you want to teach students ideal things, you are left with no choice due to lack of resources. This issue of resources is getting out of hand. At my hospital we now ask nursing colleges to provide students with basic clinical resources when coming for the placement*".

While the problem of resources is evident, inversely the number of students is also increasing. Participants pointed out that overcrowding of students is also another disturbing factor in the clinical environment. Participants' excerpts included:

"*We have too many students in a ward at the same time. Sometimes you find number of students to be double the number of patients in your ward. … for example* 23 *students taking care of* 15 *patients. Students self interest to learn becomes important during this situation. Other students leave the allocation with very little learnt due to overcrowding*".

"*… nursing colleges don't lease with each other. You find five colleges sending so many students at the same time. This really causes overcrowding and it's stressful for a preceptor to deal with so many students at the same time.*

Generally participants agreed that the clinical learning environment is a responsibility of the clinical nurses, the college teaching staff and the students themselves. Some participants reported:

"*Sometimes you meet students who are unrespectful and rude to clinical staff. Usually this type of students is not motivated to learn. With too much students in the ward, one can simply just ignore these students. However because it's our responsibility to make these students to become real nurses you try your best to deal with such students and it becomes stressing and demanding*".

Findings show that the nurses also contribute to poor clinical environment. Participants reported that there are some nurses who just expect students to work as their pair of hands. They stated that they don't give students time to learn but to work. Participants highlighted that nurses are also not receptive of the students in the sites. Some sentiments included:

"*… some nurses have show negative attitudes to students … in such cases students don't feel welcomed to a ward and they are not free to ask where they need help*".

3.2.3. Poor Competences among Nurses

Participants highlighted the need for continuous professional development among clinical nurses who support student learning. They felt that nurses working in teaching hospitals should be clinically competent in order to impart appropriate skills to students. The majority reported:

"*… how do you teach students things you are not competent yourself*".

"*Honestly speaking sometimes I don't feel confident to support students in a certain skills or procedure*". "*The majority of nurses are used to shortcuts, and you can't teach students short cuts*". *What is important I think is that if you think you are not competent to do a procedure which most nurses or even preceptors do, you should be honest with the student and refer them to someone else who could appropriately do that procedure. Unfortunately most of us don't want to look little before students*".

The discussion about competency among nurses continued:

"*I like the discussion because we are really honest with each other here … personally I have met students who were taught a procedure wrongly. It was really embarrassing for me because I confronted the student that this is not the way we do this procedure. Unfortunately the student expressed with confidence … that it was how one nurse taught him the skill. At that point I realized that I needed to appropriately correct what the student was taught without degrading my fellow nurse who taught the student. … So allow me to repeat what others already said that if you think you can't do something … refer the student to another person*".

Findings reveal that not only are skill competences lacking among nurses but also skills to teach students. Participants reported:

"*… nurses shout to students at the bedside wit patients listening. This reduces the student's confidence to approach the patient with another procedure*".

"*… when students observe that the nurses are not approachable, they rather choose to consult each other for learning. In some instances they might not teach other correct things*".

Findings reveal that nurses might be knowledgeable of clinical skills and procedures but not how to handle students. Knowledge of handling student in the clinical area is critical in creating a conducive learning environment.

3.2.4. Unsupportive Working Conditions

The study shows that the majority of the participants are dissatisfied with the conditions in which they work and operate. Frequently cited issues include shortage of staff and work overload. Common reports include:

"... in our ward we agreed to seriously make a difference in teaching students. This is part of objectives for all nurses there. Unfortunately, no matter how interested you could be to help students ... there are just too many tasks to be done by the same people. We were expecting that if you are assigned to facilitate students clinical teaching, the matron will take away some of your daily routines. But that's not the case. You find yourself still doing almost everything that you usually do".

"I was assigned to coordinate student teaching, and everybody in the ward expects me to be engaged with students all the time. ... as a preceptor will I not be relieved of some of the daily tasks then? Therefore you find that the highly overloaded tasks that I perform deny me and my fellow nurses time to interact with students".

"... My friends would agree with me that sometimes our ward could be very busy and leaves students to be my last priority".

Findings also show that participants are demotivated and stressed by lack of clear role expectations by their unit managers. One participant indicated:

"I was nominated by my unit manager to come and do this training. However her expectations on my daily program might not change. My engagement in daily meetings and other assignments do not give me an opportunity to teach students. Allow me to give you an example of my friend who came for the first training here. Since she came back I can assure you that she only interacted with students less than a week in three months. She is always up and down in workshops and meeting sent by the same manager who identified her to take up the preceptorship role".

Another participant said:

"We are not saying we should stop attending meetings, or be relieved of our daily tasks, but there should be clear expectations of our role. Teaching students should be part of our performance evaluation. I was once shouted at by a manager that why did you not do this and that.... The manager clearly told me that teaching students is not your primary role....She said so do your primary role first before you engage yourself in issues that will not contribute to your performance appraisal. I was disappointed and asked myself why am troubling myself".

Findings show that nurse managers need to be briefed on roles of clinical preceptors in the clinical area in order to clarify role expectations and task distribution among nurses.

4. Discussion

Four major themes emerged from the results of this study. The themes have actually touched almost on all areas that need to support clinical learning among nursing students. These are the faculty role, the clinical learning environment, nurses' clinical and teaching competences and nurses working conditions that included role expectations by their managers. Studies have highlighted that the preceptor role is highly satisfying, but also demanding [14].

Registered nurses identified faculty support as paramount to their performance in teaching students. Lack of faculty support really demotivates preceptors [15]. Lack of guidance from faculty becomes stressful for preceptors. Faculty members should provide direction to the overall clinical learning. O'Driscoll *et al.* (2010) named lack of faculty support as deficit in leadership of practice learning. The presence of faculty to support clinical learning is not only good for the students and their preceptors but also give faculty a chance to appreciate reality of practice [16]. Not only is the need for faculty involvement in preceptorship in nursing been reported but the need to increase their involvement has also been highlighted in literature [17].

Msiska, Smith [18] reported that students often complain of being used to cover shortage. This is true when students are not given adequate time to interact and learn from preceptors. Other studies have also agreed that high bed occupancy, shortage of staff and lack of resources exacerbate frustration and depression among nurses resulting into poor commitment and interest to spear time to teach students [19]. Preceptors expressed dissatisfaction with their inability to give students adequate engagement time. Registered nurses reported experiencing conflict between primary demands of providing patient care and performing of the preceptor role [15]. Findings clearly indicate that without proper planning and assignment of tasks within the ward, performing dual roles of both a practitioner and a preceptor could be stressful usually resulting into ineffective student teaching and supervision. The quality of clinical learning environment and the interactions between students and academic staff and preceptors directly impact on the acquisition of competences [20]. Croxon and Maginnis [21] highlighted that a constructive clinical learning environment with adequate opportunities for the development of confidence and competent is essential.

The role of clinical preceptors has universally been accepted as an approach to strengthen students' clinical learning [22]. However more studies have also reported that being a registered nurse in itself is not adequate to teach students. [23] indicates that there is a general lack of competence among some registered nurses.

The dual role of being a preceptor and a care giver is described as a serious hindrance to the fulfilment of the preceptor role [24]. In a study to investigate nurses' commitment in Finnish, findings showed that 85% of the respondents reported being committed to their profession. A number of factors tend to reduce nurses commitment and they include feeling that one's work is not meaningful or important, low level of confluence, dissatisfaction with the ways one's own abilities were being put into use, poor atmosphere at work and low quality of leadership. Preceptors would effectively discharge their role of preceptoring if nursing administrators also played their role. In view of this, preceptors would be relieved of some tasks to enable them provide an effective teaching role and student support [7].

Budgen and Gamroth [25] identified poor working conditions leading into poor retention among preceptors in their wards. Unclear role description of preceptors affects their role performance [4]. Shortage of staff is forcing the same few nurses available in the wards to be prepared as preceptors. The findings of the study show that there is a higher preceptor – student ratio than the ideal 1:10 ratio due to increased students' enrollment in colleges. This is increasing burden on the nurses.

5. Study Limitations

Focus group discussions were done with nurses coming from different clinical settings. In as much as registered nurses reported similar experiences, focus group discussions with participants from the same clinical setting would be more representative of their clinical settings.

6. Recommendations

Experiences of registered nurses of clinical teaching environment would help in the provision of appropriate learning environment for students' nurses. Registered nurses should be engaged in the improvement of clinical learning environment. Regular clinical learning and clinical teaching environment reviews should be conducted in an attempt to bring solutions to problems facing clinical environment. Clinical teaching is stressful for most registered nurses and appropriate support should be given to the nurses to maximize the benefits of students' clinical practice.

7. Conclusion

The results of the study indicate that registered nurses meet a lot challenges in clinical teaching of students. Much as the primary role of nurses in the clinical area is care provision, they acknowledge that teaching students is also a necessary role. Findings show that working as a clinical teaching and working as a clinical nurse are both stressful and demanding due to the nature of the clinical environment. It is evident that clinical nurses require adequate support from both their managers and faculty staff. Infrequent interaction between clinical nurses and faculty staff during clinical teaching fosters a sense of demotivation and lack of recognition among nurses. Lack of competence to handle students among nurses affects their willingness to manage students. Provision of clinical resources and adjustment to workload could improve the role performance of nursing during clinical teaching of students.

Acknowledgements

We extend our gratitude to all who participated in the study.

Conflict of Interest

There is no conflict of interest for this study

References

[1] Forsberg, E., *et al.* (2011) Virtual Patients for Assessment of Clinical Reasoning in Nursing—A Pilot Study. *Nurse Education Today*, **31**, 757-762. http://dx.doi.org/10.1016/j.nedt.2010.11.015

[2] Melender, H.L., Jonsen, E. and Hilli, Y. (2013) Quality of Clinical Education—Comparison of Experiences of Undergraduate Student Nurses in Finland and Sweden. *Nurse Education in Practice*, **13**, 256-261. http://dx.doi.org/10.1016/j.nepr.2013.01.003

[3] McSharry, E., *et al.* (2010) The Role of the Nurse Lecturer in Clinical Practice in the Republic of Ireland. *Nurse Education in Practice*, **10**, 189-195. http://dx.doi.org/10.1016/j.nepr.2009.08.004

[4] Meskell, P., Murphy, K. and Shaw, D. (2009) The Clinical Role of Lecturers in Nursing in Ireland: Perceptions from Key Stakeholder Groups in Nurse Education on the Role. *Nurse Education Today*, **29**, 784-790. http://dx.doi.org/10.1016/j.nedt.2009.03.014

[5] Webster, S., *et al.* (2010) Undergraduate Nursing Students' Experiences in a Rural Clinical Placement. *Australian Journal of Rural Health*, **18**, 194-198. http://dx.doi.org/10.1111/j.1440-1584.2010.01153.x

[6] Msiska, G., Munkhondya, T. and Chilemba, E. (2014) Undergraduate Students' Perceptions of the Role of the Nurse Educator during Clinical Placements in Malawian. *Open Journal of Nursing*, **4**, 12.

[7] Kalischuk, R.G., Vandenberg, H. and Awosoga, O. (2013) Nursing Preceptors Speak Out: An Empirical Study. *Journal of Professional Nursing: Official Journal of the American Association of Colleges of Nursing*, **29**, 30-38.

[8] Henderson, A., *et al.* (2011) A Framework to Develop a Clinical Learning Culture in Health Facilities: Ideas from the Literature. *International Nursing Review*, **58**, 196-202. http://dx.doi.org/10.1111/j.1466-7657.2010.00858.x

[9] Laibhen-Parkes, N., Brasch, J. and Gioncardi, L. (2014) Nursing Grand Rounds: A Strategy for Promoting Evidence-Based Learning Among Pediatric Nurses. *Journal of Pediatric Nursing*, **30**, 338-345.

[10] Killam, L.A. and Heerschap, C. (2013) Challenges to Student Learning in the Clinical Setting: A Qualitative Descriptive Study. *Nurse Education Today*, **33**, 684-691. http://dx.doi.org/10.1016/j.nedt.2012.10.008

[11] Happell, B. (2009) A Model of Preceptorship in Nursing: Reflecting the Complex Functions of the Role. *Nursing Education Perspectives*, **30**, 372-376.

[12] Giorgi, A.G. and Giorgi, B. (2004) Phenomenology. In: Smith, J.A., Ed., *Qualitative Psychology: A Practical Guide to Research Methods*, 9th Edition, Sage, London, 27.

[13] Erlingsson, C. and Brysiewicz, P. (2013) Orientation among Multiple Truths: An Introduction to Qualitative Research. *African Journal of Emergency Medicine*, **3**, 92-99.

[14] Danielsson, A., *et al.* (2009) Norwegian and Swedish Preceptors' Views of Their Role before and after Taking Part in a Group Supervision Program. *Nursing & Health Sciences*, **11**, 107-113. http://dx.doi.org/10.1111/j.1442-2018.2009.00455.x

[15] Younge, O., *et al.* (2008) Time to Truly Acknowledge What Nursing Preceptors Do for Students. *Journal for Nurses in Staff Development*, **24**, 113-116. http://dx.doi.org/10.1097/01.NND.0000300879.03061.1b

[16] Fisher, E.M. and Riley, T.A. (2005) Fostering the Scholarship of Discovery and Integration for Advanced Practice Education. *Nursing Education Perspectives*, **26**, 348-350.

[17] Gleeson, M. (2008) Preceptorship: Facilitating Student Nurse Education in the Republic of Ireland. *British Journal of Nursing*, **17**, 376-380. http://dx.doi.org/10.12968/bjon.2008.17.6.28903

[18] Msiska, G., Smith, P. and Fawcett, T. (2014) The "Lifeworld" of Malawian Undergraduate Student Nurses: The Challenge of Learning in Resource Poor Clinical Settings. *International Journal of Africa Nursing Sciences*, **1**, 35-42. http://dx.doi.org/10.1016/j.ijans.2014.06.003

[19] Moeti, M.R., van Niekerk, S.E. and van Velden, C.E. (2004) Perceptions of the Clinical Competence of Newly Registered Nurses in the North West Province. *Curationis*, **27**, 72-84. http://dx.doi.org/10.4102/curationis.v27i3.1003

[20] Brown, T., *et al.* (2011) Practice Education Learning Environments: The Mismatch between Perceived and Preferred Expectations of Undergraduate Health Science Students. *Nurse Education Today*, **31**, e22-e28. http://dx.doi.org/10.1016/j.nedt.2010.11.013

[21] Croxon, L. and Maginnis, C. (2009) Evaluation of Clinical Teaching Models for Nursing Practice. *Nurse Education in Practice*, **9**, 236-243. http://dx.doi.org/10.1016/j.nepr.2008.06.004

[22] Henderson, A., Fox, R. and Malko-Nyhan, K. (2006) An Evaluation of Preceptors' Perceptions of Educational Preparation and Organizational Support for Their Role. *Journal of Continuing Education in Nursing*, **37**, 130-136. http://dx.doi.org/10.3928/00220124-20060301-04

[23] McMurtrie, L.J., *et al.* (2014) Keeping Our Nursing and Midwifery Workforce: Factors That Support Non-Practising Clinicians to Return to Practice. *Nurse Education Today*, **34**, 761-765. http://dx.doi.org/10.1016/j.nedt.2013.08.017

[24] Hallin, K. and Danielson, E. (2008) Registered Nurses' Perceptions of Their Work and Professional Development. *Journal of Advanced Nursing*, **61**, 62-70.

[25] Budgen, C. and Gamroth, L. (2008) An Overview of Practice Education Models. *Nurse Education Today*, **28**, 273-283. http://dx.doi.org/10.1016/j.nedt.2007.05.005

6

Pressure Ulcer Prevention: Effectiveness of Heel Off-Loading Methodologies

Christopher C. Griffin[1], Tammy Dean[2], Jonathan M. Cayce[1], Mary Anne Modrcin[2]

[1]DeRoyal Industries, Powell, TN, USA
[2]Caylor School of Nursing, Lincoln Memorial University, Harrogate, TN, USA
Email: maryanne.modrcin@lmunet.edu

Abstract

Skin integrity breakdown and pressure ulcer formation on the heel are predictable and preventable healthcare occurrences. By minimizing surface contact pressures that can cause heel capillary occlusion, heel off-loading devices help mitigate the risk of decubitus ulceration. The purpose of this study is to investigate the efficacy of six off-loading methods commonly used in clinical settings to decrease heel contact pressure. Pressure mapping is used to evaluate contact pressure at the heel for underweight, normal weight, and overweight simulations. Based upon averages across four trials, it is shown that all devices reduce heel contact pressure when compared to no off-loading. The PRUventor™ boot exhibits significantly lower average pressure values than other off-loading strategies tested, suggesting that the PRUventor™ is the most effective off-loading device. From the analysis of the experimental data and comparison to similar data for respective off-loading alternatives, it is concluded that the PRUventor™ boot is an effective heel off-loading device for use in clinical settings.

Keywords

Heel Pressure Ulcer, Pressure Ulcer, Off-Loading Devices, Pruventor™ Boot, Pressure Mapping

1. Introduction

Pressure ulcer (PU) development is a serious concern in healthcare today. Patients who develop PUs are at greater risk for poor healthcare outcomes. Beginning in 2008, facilities no longer receive funds for services rendered for hospital-acquired PUs. Hospitals are focusing resources on prevention of PUs rather than treatment of PUs. Heel PU development is preventable when off-loading devices are utilized to decrease the amount of pressure exerted on the heel when a patient is on bedrest.

2. The Problem and Purpose of the Study

As a patient becomes bed-ridden for an extended duration of time, significant and constant pressure to the heel can cause capillary occlusion, eventually leading to the development of tissue ischemia and a PU. The heel is at a higher risk of occlusion due to the thin protection layers between the skin surface and calcaneus prominence and decreased resting blood perfusion levels [1]. Additionally the calcaneus has a small surface area with a large weight bearing bony prominence, which results in higher than normal pressure. VanGilder, Amlung, Harrison, and Meyer [2] studied 450,000 patients and found heel ulcers accounted for 41% of all PUs. Pressure ulceration in medical facilities are classified as never events and the incidence of a PU is commonly used as an indicator for quality of care. In fact, the US government cites the development of PUs a "serious quality-of-care issue in all settings" [3].

The significance of patients acquiring PUs while hospitalized is multi-dimensional. Patients who develop PUs experience a unique set of consequences that includes an increased length of stay in the hospital, decreased quality of life, increased morbidity and mortality rates, and increased hospital costs. The purpose of this study was to investigate the efficacy of six off-loading methods commonly used in clinical settings to decrease heel contact pressure and thus the formation of heel PUs.

3. Literature Review

The root factor for the development of a PU is the lack of pressure relief on capillaries. "The capillary pressure generally is described as being approximately 32 mmHg" [4]. If pressures higher than this are persistent, tissue ischemia and thus tissue necrosis results due to a lack of oxygen and nutrient supply to the tissues [4]-[6]. Torra I Bou *et al.* [6] concluded high pressure levels are often found in the heel area which predisposes patients to the development of a PU.

The incidence of PUs in general, and heel PUs specifically, is reported in the literature. There is a wide variation in the reported incidence of hospital acquired PUs due to various data collection methods and reporting practices. In 2009, Sanglard de Souza *et al.* [4] reported hospital units, excluding the Intensive Care Unit (ICU), had a PU occurrence rate of 3.5% to 33%. Lyder *et al.* [7] reported a PU occurrence rate of 15% but did not specify the hospital unit setting. The prevalence of PUs in patients with a fractured hip was found to be 21.3% [8]. An older study by Nicosia, Giliatta, Woodbury, and Houghton [9] reported an annual rate of 1.6 million PUs in acute care settings in the United States. The incidence of PU development is higher for patients treated in the ICU. Cooper [5] reported a PU rate ranging from 10% to 41% and Sanglard de Souza *et al.* [4] reported a range of 19.2% to 44% of patients in the ICU develop a PU.

Specifically, PUs of the heel are the most common type of hospital-acquired PU, and the rate of heel PU is higher for patients treated in the ICU, [2] [10] [11]. Various studies have been conducted to pinpoint this number as well as assist in developing best practice guidelines for prevention of heel PUs. Campbell *et al.* [11] found the PU heel incidence rate to be 13.3% in hospitalized patients. Van Gilder *et al.* [2] estimated a 12.3% overall incidence of PU in hospitalized patients and of these pressure ulcers, 18.2% to 28.9% of overall and 41% of grade III and IV ulcers occur on the heel.

The cost of treating hospital-acquired PUs is tremendous. Since 2008, insurance companies no longer reimburse hospitals for services related to these types of PUs. One study found the annual cost to hospitals to treat PUs ranged from $2.2 billion to $3.6 billion [7]. In the same year, a study by Black [10] found there were 394,699 medical insurance claims filed in the United States related to hospital-acquired PUs, at a cost of $8730 per case, for a total of $3.5 billion. The cost to treat one stage III or stage IV PU ranges between $5000 and $50,000 [5]. It has been estimated the cost to provide general prevention of PU for hospitalized patients is $54.66 per day [10].

A variety of risk factors related to the development of hospital-acquired PUs have been identified. These factors include age, ICU stays, lower extremity surgery, mechanical ventilation, decreased mobility, extended length of hospital stay, decreased level of consciousness, malnourishment, and a history of peripheral vascular disease[1] [5] [8] [9] [11]-[13].

The significance of PU development to the hospitalized patient is great. The literature mentions the more common results of PU development; increased cost, decreased quality of life, increased risk for below-the-knee amputation, limited rehabilitation, increased morbidity and mortality [11] [12]. Drake [14] reported more specific complications related to PU development as increased rates of infection, cellulitis, osteomyelitis, septicemia, limb amputation, and death. McInerney [3] found a hospital-acquired PU is one of the top three in-hospital errors that lead to death. In fact, these patients were found to have a mortality risk 2 - 6 times greater than that of a patient with intact skin.

Prevention of PUs and specifically heel PUs should be a priority for the health care team. Frain [15] determined studies designed specifically for heel ulcer prevention are rare. There are some studies in the literature aimed at determining best practice guidelines for heel ulcer prevention. These studies typically look at utilizing some form of a heel device versus standard care in the prevention of heel PUs. Heel devices have shown to significantly reduce the incidence of heel ulcer development [1] [5] [12] [16]. Campbell *et al.* [11] concluded the use of a heel off-loading device is considered best practice for the prevention of heel PUs. This study also found the characteristics of the best PU prevention device included; it was cleanable, easy to use, cost effective, comfortable according to the patient, and available. Lyman [17] compared heel PU rates before and after the adoption of a heel off-loading device retrospectively in a 550 bed facility. The study followed an interrupted time series design consisting of a 6 month pre-intervention phase, a 3 month implementation phase, and a 6 month post intervention phase. In the pre-intervention phase, 39 pressure ulcers were observed compared to 2 pressure ulcers in the post-intervention phase demonstrating a 95% reduction in pressure ulceration for the facility. The potential cost savings from this study was estimated to be $1,048,400. Donnelly *et al.* [8] conducted a randomized controlled trial to determine the difference between heel PU development for patients who were treated with a complete heel off-loading device and those receiving standard care. Of the 119 patients in the control group, 31 patients (26%) developed a PU with 8 of these PUs occurring on the heel. There were 120 patients who received a heel off-loading device and 8 of these patients (7%) developed a PU with none being a heel PU.

4. Purpose of the Study

The studies included in the literature review demonstrate the effectiveness of heel off-loading devices for preventing heel PU formation; however, heel off-loading can be achieved through a number of different techniques. The question arises if one method or device is superior in terms of reducing the pressure on the heel when compared to other devices. To answer this question, we utilized pressure mapping technology to quantify and compare the contact pressures exhibited on the heel in a model leg by 6 methods off-loading methodologies currently employed in the clinic. Our null hypothesis was that there would be no difference in the amount of contact pressure exerted on the heel when various clinical methodologies and off-loading devices were compared.

5. Method

To test the effectiveness at relieving heel contact pressure, conditions were simulated for underweight, normal weight, and overweight body mass index conditions utilizing a hollow model leg. The model leg was loaded with various weight compositions to simulate the heel and leg weight exhibited by a 5 foot, 10 inch male as defined by the National Heart, Lung, and Blood Institute [18]. The model leg is a segment comprised of the shank and calf below the knee, ankle, and foot, made from a siliconized/rubberized plastic with foam filling in the foot (**Figure 1(a)**). Weight loading was done via combinations of hollow and solid aluminum shafts, a steel shaft, copper-plated steel BBs, and sand placed inside the manikin leg. Leg, shank, and foot weights were determined via Exercise Prescription body segment data [19]. **Table 1** provides the leg weights for each simulated condition.

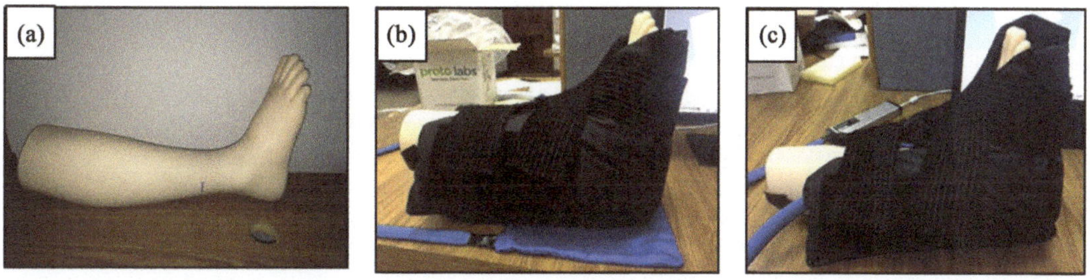

Figure 1. Orientation of control pressure mapping. (a) Manikin leg; (b) The leg is placed in the boot and set atop the Sensor Edge pressure mapping pad to gain an understanding of contact forces existing between surfaces; and (c) The sensor grid is wrapped around the heel and inserted into the boot to gain total heel contact measurements.

Table 1. Simulated model leg loading weights for simulated body mass indexes.

	Simulated Subject Weight (lbf)	Simulated BMI	Simulated Target Leg Weight (lbf)	Measured Manikin Leg Weight (lbf)
Under Weight	120	17.2	6.84	6.8
Normal Weight	170	24.4	9.69	9.15
Over Weight	220	31.6	12.54	12.25

Six popular clinical methodologies and heel off-loading devices were evaluated with pressure mapping to determine the efficacy of each condition for off-loading the heel. The conditions tested in this study included:

- Control: No off-loading of the heel;
- Pillow Condition 1: Leg and foot resting on pillow;
- Pillow Condition 2: Leg resting on pillow with heel and foot extending beyond pillow end;
- Standard Foam Heel Pillow: Egg-shell foam designed to fit on the heel;
- Off-loading Device A: Heelift Glide® off-loading boot (DM Systems Inc.; Evanston, IL);
- Off-loading Device B: Prevalon® off-loading boot (Sage; Cary, IL);
- Off-loading Device C: Pruventor™ off-loading boot (DeRoyal Industries; Powell, TN).

The initial pressure monitoring methods were based on the methods of Bush [20] where pressure mapping was used to demonstrate the off-loading efficacy of Off-loading Device B compared to no off-loading or off-loading on a pillow (Pillow Condition 1). However, testing and review of the table-top sensor arrangement shown in **Figure 1(b)** revealed that this arrangement recorded the contact pressure between the surface and the off-loading device rather than total contact pressure to the heel (**Figure 2**). This led to a new method design which provided more accurate data regarding the pressure exerted on the heel by all contact points from the heel off-loading device. The sensor grid was wrapped around the heel then either placed inside or on top of the off-loading device to obtain direct heel contact pressure readings (see **Figure 1(c)**). This arrangement allowed for a more accurate characterization of a device's heel off-loading efficacy. Pressure mapping of each off-loading methodology was measured by Sensor Edge's MeasureX software and flexible grip sensor pad (Parsippany, NJ). The MeasureX software was set to record 30 frames per second with a 100 moving average length value. The visualization palette range was set between 0 and 200. All data collected was recorded in units of mmHg.

For all conditions, the sensor grid was wrapped around the heel and ankle and secured with tape before insertion into/onto the off-loading device (**Figure 1(c)**). The leg was held in the air for several seconds before being set on the table during the initial data acquisition for calibration of the sensor grid. These initial data frame segments were subtracted out from the remaining data frames to remove the inherent contact forces that resulted from taping the sensor grid to the model leg and placing the model in or onto the off-loading device. Once the resting leg pressure readings stabilized, at least ten seconds of data was recorded for analysis. The investigator running the experiment located the center position of the heel and marked its location by indenting the pressure sensing mat. A masking grid that incorporated a 3 column by 4 row sensel array was centered on the heel location to determine heel contact pressures exerted on the heel during each condition. This grid size was chosen due to its geometric inclusion of heel contact area without significant effects of adjacent, zero-force sensel frames. The 3 × 4 grid creates a 19.35 cm^2 sensel window, meeting the recommended 9 - 10 cm^2 minimal measurement area for contact force determination on skin [21] [22]. The masking frame was used to only select data corresponding to heel to be exported from the MeasureX software.

Data analysis was performed in Microsoft® Excel® (Microsoft Corporation) to determine the average contact force over the heel from each condition. This was accomplished by averaging all pressure values recorded within the masking frame over the ten second stabilization period for each trial. Four independent trials were conducted for each condition to generate a composite average for each BMI and an overall average for each condition obtained from the 12 total trials conducted for each offloading condition. Paired t-tests were utilized to identify significant differences between study conditions for the overall average heel contact force.

6. Results

The pressure mapping following Bush's [20] method illustrated in **Figure 2** demonstrates that each of the off-loading devices effectively lift the heel off the support surface and suggests the heel is completely floated; however, this method is measuring only the contact forces between the boot and the support surface and not the contact forces between the heel and the off-loading device. **Figure 3** displays pressure mapping with the sensor grid wrapped around the model foot and leg. This data demonstrates that each off-loading method reduces heel contact forces with the heel off-loading devices being more proficient at minimizing these forces. Further, stress concentrations are noticed in the areas adjacent to the heel prominence, particularly as the loading weight (BMI) increases. This is apparent in the calf and ankle regions, as seen throughout Off-loading Device A and occasionally in Pillow Condition 2, Off-loading Device B, and Off-loading Device C. The overweight case for Off-loading Device A in particular shows the correspondence of pressure application to the Achilles tendon. These pressures are caused by the dispersion of weight-induced contact forces across the leg, necessary to off-loading the heel, to the calf region where a natural cushion exists from muscle and fat tissue decreasing the likelihood of capillary occlusion.

Heel contact forces for each condition and trial were calculated by averaging 10 seconds of data from within the region of interest. **Figure 4** visualizes the differences in off-loading efficacy between the conditions tested for each simulated BMI. Each off-loading condition was found to significantly reduce ($p < 0.05$, paired t-test) heel contact forces compared to the control condition. Furthermore, Pillow Condition 2, the foam heel pillow, and each off-loading device significantly reduced the heel contact pressure when compared to Pillow Condition 1. Interestingly, only Pillow Condition 2 and Off-loading Device C were found to significantly reduce the heel contact

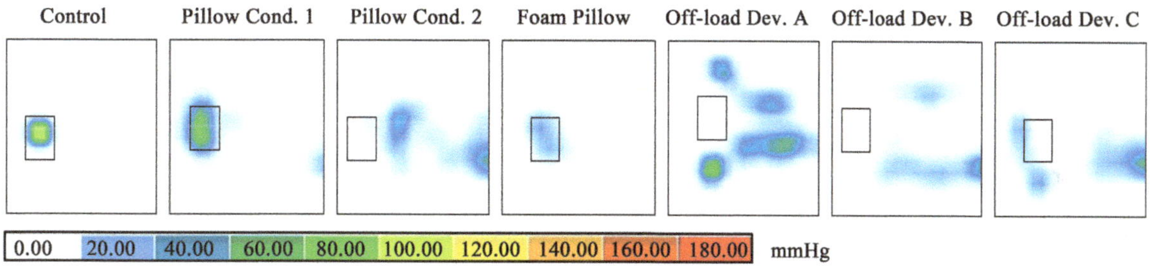

Figure 2. Pressure mapping utilizing method described by Bush 2009 [20]. Pressure maps displaying contact force distribution for each off-loading condition with pressure sensor placed between boot and table. The box indicates the location of the heel prominence. Additional external force was applied to show the orientation and location of the boot devices.

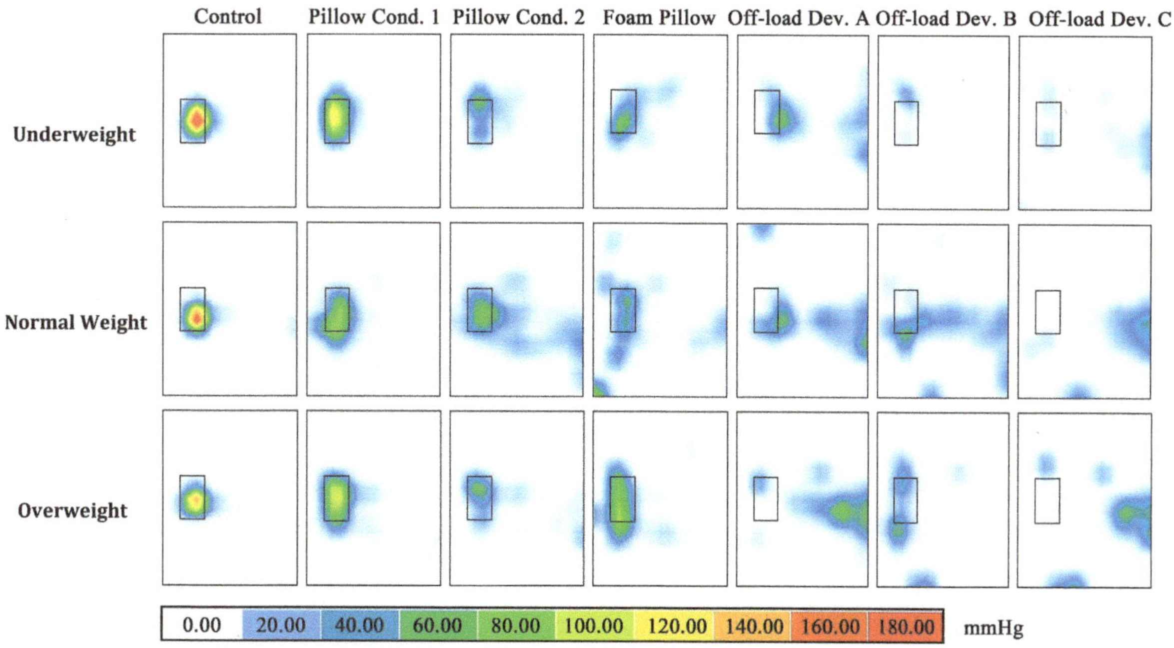

Figure 3. Pressure mapping visual comparison for pressure sensor attached to foot/leg complex. Pressure mapping visual comparison for pressure sensor attached to foot/leg complex. The rectangular box provides the location of the 3 column by 4 row sensel region of interest, as determined by heel location.

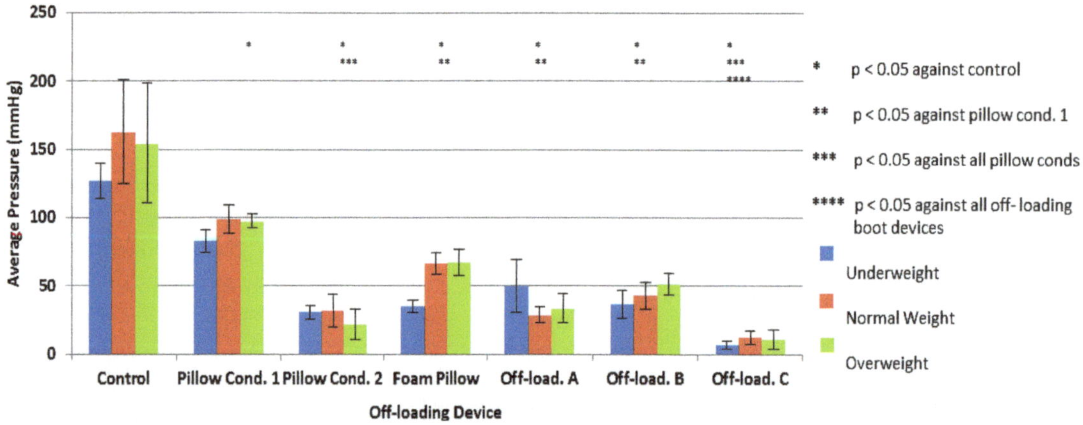

Figure 4. Data averages for each off-loading condition separated by loading amount. Standard error bars are displayed for each data set. Averages cover a twelve frame mask of heel forces averaged together over a ten second interval. Asterisks denote data significance as according to paired t-tests with a 5% significance level.

pressure compared to the heel foam pillow. No significant differences were observed between Pillow Condition 2 compared to Off-loading Device A or B. Off-loading Device C was found to significantly reduce the heel contact pressure when compared to Pillow Condition 1, Off-loading Device A, and Off-loading Device B. These observations suggest that Off-loading Device C was most effective at reducing heel-contact forces.

7. Discussion

The results of this study demonstrate the ability of each condition to reduce heel contact pressure. Off-loading Device C (PRUventor™) proved to provide the greatest amount of heel off-loading across all three simulated BMIs (**Table 1**). Pillow Condition 2 exhibited similar performance, however, it should be noted that this condition is variable depending upon pillow compressibility, leg weight, and leg position. Donnelly *et al.* [8] showed that this method is not effective in clinical practice. Additionally, Pillow Condition 2 is particularly prone to external factors, such as movement and rotation of the foot, excessive force onto the ankle, and direct blanket pressure, which could significantly affect off-loading effectiveness. Paired t-tests analysis demonstrated Off-loading Device C significantly reduced heel contact pressure when compared with all other off-loading devices and methods (p-value range: 8.92E-9 to 0.021). Both Off-loading Device A and Off-loading Device B, however, were found to be non-significant in relation to each other, the Foam Pillow, and Pillow Condition 2.

The capillary closing pressure is estimated to be at 32 mmHg in healthy individuals and can be lower in compromised patients [4]; therefore, the average contact pressure on the heel should be less than 32 mmHg for an off-loading device to be completely effective. Only Off-loading Device C averaged heel contact forces (10.00 mmHg overall), below 32 mmHg for the three simulated BMIs (6.55 mmHg underweight, 12.31 mmHg normal weight, and 11.14 mmHg over weight). Off-loading Device A and B had an overall contact force average of 37.32 mmHg and 43.75 mmHg respectively. This observation would seem to indicate that these devices are not effective at preventing heel pressure ulcers; however clinical studies have demonstrated that these devices are effective at reducing the incidence of heel pressure ulceration in at risk patients [8] [17].

Considering the massive amount of evidence related to the cause, incidence, and significance of hospital-acquired PUs, it should be a priority for the healthcare team to focus on the prevention of PUs and specifically heel PUs. Pressure ulcer development in hospitalized patients is considered a never event but according to the literature, occurs in 33% of patients outside of the ICU and up to 44% of patients in the ICU. Awareness of PU development must be a priority when considering patient safety, health care outcomes, and risk management in the hospital setting. As patients are identified as high risk for the development of PUs, the health care team should implement guidelines directed at prevention of PUs. The literature clearly validates it is cost-effective to prevent PUs rather than treat them [5] [7] [10].

8. Limitations of the Study

The primary limitation of this bench side study is that it was performed on a model leg and not in human subjects. While the model leg was viewed as an adequate surrogate for the human leg, certain limitations and inherent error existed with the model. The primary limitation was the inability to load the leg with the same weight distribution in the leg from trial to trial due to movement of the weighting elements inside the leg when the model was moved. A slight change in the distribution of weighting elements likely contributed to variability seen in the data. Latent forces due to placing the sensor pad on the foot were removed by subtracting out initial readings with the leg and boot suspended in the air. While we view this correction as adequate, it is possible that all latent forces were not removed from the analysis or latent forces were applied during the calibration phase while the leg was held in the air. A second limitation lies in the characteristics of the off-loading device itself. While the pillow produced adequate results, different pillow compressibility or leg weights can cause the heel to come in contact with the supporting surface, negating the purpose of the off-loading device. Similarly, for devices with ankle contact, particularly Off-loading Device A, off-loading the heel creates a significant resultant pressure on the ankle portion that could produce skin abrasion and pressure sores. Also, the model did not allow for the study of leg mobility and exterior weighting that would be present in a clinical setting. Foot rotation, leg movement, and additional blankets and supports can all negatively affect off-loading device performance, particularly with pillow methods [8]. These limitations motivate the need for a clinical study utilizing humans of different BMI to confirm the pressure mapping results of this study.

9. Conclusion

Based upon the results of this study, it is concluded that heel off-loading devices and techniques effectively off-loads the heel for simulated underweight, normal weight, and overweight conditions. The pressure mapping of each condition shows dispersion of contact forces in boot devices to the calf and ankle, reducing risk of capillary occlusion. Further statistical analysis of the measured heel contact forces demonstrates that all devices reduce heel pressure, with Off-loading Device C (PRUventor™) providing the greatest degree of off-loading pressure relief compared to other conditions. These data trends support the general efficacy of the PRUventor™ boot under simulated conditions and motivate the need for further clinical research.

Acknowledgements

The authors would like to acknowledge DeRoyal Industries for sponsoring this study.

Conflict of Interest

CCG was recently employed and JMC is currently employed by DeRoyal Industries. TD and MAM have no conflicts of interest to disclose.

References

[1] Langemo, D. (2014) Heel Pressure Ulcers: 2014 International Pressure Ulcer Prevention & Treatment Guidelines. 2014 National Pressure Ulcer Advisory Panel. www.npuap.org

[2] Van Gilder, C., Amlung, S., Harrison, P. and Meyer, S. (2009) Results of the 2008-2009 International Pressure Ulcer Prevalence Survey and a 3-Year, Acute Care, Unit Specific Analysis. *Ostomy Wound Management*, **55**, 39-45.

[3] McInerney, J.A. (2008) Reducing Hospital-Acquired Pressure Ulcer Prevalence through a Focused Prevention Program. *Advances in Skin & Wound Care*, **2**, 75-78. http://dx.doi.org/10.1097/01.ASW.0000305410.58350.34

[4] de Souza, T.S., Danski, M.T.R., Johann, D.A., de Lazzari, L.S.M. and Mingorance, P. (2013) Prevention's Pressure Ulcers Heel with Transparent Polyurethane Film. *Acta Paul Enferm*, **26**, 345-352.

[5] Cooper, K.L. (2013) Evidence-Based Prevention of Pressure Ulcers in the Intensive Care Unit. *Critical Care Nurse*, **33**, 57-66. http://dx.doi.org/10.4037/ccn2013985

[6] Torra I Bou, J.E., Lopez, J.R., Camanes, G., Narvaez, E.H., Blanco, J.B., Torralba, J.B., Soriano, J.V., *et al.* (2009) Preventing Pressure Ulcers on the Heel: A Canadian Cost Study. *Dermatology Nursing*, **21**, 268-272.

[7] Lyder, C.H., Wang, Y., Metersky, M., Curry, M., Liliman, R., Verzier, N.H. and Hunt, D.R. (2012) Hospital-Acquired Pressure Ulcers. *Journal of American Geriatric Society*, **60**, 1603-1608. http://dx.doi.org/10.1111/j.1532-5415.2012.04106.x

[8] Donnelly, J., Winder, J., Kernohan, W.G. and Stevenson, M. (2011) An RCT to Determine the Effect of a Heel Elevation Device in Pressure Ulcer Prevention Post-Hip Fracture. *Journal of Wound Care*, **20**, 309-318.

http://dx.doi.org/10.12968/jowc.2011.20.7.309

[9] Nicosia, G., Giliatta, A.E., Woodbury, M.G. and Houghton, P.E. (2007) The Effect of Pressure-Relieving Surfaces on the Prevention of Heel Ulcers in a Variety of Settings: A Meta-Analysis. *International Wound Journal*, **4**, 197-207. http://dx.doi.org/10.1111/j.1742-481X.2007.00333.x

[10] Black, J. (2012) Preventing Pressure Ulcers Occurring on the Heel. *Wounds International*, **3**, 58-61. www.woundsinternational.com.

[11] Campbell, K.E., Woodbury, M.G. and Houghton, P.E. (2010) Implementation of Best Practice in the Prevention of Heel Pressure Ulcers in the Acute Orthopedic Population. *International Wound Journal*, **7**, 28-40. http://dx.doi.org/10.1111/j.1742-481X.2009.00650.x

[12] Tayyib, N., Coyer, F. and Lewis, P. (2015) A Two-Arm Cluster Randomized Control Trial to Determine the Effectiveness of a Pressure Ulcer Prevention Bundle for Critically Ill Patients. *Journal of Nursing Scholarship*, **47**, 237-247. http://dx.doi.org/10.1111/jnu.12136

[13] Thorpe, E. (2015) Pressure Ulcer Prevention in Intensive Care. *Wounds UK*, **11**, 112-115.

[14] Drake, S. (2012) Implementing Evidence-Based Practice for Heel Pressure Ulcer Prevention in the Intensive Care Unit. *Critical Care Nurse*, **32**, 45-46.

[15] Frain, R. (2008) Decreasing the Incidence of Heel Pressure Ulcers in Long-Term Care by Increasing Awareness: Results of a 1-Year Program. *Ostomy Wound Management*, **54**, 62-67.

[16] Cadue, J.F., Karolewicz, S., Tardy, C., Barrault, C., Robert, R. and Pourrat, O. (2008) Prevention of Heel Pressure Sores with a Foam Body-Support Device. *La Presse Médicale*, **37**, 30-36. http://dx.doi.org/10.1016/j.lpm.2007.07.009

[17] Lyman, V. (2009) Successful Heel Pressure Ulcer Prevention Program in a Long-Term Care Setting. *Journal of Ostomy Continence Nursing*, **36**, 616-621. http://dx.doi.org/10.1097/WON.0b013e3181bd813e

[18] National Heart, Lung, and Blood Institute. Calculate Your Body Mass Index. http://www.nhlbi.nih.gov/health/educational/lose_wt/BMI/bmicalc.htm

[19] Exercise Prescription (2014) Body Segment Data. http://www.exrx.net/ Kinesiology/ Segments.html

[20] Bush, T.R. (2009) Pressure Mapping—Comparison of Unprotected Heels on a Hospital Bed vs. Heels Positioned in the Preval on Pressure Relieving Heel Protector. Sage Products. http://www.sageproducts.com/documents/pdf/education/case_studies/heel/21297.pdf

[21] Lung, C.W., Yang, T.D., Crane, B.A., Elliott, J., Dicianno, B. and Jan, Y.K. (2014) Investigation of Peak Pressure Index Parameters for People with Spinal Cord Injury Using Wheelchair Tilt-in-Space and Recline : Methodology and Preliminary Report. *BioMed Research International*, **2014**, Article ID: 508583. http://dx.doi.org/10.1155/2014/508583

[22] Davis, K. and Sprigle, S. (2008) The Science of Interface Pressure Mapping—Updates for Clinical Application. http://hdl.handle.net/1853/36795

7

Reducing Hospital Stays through Subacute and Complex Care Programs

Ronald Lagoe[1*], Louise Pernisi[2], Shelly Littau[1]

[1]Hospital Executive Council, Syracuse, NY, USA
[2]Upstate University Hospital, Syracuse, NY, USA
Email: *Hospexcl@cnymail.com

Abstract

The needs of patients who can stay for extended periods in hospitals generate large amounts of health care expenses. They usually experience multiple diagnoses and their needs are not easily understood or served. This study described the efforts of the acute hospitals in Syracuse, New York to address the needs of these Complex Care patients. The hospitals developed a series of Subacute Programs, each of which addressed a single care need, which might have helped restrain the growth of adult medicine stays during a five-month period. The study demonstrated that reductions in adult medicine stays were associated with the introduction of Complex Care Programs that addressed multiple care needs, in 2015. The association between the implementation of the Complex Care Programs and length of stay reduction for adult medicine was present at the combined and individual hospital levels. The study suggested that the amount of Program Development Funds invested in these programs saved 2000 adult medicine days or $1,600,000 compared with total expenses of $292,000 during a five-month period. The experiences of the Syracuse hospitals suggested that small programs with simple structures could have a positive impact on health care efficiency at the community level.

Keywords

Hospitals, Long Term Care, Hospital Lengths of Stay

1. Introduction

In recent years, the importance of efficiency in the movement of patients among health care services has increased. The need for efficiency has been supported by limitations in resources for major health care payors. It

*Corresponding author.

has become especially important for health care organizations that provide episodic care, such as hospitals and physicians [1] [2].

From a financial perspective, efficiency is important because extended stays in hospitals result in large expenses related to patient care. Limitations in reimbursement from health care payors have not covered the cost of care for outlier patients with multiple diagnoses. The impact of these limitations has been heightened by programs such as Accountable Health Care and Bundling [3]-[5].

Efficiency is also important from the perspective of patient outcomes. Patients who stay for extended periods in hospitals have a greater risk of developing inpatient complications than those with shorter stays. Patients whose care needs are addressed fully on inpatient admissions have lower probability of being readmitted [6].

In the United States, one of the greatest challenges to efficiency in hospitals is the complex care or long term acute population. These individuals have clinical conditions that generate extended adult medicine stays, and in some cases, long post operative surgical stays which reduce the efficiency of care at the provider and community levels [3] [7]-[9].

A number of states have developed Long Term Acute Care Programs that provide specific reimbursement to nursing homes and other providers of care of these patients. In some areas, however, these programs are not available. As a result, hospitals and other providers must develop alternatives or provide care to these patients themselves, or they can stay for extended periods and compromise access to hospitals [10]-[12]. This process has frequently required that they develop the resources necessary to support those programs [13].

In this context, relationships between hospitals and nursing homes have become more important than ever. As facilities that provide residential health care on a 24 hour/seven day basis, nursing homes are the only facilities that can provide care for many types of patients who will otherwise remain in hospitals for extended periods of time [14] [15].

2. Population

This study evaluated the development of programs addressing long term acute care patients in the metropolitan area of Syracuse, New York. This area includes three acute care facilities (numbers of inpatient discharges for 2014 in parentheses), Crouse Hospital (19,919), St. Joseph's Hospital Health Center (25,532), and Upstate University Hospital (26,649). These hospitals provide primary and secondary services to a service area of approximately 600,000 and referral center services to the eleven county Central New York Health Service area, with a population of 1,400,000.

Historically, the Syracuse hospitals have worked cooperatively to improve the efficiency and outcomes of care in the local acute care system. A number of these efforts have been undertaken through their planning organization, the Hospital Executive Council [16].

A number of these efforts have focused on reduction of lengths of stay, especially for patients who remain in hospitals for extended periods of time. The hospitals have not developed ownership of large numbers of nursing home beds. Only 14 percent of nursing home beds in the community are hospital owned. Most importantly, New York State has no dedicated program for support of long term acute care patients, such as the programs that exist in a number of states.

3. Methods

Between 2003 and 2012, the Syracuse hospitals developed a number of Subacute Programs to support the movement of long term acute care patients from hospitals to nursing homes. The project included the three hospitals and five nursing homes with an interest in caring for these patients. Each of these programs focused on provision of a single service in the participating nursing homes in order to reduce hospital stays. They have included the following.

- Intravenous Medications, including generic, low cost medications;
- Enhanced Medications, including higher cost specific medications;
- Enhanced Plus Medications, including higher cost specific medications and dosages;
- Wound Vac, including extensive wound care equipment;
- Offsite Transport, including transportation for services such as dialysis;
- Bariatric, including support for care of high Body Mass Index patients.

The Subacute Programs have been implemented through agreements between the Syracuse hospitals, local nursing homes, and the Hospital Executive Council. These agreements include the following components.

- Certification by an Access Coordinator at each hospital that the need for the program in the community is the principal barrier to discharge;
- A Community Wide Pool of Program Development Funding to support some expenses of care in nursing homes maintained by the Hospital Executive Council;
- Distribution of Program Development Funds for specific types of care, rather than the needs of each patient.

Implementation of the Subacute Programs between 2003 and 2012 were useful in restraining the growth of lengths of stay for adult medicine and adult surgery patients in the Syracuse hospitals. At the same time, the impacts of these programs were limited because they focused on a single patient need, rather than multiple issues. To address this need, an additional series of programs addressing multiple Long Term Acute Care or Complex Care requirements were developed and implemented in 2015. These programs have included the following.

- Multiple Intravenous Antibiotics;
- Extensive Wound Care (Wound Vac) Plus Antibiotics;
- Other Combinations of Medications;
- Behavioral Issues Requiring One on One Care;
- Care for Specific Disabilities.

The Complex Care Programs were implemented with the same agreement and components that were used for the Subacute Programs. Program Development Funds included larger amounts of expenses because of the higher care needs of the patients. All of these expenses were funded by the Syracuse hospitals through the Hospital Executive Council.

This study evaluated the impact of the Subacute and Complex Care Programs in the hospitals of Syracuse, New York between March and July 2013 and 2015. This was the most recent three year period for which complete data were available concerning utilization of the programs and their impacts on hospital lengths of stay.

The initial component of the analysis focused on utilization of the individual Subacute and Complex Care Programs during the three five month periods. This analysis included the Subacute Programs in 2013, 2014, and 2015, and the implementation of the Complex Care Programs in 2015. The study data included numbers of patients admitted to nursing homes for the combined hospitals for each individual program as well as for the combined Subacute and Complex Care Programs. This information also included total Program Development Funds expended for the Subacute and the Complex Care Programs combined.

The second component of the analysis focused on the impact of the Subacute and Complex Care Programs on lengths of stay for adult medicine patients discharged to nursing homes from the Syracuse hospitals during March-July 2013, 2014, and 2015. Adult medicine patients were defined as those aged 18 years and over assigned to medicine All Patients Refined Diagnosis Related Groups. The study data included the adult medicine mean length of stay and the severity adjusted All Patients Refined Case Mix Index for each hospital in each five month period.

The third component of the analysis focused on the impact of the Subacute and Complex Care Programs on lengths of stay for adult surgery patients discharged to nursing homes from the Syracuse hospitals during January-June 2013, 2014, and 2015. Adult surgery patients were defined as those aged 18 years and over assigned to surgical All Patients Refined Diagnosis Related Groups. The study data included the same indicators used in the analysis of adult medicine patients.

4. Results

The first component of the study focused on utilization of the Subacute and Complex Care Programs in the Syracuse hospitals between March and July 2013 and 2015. Relevant data are summarized in **Table 1**.

This information demonstrated that the utilization of the Subacute Programs, each of which included a single service, such as a medication or wound care, increased from 35 to 60 between March and July 2013 and 2014, and then remained relatively constant at 60 - 62 patients between March and July 2014 and 2015. Much of the Subacute Program use involved patient medications, including the Intravenous Therapy, Enhanced Medications, and Enhanced Plus Medications.

Utilization of the Subacute Programs for these time periods was reflected in Total Program Development expenses, which more than doubled between March and July 2013 and 2014, then remained relatively constant between the same periods in 2014 and 2015. At the March-July 2015 level, the annualized amount of Subacute Program Expenses would have been $ 225,840.

Table 1. Subacute and complex care program utilization, Syracuse hospitals, March-July 2013-2015.

	Number of Patients		
	2013	2014	2015
Subacute Programs			
Oral Medications	6	0	0
IV Medications	11	18	17
Enhanced	4	9	8
Enhanced Plus	2	6	8
Wound Vac	5	12	13
Offsite Transports	4	12	13
Bariatric	3	3	3
Complex Care Programs			
Multiple IVs	0	0	8
Wound Vac w Meds	0	1	4
Behavioral	0	0	15
Combined Medications	0	0	4
Disability	0	0	1
Total Subacute Patients	35	60	62
Total Complex Care Patients	0	1	32
Total Subacute & Complex Care Patients	35	61	94
Total Subacute Expenses	$ 44,850	$ 98,550	$ 94,100
Total Complex Care Expenses	$ 0	$ 2800	$ 98,000
Total Expenses	$ 44,850	$ 101,350	$ 192,100

The data in **Table 1** demonstrated that the introduction of the Complex Care Programs in the Syracuse hospitals resulted in a significant increase in program utilization and costs between March and July 2015. When compared with use of the Subacute Programs, this amounted to a 52 percent rise in total program utilization and an 89.5 percent increase in Program Development expenses. The disproportionate increase in Program Development Expenses resulted from multiple services and resources addressed by the Complex Care Programs.

The data suggested that most of the programs and resources addressed by the Subacute and Complex Care Programs involved adult medicine. The only programs with some involvement for surgical patients were the Wound Care (wound vac) services, where the patient volumes were approximately 50 percent medicine patients and 50 percent surgical patients.

The second component of the analysis focused on the impact of the Subacute and Complex Care Programs on lengths of stay for adult medicine in the Syracuse hospitals. Relevant data are summarized in **Table 2**.

This information demonstrated that the mean adult medicine length of stay for discharges to nursing homes for the combined hospitals increased from 8.05 to 9.15 days between March and July 2013 and 2014, then declined from 9.15 to 8.32 days between March and July 2014 and 2015. The 2014-2015 decline resulted in a reduction of 2,000 inpatient days. The decline in stays occurred during the period when the Complex Care Programs were implemented. The data also indicated that the severity of illness for this population increased during the three year period.

The information in **Table 2** also indicated that the mean adult medicine lengths of stay for discharges to nursing homes for each of the three hospitals increased between March and July 2013 and 2014, then declined between March and July 2014. The largest reductions in stays occurred at Upstate University Hospital where the mean length of stay declined by 2.16 days, resulting in a reduction of 1762 patient days. These declines occurred as the clinical severity of illness for Upstate University Hospital was increasing.

The data suggested that most of the reductions in adult medicine stays for discharges to nursing homes were associated with the implementation of the Complex Care Programs in the Syracuse hospitals during 2015. During this period, most of the increases in stays for this population that occurred between March and July 2013 and 2014 were reversed at each of the three hospitals. The largest reductions in stays occurred at Upstate University Hospital where utilization of the Complex Care Programs was highest. Of the 32 patients admitted to these programs during 2015, 20 were discharged from that hospital.

The data in **Table 2** concerning total adult medicine discharges also identified the impact of shorter stays for discharges to nursing homes on stays for total discharges for this service. They indicated that the reductions in total adult medicine mean stays for the combined hospitals that occurred between March and July 2014 and 2015 were probably related to the reductions in mean stays for discharges to nursing homes.

The third component of the study evaluated the association between the Subacute and Complex Care Programs on adult surgery lengths of stay in the Syracuse hospitals. Relevant data are summarized in **Table 3**.

This information demonstrated that the mean adult surgery lengths of stay for discharges to nursing homes for the combined hospitals declined slightly from 10.46 to 10.30 days between March and July 2013 and 2014, then increased slightly from 10.30 to 10.72 days between March and July 2014 and 2015. The increase in stays that occurred during the implementation of the Complex Care Programs, between 2014 and 2015, was associated with an increase of 627 patient days. This compared with the reduction of 2000 adult medicine patient days that occurred during the same period.

The data also indicated that there was no consistent direction in adult surgery stays for discharges to nursing homes from the three hospitals. Lengths of stay for discharges to nursing homes at St. Joseph's Hospital Health Center increased throughout the period, while stays at Upstate University Hospital declined then increased and stays at Crouse Hospital decreased throughout the period.

The data in **Table 3** also indicated that, between March and July 2014 and 2015, adult surgery patient days increased by 62.73 at St. Joseph's Hospital Health Center and by 136.53 at Upstate University Hospital while declining by 59.92 at Crouse Hospital. The numbers of these days, both increases and decreases, were considera-

Table 2. Inpatient mean lengths of stay, adult medicine, Syracuse hospitals, March-July 2013-2015.

	Number of Discharges			Mean Length of Stay			Length of Stay Difference	Patient Days Difference	Severity Adjusted Case Mix Index			Severity Adjusted Case Mix Difference
	2013	2014	2015	2013	2014	2015	2014-2015	2014-2015	2013	2014	2015	2014-2015
Discharges to Nursing Homes												
Crouse Hospital	527	582	675	7.16	7.83	7.56	−0.27	−182.25	1.3273	1.2982	1.3535	0.0553
St. Joseph's Hospital Health Center	817	804	919	7.96	8.10	7.61	−0.49	−450.31	1.1952	1.2198	1.1881	−0.0317
Upstate University Hospital-SUNY UMU	636	584	816	8.90	11.91	9.75	−2.16	−1762.56	1.4029	1.3365	1.4582	0.1217
Total	1980	1970	2410	8.05	9.15	8.32	−0.83	−2000.30	1.2971	1.2775	1.3259	0.0484
Total Discharges	14,589	14,148	14,452	5.09	5.41	5.32	−0.09	−1300.68	1.0734	1.0690	1.1317	0.0627

Table 3. Inpatient mean lengths of stay, adult surgery, Syracuse hospitals, March-July 2013-2015.

	Number of Discharges			Mean Length of Stay			Length of Stay Difference	Patient Days Difference	Severity Adjusted Case Mix Index			Severity Adjusted Case Mix Difference
	2013	2014	2015	2013	2014	2015	2014-2015	2014-2015	2013	2014	2015	2014-2015
Discharges to Nursing Homes												
Crouse Hospital	263	395	428	7.62	6.94	6.80	−0.14	−59.92	2.5131	2.2367	2.4043	0.1676
St. Joseph's Hospital Health Center	736	673	697	9.02	10.10	10.19	0.09	62.73	2.8343	2.9099	3.1657	0.2558
Upstate University Hospital-SUNY UMU	243	261	369	17.88	15.88	16.25	0.37	136.53	3.7826	3.2250	3.4359	0.2109
Total	1242	1329	1494	10.46	10.30	10.72	0.42	627.48	2.9518	2.7717	3.0143	0.2426
Total Discharges	8596	8656	8711	5.87	6.22	6.31	0.09	783.99	2.3192	2.3137	2.4072	0.0935

bly smaller than the reductions in adult medicine patient days during the same period.

These data suggested the implementation of the Complex Care Programs in the Syracuse hospitals during 2015 were probably not associated with a reduction in adult surgery lengths of stay and patient days. The only facility where reductions in these indicators occurred, Crouse Hospital, admitted six patients to the wound vac programs during this period. The mean length of stay for total discharges to nursing homes also increased throughout the three year period.

5. Discussion

The need for efficiency in the delivery of health care continues to increase, especially for providers of short duration care, such as acute hospitals. In this context, the needs of patients who can stay for extended periods present a considerable challenge, both economically and clinically.

The economic challenges of Complex Care or Long Term Acute Care patients are well known in United States hospitals. These patients, through no fault of their own, generate larger amounts of health care expenses than the revenue that they generate. They can also result in costly adverse outcomes such as inpatient complications and readmissions.

At the same time, these patients present a major human challenge to health care providers at the community level. Because they usually experience multiple diagnoses, rather than a single one, their needs are not easily understood or served by a society that tends to deal with health care one need at a time. They are, arguably, the most disadvantaged members of the population.

A number of states have developed Long Term Acute Care Programs to help address the needs of these patients. In areas where these programs are not available, however, individual hospital providers are left to develop their own programs, usually with their own resources, to address their needs.

This study described the efforts of the acute hospitals in Syracuse, New York to address the needs of Complex Care patients without a Long Term Acute Care Program. It described how those hospitals and nursing homes developed a series of Subacute and Complex Care Programs in nursing homes to support shorter stays in hospitals and residential care in a number of nursing homes. These programs were based on relatively simple structures and modest levels of funding.

The results of the study suggested that the Subacute Programs, each of which addressed a single care need, which were developed by the Syracuse hospitals, might have helped restrain the growth of adult medicine stays for discharges to nursing homes between March and July in 2013 and 2014, but were not associated with reductions of these stays. Most of this impact was probably related to the transfer of patient days for individuals receiving intravenous medications from hospitals to nursing homes.

The study data demonstrated that reductions in adult medicine stays for this population were associated with the introduction of the Complex Care Programs, which addressed multiple care needs, in 2015. The association between the implementation of the Complex Care Programs and length of stay reduction for adult medicine was present at the combined and individual hospital levels. The provider with the largest volume of Complex Care patients, Upstate University Hospital, experienced the largest reduction in stays and the largest number of patient days for this service.

The study data suggested that, for the amount of Program Development funds invested in these programs by the Syracuse hospitals, area nursing homes, and the Hospital Executive Council, the return on investment was impressive. At an average per diem expense of $ 800 for a late length of stay day, these programs saved 2000 adult medicine patient days or $ 1,600,000 between March and July in 2015. The total Program Development Funds expended by the Subacute and Complex Care Programs during this period was $ 192,100. Adding another $ 100,000 for staffing the programs at the hospitals, nursing homes, and the Hospital Executive Council, total expenses were still only $ 292,000.

The study data also suggested that the impact of Complex Care Programs implemented in Syracuse was largely limited to adult medicine. This probably resulted from the types of therapies, many of which involved medications, included in the programs. No clear association between these programs and reduction of hospital stays for adult surgery could be identified in the study data.

Moving forward, the Syracuse hospitals and the Hospital Executive Council are interested in building on their experience with the Subacute and Complex Care Programs to make further progress in length of stay reduction for adult medicine patients. These efforts will probably include additional Complex Care Programs for total parenteral nutrition and low level chemotherapy patients. An important component of these efforts is identification of long term care partners who can support these services. These initiatives could reduce the combined hospital stays for adult medicine stays for discharges to nursing homes below eight days. The development of Complex Care Programs for adult surgery patients is also a challenge that will require long term care partners who can support these services.

The need for efficiency in the delivery of health care services will probably continue to shift responsibility for development of these programs to hospitals and other providers. Patients requiring Subacute and Complex Care services will continue to challenge these efforts at the community level. The experiences of the Syracuse hospitals suggest that small programs with simple structures can have a positive impact on efficiency at the community level.

References

[1] Keehan, S.P., Cuckler, G.A., Sisko, A.M., Madison, A.J., Smith, S.D., Stone, D.A., Poisal, J.A., Wolfe, C.J. and Lizonitz, J.M. (2015) National Health Expenditure Projections, 2014-24: Spending Growth Faster than Recent Trends. *Health Affairs*, **34**, 1407-1417. http://dx.doi.org/10.1377/hlthaff.2015.0600

[2] Dentzler, S. (2011) Urgent Measures for an Old Problem. *Health Affairs*, **30**, 1626. http://dx.doi.org/10.1377/hlthaff.2011.0961

[3] Joynt, K.E., Gawande, A.A., Orav, E.J. and Jha, A.K. (2013) Contribution of Preventable Acute Care Spending to Total Spending for High Cost Medicare Patients. *JAMA*, **309**, 2572-2578. http://dx.doi.org/10.1001/jama.2013.7103

[4] Evans, M. (2012) The Early Returns on Accountable Care. *Modern Healthcare*, **42**, S1-S5.

[5] Fisher, E.S., Shortell, S.M., Kriendler, S.A., Van Citters, A.D. and Larson, B.K. (2012) A Framework for Evaluating the Formation, Implementation, and Accountable Care Organizations. *Health Affairs*, **31**, 2368-2378. http://dx.doi.org/10.1377/hlthaff.2012.0544

[6] Weil, A.R. (2015) Hospital Costs and Quality. *Health Affairs*, **34**, 1263.

[7] Gawande, A.A. (2011) The Hot Spotters: Can We Lower Costs by Giving the Neediest Patients Better Care? *New Yorker*.

[8] Johnson, T.L., Rinehart, D.J., Durfee, J., Brewer, D., Batal, H., Blum, J., Oronce, C.J. and Melinkovich, P. (2015) For Many Patients Who Use Large Amounts of Health Care Services, The Need Is Intense Yet Temporary. *Health Affairs*, **34**, 1312-1323. http://dx.doi.org/10.1377/hlthaff.2014.1186

[9] Riley, G.F. (2007) Long Term Trends in the Concentration of Medicare Spending. *Health Affairs*, **26**, 808-816. http://dx.doi.org/10.1377/hlthaff.26.3.808

[10] Hasselman, D. (2013) Super Utilizer Summit: Common Themes from Innovative Complex Care Management Programs. Center for Health Care Strategies, Princeton.

[11] Hong, C.S., Siegel, A.L. and Ferris, T.G. (2014) Caring for High Need, High Cost Patients: What Makes for a Successful Care Management Program? Commonwealth Fund, New York.

[12] Bodenheimer, T. (2013) Strategies to Reduce Costs and Improve Care for High Utilizing Medicaid Patients: Reflections on Pioneering Programs. Center for Health Strategies, Princeton.

[13] Lagoe, R., Pernisi, L., Haag, D. and Drapola, B. (2015) Evolution of Programs to Improve Transfers Between Hospitals and Nursing Homes at the Community Level. *Open Journal of Nursing*, **5**, 587-595. http://dx.doi.org/10.4236/ojn.2015.57062

[14] Marek, K.D. and Rantz, M.J. (2000) Aging in Place: A New Model for Long Term Care. *Nursing Administration Quarterly*, **24**, 1-11. http://dx.doi.org/10.1097/00006216-200004000-00003

[15] Wagner, E.H., Austin, B.T., Davis, C., Hindmarsh, M., Schaefer, J. and Bonomi, A. (2001) Improving Chronic Illness Care: Translating Evidence into Action. *Health Affairs*, **20**, 64-78. http://dx.doi.org/10.1377/hlthaff.20.6.64

[16] Lagoe, R., Pasinski, T., Kronenberg, P., Quinn, T. and Schaengold, P. (2005) Linking Health Services at the Community Level. *Canada Healthcare Quarterly*, **9**, 60-65. http://dx.doi.org/10.12927/hcq..18229

8

The Effect of a Psycho-Educational Intervention on Quality of Life of Patients with Advanced Lung Cancer Undergoing Chemotherapy

Yanli Zhao[1*], Ruifang Zhu[2]

[1]Shanxi Cancer Hospital, Taiyuan, China
[2]The First Hospital of Shanxi Medical University, Taiyuan, China
Email: [*]zhaoyanli7832395@163.com

Abstract

Objective: Cancer patients undergoing chemotherapy commonly experience depression and anxiety, which, along with adverse effects of chemotherapy, inevitably compromise quality of life (QOL) of the patients. The aim of this study was to investigate the effect of a psycho-educational intervention on the quality of life (QOL) of patients with advanced lung cancer undergoing chemotherapy. Methods: Two hundred in-patients with unresectable advanced lung cancer undergoing chemotherapy in Shanxi Cancer Hospital from January to October 2013 were randomized into the intervention group (n = 100) and the control group (n = 100). Patients in the intervention group received a purposely designed and nurse-delivered psycho-educational intervention in addition to routine caring and chemotherapy, whereas those in the control group underwent chemotherapy and routine caring only. QOL of patients was assessed according to QOL instrument for lung cancer (QLICP-LU). The impact of the psycho-educational intervention on QOL was analyzed using independent-sample *t* test and χ^2 test. Results: The psychological, physical, and social function, and the overall QOL scores were significantly improved in patients who received the psycho-educational intervention compared with those in the control group. Conclusions: A nurse-delivered psycho-educational intervention is a useful strategy to improve QOL of patients with advanced lung cancer undergoing chemotherapy.

Keywords

Psychological Intervention, Psycho-Educational Intervention, Lung Cancer, Quality of Life

[*]Corresponding author.

1. Introduction

Lung cancer is a leading cause of cancer-related mortality in men and women all over the world. In particular, the incidence of lung cancer is rapidly increasing in China with the crude incidence rate being 46.08 per 100,000 in 2010 [1]. In the same year, 605,900 patients were diagnosed and 486,600 patients died of lung cancer in the country [1]. This is closely related to the rapid increase in aged population, environment pollution, and cigarette smoking [1].

Despite recent advances in molecularly targeted therapy and immunotherapy, conventional chemotherapy remains one of the major therapeutic approaches in the treatment of patients with advanced lung cancer [2]. Nevertheless, these patients commonly experience depression and anxiety, which, along with adverse effects of chemotherapy, inevitably compromise their quality of life (QOL) [3] [4]. Effective interventions to improve the psychological, physical, and social function of patients with advanced lung cancer undergoing chemotherapy are urgently needed.

In this study, we have examined the effect of a purposely designed and nurse-delivered psycho-educational intervention on QOL of patients with advanced lung cancer undergoing chemotherapy. We report here that the psycho-educational intervention significantly improves the psychological, physical, and social function, and overall QOL of the patients, and that it reduces common symptoms associated with chemotherapy. These results suggest that nurses can play an important role in assistance of patients in improving their QOL through delivering psycho-educational interventions.

2. Materials and Methods

2.1. Patients and Inclusion and Exclusion Criteria

In-patients (n = 200) with unresectable advanced lung cancer undergoing chemotherapy in Shanxi Cancer Hospital from January to October 2013 were enrolled in this study according to the following criteria: 1) they met the lung cancer diagnostic criteria of the Chinese Common Malignancy Norms; 2) Advanced lung cancer (Stage IIIB to IV) was diagnosed according to the International Union Against Cancer TNM classification in 1997; 3) they were prescribed for chemotherapy; 4) they had accepted at least primary school education; 5) they did not have any heart diseases, liver diseases, kidney disease, systemic infection, severe anemia, and cachexia, and were not complicated with other chronic diseases at the time of commencement of chemotherapy; 6) they agreed to participate in the study and signed informed consent forms. According to the completely randomized grouping design, the patients were numbered chronologically from 1 to 200. Patients with odd numbers were assigned into the intervention group, whereas those with even numbers were assigned to the control group. There were 70.75% males and 29.25% females, which ages ranging from 61 to 70 years old. 70.25% of the enrolled patients had a smoking history longer than 10 years. Chi-square analysis showed that the differences in the general demographic characteristics were not statistically significant between the intervention and control groups.

2.2. Tools of Quality of Life Instruments for Cancer Patients: Lung Cancer (QLICP-LU)

The one-scale method developed by Wan Chong Hua, *et al.* was used to measure the QOT of cancer patients [5], which includes common modules (the physical function, the psychological function, the social function, common symptoms, and side effects) and a specific module that contains eight entries. The reliability of this scale was above 0.7 and its validity was 0.82 [4]. QOL was assessed once one week for each patient throughout the hospitalized period.

2.3. Therapies

Patients in both the control group and the intervention group were treated with conventional chemotherapy. At the same time, patients in the control group received routine caring while those in the intervention group received an additional nurse-delivered psycho-educational intervention.

2.4. Psycho-Educational Intervention

A three-stage measure was taken according to general psychological conditions of patients: 1) the establishment of a nurse-patient communication platform to assist patients in relieving tensions and fears (nurses are readily available to listen and respond to narrations of patients with a sincere attitude); 2) Assistance of patients in establishing a positive attitude towards the disease (nurses respect patients' beliefs, provide guidance, and meet the requirements of the patients); 3) provision of educational counseling to patients and caregivers (nurses explain the disease and the therapeutic process to patients and their caregivers).

2.5. Statistics

EpiData Software was used to establish a database. Statistical analysis was performed using SAS 8.0 and SPSS 13.0 software. Independent-sample t test and χ^2 test was used to compare the difference between groups.

3. Results

3.1. The Psycho-Educational Intervention Improves QOL of Patients with Advanced Lung Cancer Undergoing Chemotherapy

We used the one-scale method to measure QOT of cancer patients before and after they recieved the psycho-educational intervention [4]. The results showed that the physical function, the psychological function, and the social function were all significantly improved by the intervention (**Table 1**). Similarly, the scores for overall QOL were also increased (**Table 1**). In addition, common symptoms and adverse effects associated with chemotherapy that were included in the specific module domain such as nausea, vomiting, and fatigue were markedly reduced after the intervention (**Table 1**). Of note, scores for cough was also reduced, although whether this was due to the psycho-educational intervention remains to be determined.

3.2. QOL of Patients in the Intervention Group Is Significantly Improved Compared with Those in the Control Group

We also compared QOL of patients in the intervention group and those in the control group. As shown in **Table 2**, the scores of the physical function, the psychological function, and the social function for patients in the intervention groups were significantly higher than those in the control group. Consistently, the scores of overall QOL were also higher for patients in the intervention group. In contrast, the scores of common symptoms and side effects were lower for patients in the intervention group (**Table 2**). Taken together, these results suggest that the psycho-educational intervention improves the psychological, physical, and social function in patients with advanced lung cancer undergoing chemotherapy, and that it also lessen common symptoms and side effects associated with chemotherapy.

4. Discussion

To maintain high QOL is an important objective of treatment of patients with advanced cancer.

In this study, we have demonstrated that a purposely designed, nurse delivered psycho-educational intervention significantly improves QOL of patients with advanced lung cancer undergoing chemotherapy. This was not only revealed by the improved physical, psychological, and social function, and overall QOL scores, but was also

Table 1. Comparison of QOL of patients in the intervention group before and after the psycho-educational intervention[1].

Variables	Before the intervention		$\overline{X} \pm S$	After the intervention		$\overline{X} \pm S$	t	p[4]
	Min[2]	Max[3]		Min	max			
Physical function	13.00	34.00	22.03 ± 3.48	12.00	35.00	26.01 ± 3.52	4.347	0.026
Psychological function	21.00	55.00	37.49 ± 5.79	19.00	50.00	30.38 ± 6.03	10.034	0.002
Social function	15.00	28.00	21.07 ± 2.51	14.00	30.00	22.29 ± 2.74	1.049	0.549
Common symptoms and side effects	22.00	34.00	28.77 ± 2.08	23.00	34.00	28.06 ± 2.39	1.982	0.380
Specific module	25.00	37.00	30.92 ± 2.35	20.00	33.00	26.29 ± 2.61	6.168	0.019
Total quality of life scores	104.00	176.00	150.48 ± 15.41	115.00	193.00	170.23 ± 15.88	11.493	<0.000

[1]QOL was measured using the one scale method developed by Wan *et al.* [5];
[2]Minimal values; [3]Maximal values;
[4]χ^2 test was used to compare the difference between groups. A p value < 0.05 was considered statistically significant.

Table 2. Comparison of QOL of patients with advanced lung cancer undergoing chemotherapy with or without the psycho-educational intervention[1].

Variables	Intervention group			Control group			t	p[4]
	Min[2]	Max[3]	$\bar{X} \pm S$	min	max	$\bar{X} \pm S$		
Physical function	12.00	35.00	26.01 ± 3.52	10.00	33.00	22.47 ± 2.49	5.948	<0.01
Psychological function	19.00	50.00	30.38 ± 6.03	21.00	53.00	36.29 ± 7.19	6.034	<0.01
Social function	14.00	30.00	22.29 ± 2.74	10.00	25.00	17.87 ± 2.42	7.049	<0.01
Common symptoms and side effects	23.00	34.00	27.06 ± 2.39	25.00	38.00	31.88 ± 2.51	6.367	<0.01
Specific module	20.00	33.00	26.29 ± 2.61	22.00	38.00	30.43 ± 3.09	8.741	<0.01
The total quality of life scores	115.00	193.00	170.23 ± 15.88	103.00	168.00	142.47 ± 13.01	23.49	<0.01

[1]QOL was measured using the one scale method developed by Wan *et al.* [5];
[2]Minimal values; [3]Maximal values;
[4]χ^2 test was used to compare the difference between groups. A p value < 0.05 was considered statistically significant.

shown by reduced common symptoms and adverse effects associated with chemotherapy. Noticeably, scores for cough also appeared lower in patients after the psycho-educational intervention, but whether this was due to implementation of the intervention or other factors remains to be further clarified. Regardless, Results from this study suggest that nurses can play an important role in improving QOL of patients with advanced lung cancer who undergo chemotherapy by providing systemic psycho-educational interventions.

Although psychological interventions to improve QOL of lung cancer patients has received increasing attention in recent years, there have been only limited numbers of reports in the literature about QOL of lung cancer patients in China, where lung cancer is becoming the leading cause of cancer-related death [5]-[7]. This is conceivably related to the large population and relatively few psychologists specialized in the field of QOL of cancer patients in China. The results from this study showing that a psycho-educational intervention can be delivered by trained nurses to late-stage lung cancer patients undergoing chemotherapy have important practical implications, in that this is a highly feasible and cost-effective way that can be carried out in large scales independently of the availability of specialized psychologists. In addition, this approach can be readily adapted to the management of patients with other types of cancers who undergo systemic treatment.

5. Conclusion

Psycho-educational interventions delivered by nurses are a useful strategy to improve QOL of late-stage lung cancer patients undergoing chemotherapy, which are also conceivably applicable to patients with other types of advanced cancers.

Conflicts of Interest

The authors declare no conflict of interest.

References

[1] Chen, W., Zheng, R., Zeng, H. and Zhang, S. (2015) Epidemiology of Lung Cancer in China. *Thoracic Cancer*, **6**, 209-215. http://dx.doi.org/10.1111/1759-7714.12169

[2] Lemjabbar-Alaoui, H., Hassan, O., Yang, Y.W. and Buchanan, P. (2015) Lung Cancer: Biology and Treatment Options. *Biochimica et Biophysica Acta*, **1856**, 189-210. http://dx.doi.org/10.1016/j.bbcan.2015.08.002

[3] Gerber, D.E. and Schiller, J.H. (2013) Maintenance Chemotherapy for Advanced Non-Small-Cell Lung Cancer: New Life for an Old Idea. *Journal of Clinical Oncology*, **31**, 1009-1020. http://dx.doi.org/10.1200/JCO.2012.43.7459

[4] Wang, D. and Fu, J. (2014) Symptom Clusters and Quality of Life in China Patients with Lung Cancer Undergoing Chemotherapy. *African Health Sciences*, **14**, 49-55. http://dx.doi.org/10.4314/ahs.v14i1.8

[5] Wan, C., Zhang, C., Li, G., Shen, L., Luo, J., Yang, Z. and Meng, Q. (2007) Development and Psychometric Properties of the System of Quality of Life Instruments for Cancer Patients: Lung Cancer QLICP-LU. *Bulletin of Chinese Cancer*, **11**, 858-861

[6] Geater, S.L., Xu, C.R., Zhou, C., Hu, C.P., Feng, J., Lu, S., Huang, Y., Li, W., Hou, M., Shi, J.H., Lee, K.Y., Palmer,

M., Shi, Y., Lungershausen, J. and Wu, Y.L. (2015) Symptom and Quality of Life Improvement in LUX-Lung 6: An Open-Label Phase III Study of Afatinib Versus Cisplatin/Gemcitabine in Asian Patients With EGFR Mutation-Positive Advanced Non-small-cell Lung Cancer. *Journal of Thoracic Oncology*, **10**, 883-889. http://dx.doi.org/10.1097/JTO.0000000000000517

[7] Ma, Y., Yang, Y., Huang, Y., Zhao, H., Hou, X., Tian, Y., Zhao, Y., Xue, C., Fang, W., Wu, X., Hu, Z., Liang, W., Zhou, T., Qin, T. and Zhang, L. (2014) An Investigation of Symptom Burden and Quality of Life in Chinese Chemo-Naïve Advanced Lung Cancer Patients by Using the Instrument-Cloud QOL System. *Lung Cancer*, **84**, 301-306. http://dx.doi.org/10.1016/j.lungcan.2014.01.027

9

Individualism and Partnership: A Descriptive Qualitative Analysis of the Chronic Disease Phenomenon as Perceived by Older Adults

Elaine Amella[1], Martina Mueller[1], Jeannette Andrews[1], Joy Wachs[2], Kimberly Sell[2]

[1]Medical University of South Carolina, Charleston, USA
[2]East Tennessee State University, Johnson City, USA
Email: amellaej@musc.edu, muellermm@musc.edu, JANDREWS@mailbox.sc.edu, WACHS@mail.etsu.edu, sell@etsu.edu

Abstract

With the older adult population projected to increase substantially in the next 10 years, the incidence of chronic disease will become a significant factor in the burden of disease both globally and within the United States. The chronic disease state has been shown to decrease quality of life and the life expectancy of those individuals. In Tennessee the incidence of chronic disease, lower incomes, and education levels increases the risk of decreased quality of life and increased mortality in the older adult population. A review of literature by the researcher reveals that scant research has focused upon the older adult's perspective toward chronic illness and making changes to their health routine. As part of a mixed-method correlational study, focus groups used a descriptive qualitative approach to increase understanding of the phenomenon of chronic illness. The purpose of this qualitative study was to determine the attitudes and perceptions of older adults in East Tennessee towards behavior change and health maintenance in chronic disease.

Keywords

Qualitative, Chronic Disease, Older Adults

1. Introduction

Due to changes in medical care, the older adult population is living longer and the proportion of older adults will continue to grow until one in every five Americans will be over the age of 65 by the year 2050 [1]. While life expectancy is increasing, the number of chronic diseases also continues to grow necessitating further understanding of the chronic disease phenomenon as perceived by the older adult. The aim of this current study is to develop an understanding of the perceptions of older adults towards the chronic disease phenomenon using a descriptive qualitative method. This study is part of a mixed-method study in which 29 older adults from Northeast Tennessee participate in focus groups. The analysis of qualitative data revealed that older adults desired individualized care and wanted to be an active partner in the healthcare team. As the participants felt like this is a current gap in healthcare, knowledge of this desire by older adults can be beneficial to clinical approaches in chronic disease care.

1.1. Background

Chronic disease is a burden for all involved including the individual, family, healthcare provider, and healthcare systems. For individuals with chronic disease, there is a significant risk of premature death, prolonged disability, and an overall decreased quality of life [1] [2]. For those living with chronic disease, 25% have daily limitations [3]. For healthcare providers, the burden is to deliver care to complex patients with co-morbidities in a cost-effect manner. For example, for individuals with one chronic disease, the average number of physician visits is 13 times per year and this number increases drastically as the number of chronic diseases increases [4]. Healthcare systems struggle to find ways to efficaciously manage patients and control costs. Presently, for those with chronic disease 95% of healthcare costs are related to healthcare visits [1] and as a result of the increased numbers of older adults, by 2020 the cost will increase by 25% to a total of 903 billion spent on chronic disease care (CDC, 2013).

Not only are the prevalence and impact of disease changing, but also the inherent characteristics of the population are changing. The silent generations are those who have experienced the great depression and war [5]. These are individuals who, as a result of their experiences, learn to be conservative, frugal, and to focus on community instead of self [5]. For those born between 1946 and 1964, they have become the baby boomer generation. They are a unique generation that contrasts sharply in viewpoints from those generations before them. They have grown and developed during a period of an increased wealth, spending [6], and increased consumerism [6] which is a stark contrast to previous generations. The boomers are more likely to challenge processes, focus more on individuality than collectivism [6], and communicate opinions openly and unreservedly [5]. The baby boomers are a generation of consumers with high expectations and demands, and are less likely to accept physical changes as natural components of aging [6] but instead more likely to seek health interventions to address them. They are the generations who change the expectation of the career purpose from working to provide to one of working towards retirement [6]. As the previous generations are viewed as conformists, who are conservative, respectful of authority and the systems with which they interact [5], the baby boomer population displays significant contrasts through avid consumerism. This dissimilarity with past healthcare consumers results in a healthcare consumer who may very likely change the way that healthcare is delivered and therefore signals an imminent need to understand the perspective of the older adult population towards chronic disease and managing the chronic disease process.

1.2. Theoretical Framework

The Social Cognitive Theory is a theoretical framework that encompasses a broad spectrum of characteristics affecting the ability of individuals to change such as setting goals, identifying barriers, and beliefs [7]. This theory supports both internal and external factors for behavior change [8] and provides the structure for the focus group questions. The key concepts within the social cognitive theory are reciprocal determinism, outcome expectations, observational learning, incentive motivation, facilitation and moral disengagement [8]. The social cognitive theory also recognizes the impact that the environment can have on an individual as well as the effect the individual can have on the environment. Reciprocal determinism is the three-way (triadic) interaction among these variables [8] [9]. In this process, the individual, social factors, and the environment facilitate the type of reaction an individual may have in a given situation [9]. Understanding the process of reciprocal determinism in behavior change enhances understanding of potential barriers and social norms of learner self-management [8]. With the Social Cognitive Theory, the individual's expectations and perceptions of both the self-management process and disease status are addressed as well as environmental and social obstacles to changing health behaviors.

2. Method

A qualitative study using focus groups was completed as part of convergent-parallel mixed method study.

2.1. Study Design

The descriptive qualitative study was part of a larger mixed method study in which thematic analysis was used to correlate the quantitative data in a convergent-parallel design. The theoretical framework that was used for the study was the Social Cognitive Theory. Participants were recruited from area churches using parish nurses as community liaisons. Those participants were then given lunch and invited to participate in a focus group consisting of 5 - 8 individuals. The individual participated in a focus group at their home church. Prior to beginning the focus group, the participants were instructed about the purpose of the study and consent was obtained. Rules for the group interaction were reviewed before beginning the discussion. The focus group utilized 13 prepared questions (**Appendix 1**) and was conducted using a semi-structured format that allows for evolution of the conversation as the themes emerge [10]. These questions were derived from the concepts within the Social Cognitive Theory to obtain insights into the perception regarding behavior change, goal attainment, internal and external barriers to change.

The Krueger focus group methodology [11] was used to structure the interaction. The data collection process was completed within the one meeting to reduce burden and attrition of the participants. The interaction was recorded to verify field notes, and field notes were collected by a second member of the research team.

2.2. Sample

Qualitative analysis was completed as part of a mixed method study in which focus groups were held using purposive sampling [12] to collect data. Stratified purposive sampling was used in faith based organizations in the Appalachian Region of Northeast Tennessee to recruit older adults diagnosed with diseases reflective of the regional population where chronic disease ranks in the top six for mortality [13]. All individuals who were age 55 (or greater) and had been diagnosed with hypertension, Type 2 diabetes, or chronic obstructive pulmonary disease were included. If the individual had been hospitalized within 30 days prior to the study or non-English speaking, they were excluded. Individuals who had cognitive disorders were also excluded from the study. A total of 29 participants were eligible and enrolled in the study.

2.3. Ethical Consideration

The study received approval from the Internal Review Board (IRB) at the Medical University of South Carolina as well as the IRB from East Tennessee State University.

2.4. Data Collection

For data collection, 5 focus groups were held consisting of 5 - 8 participants. During the research study, the participant participated in a focus group to evaluate their perceptions of self-management in chronic disease, attitude to self-management and behavior change, as well as barriers and facilitators to the change process. For data collection, a semi-structured discussion format was utilized in the focus groups. The focus group setting allowed for conversation to evolve from multiple perspectives. Data saturation was achieved in each focus group and at that time the focus groups were ended.

2.5. Analysis

Once the focus groups concluded, the audio recordings were then transcribed verbatim and compared to the field notes. For qualitative data analysis, the six phase of thematic analysis [14] was used. Substantive coding was used to determined themes in relation to the chosen theoretical framework. The thematic analysis occurred in a sequential fashion with first the data being, transcribed, read, and then re-read by two investigators (KS, JW); once the data had been reviewed twice, the data set was coded and organized into potential themes as determined by the investigators (KS, JW); these themes were then organized into an table for analysis. In addition to theme analysis, coding was accomplished through the use of QRS NVivo 10 software [15]. In addition to coding for identification of prevalent themes [16], the analysis format also supported the purpose of data merging in the mixed method feasibility study [17].

2.6. Qualitative Rigor

The rigor of the thematic analysis is important in providing accurate and valid results in the qualitative analysis. The repetitive nature of thematic analysis provides richness to descriptions and a deeper understanding of each theme; the use of particular quotes from the focus group substantiate the findings relative to the research question [14].The use of selective coding allowed for identification of the over-arching themes related to perceptions and attitudes toward the chronic disease phenomenon. The use of several stages addressed reflexivity and recursiveness [14] [18]. Member checking was also used with several study participants further validating deducted themes [19].

There are four criteria to ensure trustworthiness of data: credibility, confirm ability, transferability, and dependability. Credibility was addressed during the focus group interview which took approximately 45 - 90 minutes to ensure prolonged engagement with the participants. The prolonged interaction was designed to build trust and to provide an opportunity to identify distortions created by the participants or researcher that could affect interpretation of the data [20]. Merging of quantitative and qualitative data achieved triangulation of data. For peer debriefing, the study investigator met with an experienced researcher who was not associated with the research study to ensure that integrity of the process was maintained. In addition, the number of individuals involved as well as data saturation was used to achieve credibility in the study.

Dependability refers to the consistency of results over time. The use of multiple focus groups and consistent protocol use addressed dependability [10]. Confirm ability ensures objectivity and removes bias from the process. In order to establish both of these criteria, the use of an audit trail was utilized [10] and documented the research process and provide documentation of each step during the study. The audit trail included documentation of data collection, analysis, coding, and memos utilized during the study, as well as consistent documentation in field notes. Transferability was addressed through the use of purposive sampling in order to provide sufficient information so that the data could possibly be taken and used with other cases [10].

During the research process, bias was addressed. The researcher clarified personal beliefs and internal biases [21]. The nature of qualitative research places the researcher within the lived experience so that subjective bias is present. To minimize the possibility of bias, prior identification of beliefs and biases should be determined to increase the principal investigator's awareness.

3. Results

A total of 33 individuals expressed interest in the study and 29 were included by established criteria. Of the 29 participants in the focus groups, 76% were female (n = 22), 90% white (n = 26), and 55% had completed high school. A majority had been diagnosed with hypertension (83%), followed by diabetes (31%), and COPD (14%). All participants had an average length of time since diagnosis of 10 years or greater (see **Table 1**).

Thematic Analysis

In reviewing the focus group interactions, two themes were most significant. Those themes were *individualization* and *partnership*. Individualization was seen in their perception of the disease experience; relationship with the healthcare provider; and interactions with the insurance health coach. Partnership was expressed as a desire to take more active role in healthcare decisions and increased their role as a team member. Something that at the time of the focus group, the participants felt was lacking in their care.

Perceptions of Chronic Disease

In each focus group, individuals were asked to describe how they felt about being diagnosed and how their lives had changes since diagnosis. Clearly, in the analysis of the themes, there were three distinct impressions that were consistent with diagnosis. These revealed three sub themes that supported the individuality of the disease phenomenon and how it is experienced. These sub-themes appeared to reflect the individual's perception of control in the disease process and awareness of the symptoms.

Hypertension

Those individuals who were diagnosed with hypertension expressed feelings associated with the most control over the disease process while at the same time expressing that the subtle symptoms allowed the individual to forget they had been diagnosed with hypertension.

Hypertension: Intangible

Table 1. Means and standard deviations for demographic variables.

Variable	N = number	Mean and Standard Deviation
Gender		
Male	7 (24%)	
Female	22 (76%)	
Race		
White	26 (90%)	
Native American or Alaskan Native	2 (6.8%	
Spanish Ethnicity	1 (3.4%)	
Age		M = 69.8 (SD ± 8.3)
Education		
Completed High School	N = 16 (55%)	
Completed College	N = 13 (45%)	
Marital Status		
Married	N = 19 (65.5%)	
Single/divorced	N = 6 (20.7%)	
Widow/Widower	N = 4 (13.8%)	
Diagnosis		
Hypertension	N = 24	
Years since diagnosis		M = 22 (SD ± 10.3)
Diabetes Mellitus	N = 9	
Years Since Diagnosis		M = 16 (SD ± 10.6)
COPD	N = 4	
Years Since Diagnosis		M = 10 (SD ± 13.49)
Number of medications per day		M = 4.97 (SD ± 2.54)
Average annual physician visits		M 3.07 (SD ± 2.14)
Time since last visit	1 - 3 months	
Health Rating		M = 3.13 (SD ± 0.63)
Very Good	N = 6 (8%)	
Good	N = 14 (55%)	
Fair	N = 3 (13.8%)	
Physiologic Data		
Blood Pressure		
SBP		M = 133 (±14.3)
DBP		M = 75 (±8.9)
Oxygen Saturation		M = 96.6 (±2.11)
HgbA1C (n = 7)		M = 7.0 (±0.59)
BMI		M = 30.35 (±8.32)
Shortness of Breath (n = 12)		M = 2.75 (±0.45)

"You really don't see symptoms and it is hard to remember to take your medications.", "Having hypertension doesn't really affect me.", "Forget you have it; I can do just about anything I want too.", "Until you (researcher) said it, I really had not thought about it as a chronic condition."

Hypertension is seen to have few symptoms, manageable by medications, and least disruptive to their lives. As the individuals indicated the diagnosis of hypertension was not seen to have many effects on the individual and the impact was that the disease was not seen as a chronic condition that could cause multiple serious complications.

Diabetes

The perception of the diagnosis of diabetes was expressed differently by those in the group. The presentation of the disease was swift and the chronicity of the disease is readily apparent. The individuals verbalize that there was a constant awareness of the disease presence and the need to make changes was always foremost in the mind of the individual.

Diabetes: Unforgettable

> It was a surprise, a shock, I was really anxious. You know I am going to have it forever. You are always aware. You have to make a lot of changes. It's not like you can forget you have it.

Most individuals in the focus groups expressed surprise at the suddenness and severity of the diabetes when initially diagnosed. The symptoms of the disease are prevalent and the care required was more disruption to their normal life pattern. But, the individuals were well versed in the disease process and felt that they had acquired sufficient knowledge to manage the disease.

With the diabetic, there was a consistent overshadowing of the possible complications.

> "It's scary when you blood sugar drops. It's scary for you and your family. Your blood sugar is 40 and 340 and you wonder am I going to be able to do this?"

As suggested by this individual, the presence of diabetes and the adverse effects promoted a feeling of uncertainty and constant vigilance to prevent complications.

COPD

Those diagnosed with chronic obstructive pulmonary disease expressed a loss of control and a feeling of helplessness in the care process. Symptoms of the disease are significant in presentation. The disease was seen as causing limitations on daily activities of life.

Chronic Obstructive Pulmonary Disease (COPD): Daily Limitation

> "It slows me down.", "You just have to do what you can do and leave the rest.", "My hypertension is controlled, but my COPD will never be controlled.", "I battle it, it is always on edge.", "I can't do things like I used too.", "It's not that you can't control it, you can with medications and I do pretty good", "If I am just sitting, I am fine …. I am perfect. But, if I try to do something then I get short of breath.", "If it's too cold, too hot, raining, … a lot affects it".

Those with COPD are acutely aware of the status of their breathing and confer significant restrictions on activities such as walking, exercising, and socialization. The perception was that it was well controlled as long as they could sit and not be short of breath and yet any normal daily activity was limited in that shortness of breath occurred with activation. With this disease, an attitude of acceptance toward what they saw as the inevitable outcome from an incurable disease, death.

> "What good would it do to quit smoking now? In what years I have left, I won't see any reversal in the disease if I quit now. I will be dead before the changes take place." "But, you know it is never going to get better, there's no cure."

There was a perceived helplessness in this group resulting from the understanding that the disease process was a continual downward progression and that maintaining the best control they can was the focus of management.

The phenomenon of the disease experience is individualized as seen in the focus group discussions. The disease experience varies from barely being aware of the diagnosis to being very limited in basic daily functioning causing a significant impact on quality of life.

In looking at the perception of chronic disease, an overarching theme of individuality reigns as each individual expresses the personalized impact the disease has on one's life.

Perceptions towards Making Health Behavior Changes

As the attitude toward the actual disease process varies, the analysis also demonstrated a variety of attitudes that varied by individual. Each focus group was asked to describe how they felt about making changes as a result of being diagnosed. These changes included diet and exercise as well as medication management. The responses discussed making changes, and also focused upon motivators and de-motivators of change.

> "I am just grateful they have medications for it." "At first I didn't make any changes, I was probably in denial.". "I want to lose weight." "If I lost forty pounds, I don't think I would have to take blood pressure medications.", "I have always been very active, so up until this point I have not had to exercise." "I try to be compliant, but there are things I am not compliant with like exercise. I just hate to exercise." "It's hard,

it's not like you can quit eating (diabetic)."

As the themes were further explored subcategories of themes were identified. Motivators for change could be further divided into *internal* and *external* foci that motivated change. A motivating internal focus for change focused on the rewards that an individual could receive if changes were successfully maintained and maintaining quality of life.

Internal Foci:

"Encouraged when you see the changes work (decreased weight, blood sugar, blood pressure).", "I like feeling good. I want a good quality of life. I don't want to be put into a nursing home.", "Seeing others having complications, I don't want to end up like that."

External foci:

"I want to be able to do things with my family.", "My husband is very active and I want to be able to keep up with him.", "My grandchildren, I want to be around to see them grow up.", "I want to be able to do things with my grandchildren.", "I want to be able to go to church. If I can't go to church, you might as well bury me.", "I want to see my grandchildren graduate, get married and have babies."

In this study, the older adult with chronic disease focused not only on longevity, but on quality of that longer life. Reasons expressed that encouraged the individuals to make change, centered on spousal/partner and the family interactions. Not only were the interactions important but the quality of those interactions were significant to the individuals and supporting the theme of each person having their own motivation for changing and should be seen as an individualized process. The individuals saw themselves as continually being an active participants in future relationships if successful health behavior change was to be made.

In changing behaviors, the emphasis on individualization was found when an individual was learning about or attempting change. Whether based on disease process or level of learning, individuals felt that being recognized as a person and not a disease was important.

Not only were the groups asked about current relationships, they were asked to visualize a situation in which they were required to change and to describe what format that they would most likely participate in. The types of social support that they preferred to help with change varied. The groups were asked about how they would be most likely to initiate a health behavior change and the methods of change varied among individuals as well:

"I couldn't keep up with a support group.", "It depends on the support group as to whether I would attend.", "I think coaching would be ok.", "Yea, having a coach would be good.", "I don't think I would like internet. I don't know much about the internet. I would have to look at it.", "I like to do things with (spouse), we do pretty good together.", "It makes it better to have someone to do it with.", "I've taken classes, but it is hard when you don't know anyone and if your late you are definitely not going to go in."

Each individual had different concerns and needs to be addressed in the health behavior change process. In making changes in behaviors to manage the chronic disease process, the individuals felt that family was most preferred while coaching was also of interest to them.

At the same time, the participants recognized that there were de-motivators for behavior change. The reasons for being unable to make behavior changes consistently varied and were based upon either physical limitations or psychosocial issues. Physical de-motivators tended to be consistent within the groups and reflected interference or impedance caused from pain or complications of another disease. The psychosocial barriers were related to loneliness and self-consciousness. These conversations took place using exercise and diet the behavioral changes needed for successful self-management.

While many understood that their disease management required them to incorporate exercise into the plan of care, many expressed a reluctance or inability to exercise.

"I have COPD, I can't exercise. I would like to lose weight, but I can't do those things.", "I can't because of my COPD. If it's humid, hot, or too cold, it makes my breathing worse.", "I can't because of my pain (arthritis).", "I hate to exercise, I just hate it. You get sweaty and have to change your clothes, makeup, hair… I just hate it. I know it works, but I am just as glad when it's over."

For those who participated in organized classes, lack of knowledge of other participants deterred participation.

"You know if you go to a class and you don't know anyone its hard or if you're late, you sure are not going to go in there."

The lack of rewards for maintaining the behavior change was also hindrance to behavior change.

"It's unfair I can exercise and do all the right things and I don't get the results that others do. It's frustrating.", "It would be easier if you saw some kind of reward." "Well it's hard because they keep changing the goal. You work to get our blood pressure down to where they want it and then they change it on you."

For dietary changes, psychosocial factors were prevalent from self-consciousness in not eating foods that were not on their diet or loneliness.

"It's hard eating for one.", "You can't cook for just one person. I don't sit at the table if it's just me. I just don't like to sit there by myself.", "I get self-conscious when I am eating with others...what if I offend someone by not eating what they have fixed. They don't understand I may not be able to have it. I just do the best I can, but I hate to offend them."

Psychosocial and physical barriers were prevalent in the conversations. These were all cited as reasons that would prevent an individual for initiating and maintaining an exercise routine or maintaining diet changes. A need to see improvement based upon the behavior change was measures in blood pressure, weight, or blood glucose values by the participants relative to their respective diseases. The individuals with COPD saw little opportunity to make changes based upon the limitations of their disease.

"I don't know what I could do to control it (COPD)."

In looking at each person's perception towards the disease process and behavior change, it is determined that each disease is inherently different in the impact on an individual's life.

Partnership with Healthcare Providers

Having established that individuality is important in the chronic disease process, another theme became prevalent during analysis. The person not only wants to be treated as an individual, but also as an equal member, a partner, in the care process. The relationship with the provider was seen as a support mechanism in which partnership was considered important and perceived lacking by the participants. As for the provider, the participants expressed trust and satisfaction with the level of knowledge of the provider, but greater dissatisfaction with the lack of time, lack of input into goal setting, and quality of the relationship.

The participants described the current relationship as one with parental overtones.

"He'll fuss. I don't want to be fussed at.", "He fussed at me the last time I was there too", "I lost weight and my blood pressure got low. So, I stopped taking my medicine, but I didn't tell my doctor.", "Mine fussed at me and I finally told him that when I got ready to talk about it (smoking) I would let him know. Otherwise he was not to bring it up again."

The participants are reluctant to engage the provider to avoid being treated as if they have done something wrong.

"I am heading him off today and presenting him with what I see as the plan."

A plan of action is seen as an appropriate mechanism for changing the healthcare providers' response to their visit. At the same time, the participants felt that there were other inhibitors to the interaction.

"Not like it used to be, they used to know you and your family.", "Time is limited to answer your questions.", "They only have so much time, who is going to answer your questions?", "I feel sorry for them because they have only a certain amount of time to spend with you, but it's their job to answer my questions.", "I trust him. He provides good care and is very knowledgeable.", "He should send me to someone who can answer my questions.", "I want someone, a coach, to teach me what I need to know.", "I want a partnership, I don't want to be fussed at.", "I am the one taking care of this every day.".

The care of the disease process is a team approach in which the individual is the center. The results of the analysis demonstrated that older adults want to work together with their provider, not be told what to do and not be "fussed at" as if a small child. The individuals wants input and to be heard in the decision making and care process recognizing that they will be the one actively addressing change.

The participants also expressed the need to have the opportunity to ask questions and to improve their knowledge about the disease process.

> "I am on this new medicine. They gave me a brochure and a DVD. That was all good, but who is going to answer my questions?", "I need someone who will teach me! What do I do if my blood sugar drops? I need to know what to do.", "When I was diagnosed they sent me home with insulin. Insulin! I didn't know anything about it, I just wanted to cry.", "I have diabetes, but I would like to lose weight. I know it's hard to and I told my doctor that I wanted to lose weight. He looked at me and said, 'well go ahead.' Now what kind of help is that?" "I need somebody, who will teach me what to do".

Acquiring knowledge seems to be lead predominately by those with diabetes who have an increased number of activities to complete to manage the disease process. Those with hypertension expressed interest in more education, while those who were diagnosed with COPD had no input into the conversation.

An unexpected finding in the conversation was revealed in the evolution of the discussion. Most participants voiced similar opinions towards the current status of health insurance and the use of what is being called "the health coach". The insurance health coach is someone who calls based upon screening of health documents. The content of the call can vary from individual to individual based upon the insurance companies chosen focus. The perception of the "health coaching" role in self-management was perceived negatively.

> "I am so angry (slams hand down on table).", "The insurance company is telling me what to do and if I don't… what are they going to do? Raise my premiums.", "They have this health coach call you and they ask you questions. It's not individualized, it's based upon your disease.". "Everybody treated the same.", "It's a waste of time, what are they going to tell me that I don't already know?" "The person is simply asking a question that is on the computer screen.", "I am not going to let the insurance company (health coach) get credit for what I am doing. I got my shot, and they check a box off and they get credit for me doing it.", "In some cases, I know more than they do. They can't even tell me why the insurance company flagged me.", "I asked a question and they tell me that they will have to find someone who can help me.", "they were at least trying to help me, but shouldn't someone know about my condition?", "I don't have time to sit there and chit chat. It makes you… I am sitting there smoking and I wouldn't be if they would get off there."

Individuals with chronic disease, expressed frustration over being required to participate in a process in which there appears to be no inherent benefit to them (other than keeping their premium down) and one in which they have no input. The insurance company's utilization of the "health coach" is perceived as a waste of time and of little benefit to the individual.

4. Discussion

Self-management is an important method of managing chronic disease, but over time self-management programs have not sustained lasting change. Most programs are group activities that may be beneficial for some, but as found in this qualitative study not all individuals may respond the same to behavior change intervention.

For those individuals participating in the study, two overall themes could be identified *individualism* and *partnership*. Each person described a unique experience with the chronic disease process and a preference for a treatment plan that was individualized to their needs. A person with chronic disease is still an individual and does not want to become simply the face of a specific disease. Partnership was a prevalent theme with the participants verbalizing the desire to take a more active role and have a voice in healthcare decisions. The clients desired to have the team work together to develop goals that not only addressed the disease, but allowed them to meet their own personal goals. The older adult recognized that ownership of the disease rests with them and that the services of the healthcare provider should be driven by the needs of the consumer.

For health behavior change to occur, an individual must participate in setting goals, while addressing barriers to change. In these focus groups, a desire to be treated as a member of the team and develop mutually agreeable goals seems to be at the forefront of concern. At present, as perceived by the participants, the locus of control in the self-management process is driven by healthcare providers and health policy (**Figure 1**), yet the older adult desires to have individualized relationship that is in partnership with the treatment team (**Figure 2**).

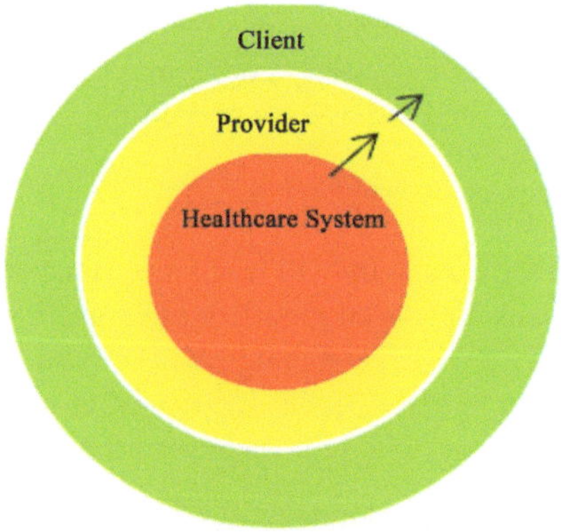

Figure 1. Locus of control in health management as perceived by adults.

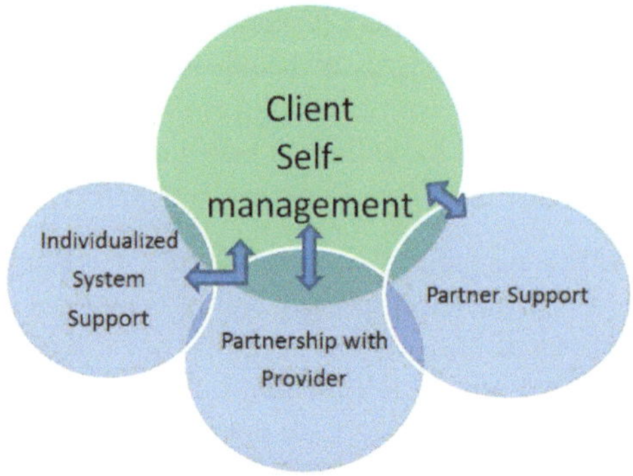

Figure 2. Older adult desired health management model.

They do not want to be told what to do… they want to be asked what they would like to do. In most aspects of life, an individual has the right of opinion, right to know, and autonomous decision making and yet in chronic disease management, healthcare is falling short of meeting the needs of the consumer. As seen in this study, many felt that their educational needs were not being met and expressed a desire for increased education and opportunities to ask their specific questions from someone knowledgeable in the disease process. **Figure 2** shows a self-management model in which the stakeholders in the process have an overlapping and reciprocal relationship. The client, provider, partner, and health entities work together with the central focus being the older adult and their desire for health behavior change.

Inclusion of social support was a subtheme of the focus group discussions and evolved around the important of social support systems. Spouses/significant other appeared to be most likely utilized as a support system in the change behavior process, but as the discussion evolved the healthcare provider and insurance support was highlighted. Little information was uncovered regarding the role of children in social support, but the role of spouses/significant other and close friends appears to influence an individual's attitude towards health behavior change. Of those couples that participated in the study, all verbalized strong spousal/significant other support with medication, diet, and exercise change. There was an overall feeling that having good spousal participation was beneficial while one individual shared a lack of spousal/significant other support and reflected on preferring a greater amount of support to be successful.

The barriers and motivators to health behavior change were also individualized as to what could help them be most successful in making health behavior change and also to help healthcare providers understand that non-adherence may not simply be a matter of refusal but may be motivated by physical or psychosocial barriers such as pain and loneliness. Many of the participants expressed an interest in making changes, yet could not in the face of barriers.

5. Limitation of Study

Sampling for the study used purposive sampling which limits generalizability of findings to the population. The focus groups were held in faith based organizations and most individuals already knew each other prior to participation. The composition of the focus group could have altered responses to socially appropriate answers. In addition, the severity of illness and number of chronic diseases diagnosed could also have impacted the individual response.

6. Conclusion

Results of this qualitative descriptive study indicate that there is a disconnect between the perceptions of the older adult towards chronic disease care and behavior change in comparison to what is presently being experienced in healthcare interactions. This disconnect suggests that further research regarding healthcare providers' attitudes towards the older adults' role in chronic disease care should be explored. The preference for older adults to include spouses in the change process or immediate family suggests that developing a plan that includes this support system may be beneficial. The themes of individualization and partnership suggest that a method of health behavior change that addresses these two main concerns should be explored to enhance the older adult's satisfaction and success in chronic disease care. Understanding the perceptions of the older adult towards the chronic disease phenomenon can provide healthcare providers with insight that can be valuable in providing specific care to this unique population.

References

[1] Centers for Disease Control and Prevention (2013) The State of Aging & Health in America. C.f.D. Control, Editor, US Department of Health and Human Services, Atlanta.

[2] Whittemore, R. and Dixon, J. (2008) Chronic Illness: The Process of Integration. *Journal of Clinical Nursing*, **17**, 177-187. http://dx.doi.org/10.1111/j.1365-2702.2007.02244.x

[3] Centers for Disease Control (2009) Chronic Disease: The Power to Prevent, the Call to Control. U.S.D.o.H.a.H. Resources, Editor, Atlanta.

[4] Centers for Medicare and Medicaid Services (2010) National Expenditure Projections 2010-2020: Forecast Summary. Centers for Medicare and Medicaid Services, Woodlawn.

[5] Dunn-Cane, K., Gonzalez, J. and Stewart, H. (1999) Managing the New Generation. *American Journal of Operating Room Nurses*, **69**, 930-940. http://dx.doi.org/10.1016/S0001-2092(06)62292-8

[6] Phillipson, C., *et al*. (2008) Social and Cultural Constructions of Ageing: The Case of the Baby Boomers. *Sociological Research Online*, **13**, 5. http://dx.doi.org/10.5153/sro.1695

[7] Bandura, A. (2004) Health Promotion by Social Cognitive Means. *Health Education & Behavior*, **31**, 143-164. http://dx.doi.org/10.1177/1090198104263660

[8] Glanz, K., Rimer, B.K. and Viswanath, K., Eds. (2008) Health Behavior and Education. 4th Edition, Jossey-Bass, San Francisco.

[9] Bandura, A. (1986) Social Foundation of Thoughts and Action: A Social Cognitive Theory. Prentice-Hall, Inc., Upper Saddle River.

[10] Polit, D.F. and Beck, C.T. (2012) Nursing Research: Generating and Assessing Evidence for Nursing Practice. 9th Edition, Lippincott, Williams & Wilkins, Philadelphia.

[11] Krueger, R.A. (2009) Focus Groups: A Practical Guide for Applied Research. Sage Publications, Thousand Oaks.

[12] Sandelowski, M. (2000) Combining Qualitative and Quantitative Sampling, Data Collection, and Analysis Techniques in Mixed-Method Studies. *Research in Nursing & Health*, **23**, 246-255. http://dx.doi.org/10.1002/1098-240X(200006)23:3<246::AID-NUR9>3.0.CO;2-H

[13] Tennessee Department of Health (2008) Tennessee Deaths 2007.

[14] Braun, V. and Clarke, V. (2006) Using Thematic Analysis in Psychology. *Qualitative Research in Psychology*, **3**, 77-101. http://dx.doi.org/10.1191/1478088706qp063oa

[15] QRS International (2012) NVivo. http://www.qsrinternational.com/products.aspx

[16] Sandelowski, M. and Leeman, J. (2012) Writing Usable Qualitative Health Research Findings. *Qualitative Health Research*, **22**, 1404-1413. http://dx.doi.org/10.1177/1049732312450368

[17] Plano Clark, V.L. and Creswell, J.W. (2008) The Mixed Methods Reader. Sage Publications, Thousand Oaks.

[18] Fereday, J. and Muir-Cochrane, E. (2006) Demonstrating Rigor Using Thematic Analysis: A Hybrid Approach of Inductive and Deductive Coding and Theme Development. *International Journal of Qualitative Methods*, **5**, 80-92.

[19] Creswell, J.W. and Plano Clark, V.L. (2011) Designing and Conducting Mixed Methods Research. 2nd Edition, Sage Publications, Los Angeles.

[20] Lincoln, Y. and Guba, E. (1985) Naturalistic Inquiry. Sage Publications, Newbury Park.

[21] Specialze, H.J. and Carpenter, D.R. (2007) Qualitative Research in Nursing. 4th Edition, Lippincott, Williams & Wilkin, Philadelphia.

Appendix 1

Focus Group Questions

1. **Each one of you has been diagnosed with a chronic illness such as hypertension, Chronic Obstructive Pulmonary Disease, or Diabetes. When you think about what has happened since you were diagnosed, can you tell me….**
   What is it like living with (COPD, HTN, DM)?

2. **When you were diagnosed you were asked to make changes so that you could better control you illness. Can you describe…………….**
   How do you take care of your (COPD, HTN, DM)?

3. **When you think about what has happened since you diagnosis, can you tell me…..**
   a. What changes have you had to make in your everyday life since diagnosed with (COPD, HTN, DM)?

   You have described some changes…….
   b. How do you feel about those changes that you had to make?

4. **What things could you do better to manage your (COPD, HTN, DM)?**

5. **In looking at your health and diagnosis,**
   What keeps you from managing these better?

6. **When you think about your health,**
   What are you doing well in managing your (COPD, HTN, DM)?
   How do you feel about the things that you still need to change?

7. **In looking at having a chronic illness…….**
   What motivates you to make change and manage your (COPD, HTN, DM)?

8. **In order to take care of yourself and manage your illness, …..**
   a. can you tell me how you feel about setting goals? Do you?

9. **If you do set goals or thought about setting goals, describe…………**
   b. How do think that you setting goals would or does impact managing your illness?
   c. Can you give me an example of goals you set?

10. **Thinking about the things that you have been asked to do related to taking care of yourself and your illness,**
    What could you use more help with in managing your illness?
    In managing your illness, it is important to have support.
    Can you describe the support that you have with taking care of your illness?
    Who could help you more with managing your illness? (family, friends, nurse, doctor)

11. **In thinking about improving the support you get, ……………………………**
    How do you feel that they could give you more support?

12. **If the amount of support you had improved, …………………………………..**
    What might be some benefits to you with getting more support to manage your illness?

13. **There are different ways to offer support for your illness from a healthcare provider,**
    Can you describe………………..
    How do you feel about the different ways of support to manage your illness and make change such as groups, (support) internet, (information or education modules) and working with a health coach? (one on one meeting)

10

Developing a Scale for Measuring Uncertainty in Patients with Unruptured Intracranial Aneurysms Undergoing Endovascular Coiling

Mitsumi Masuda[1], Hidenori Ohishi[2], Noriko Terunuma[3], Ikuko Tojima[3]

[1]Department of Critical Care Nursing, Graduate School of Nursing, Kitasato University, Tokyo, Japan
[2]Department of Medical Science, Graduate School of Medicine, Juntendo University, Tokyo, Japan
[3]Nursing Department, Juntento University Hospital, Tokyo, Japan
Email: mitsumi_0323@yahoo.co.jp, ohishi@juntendo.ac.jp, terunuma@juntendo.ac.jp, itojima@juntendo.ac.jp

Abstract

A measure called the Uncertainty in Unruptured Intracranial Aneurysm Patients Undergoing Endovascular Coiling Scale (UUIACS) was developed and its validity and reliability were examined. The 49 questions that comprised the original draft of the UUIACS were created based on interview data. Based on data from 172 participants, exploratory and confirmatory factor analyses were conducted. As a result of exploratory factor analysis, the UUIACS e retained 17 items and extracted four factors ("Lack of decision-making cues", "Lack of information and complexity of information interpretation", "The ambiguous nature of the disease", and "The unpredictable living with UIA"). All of the UUIACS items showed adequate internal consistency. Between the UUIAC scale and the Universal Uncertainty in Illness Scale (UUIS), the Health Locus of Control (HLC) scale, and the SF-36v2® (Japanese version), positive correlations were found between the UUIACS and UUIS, and the HLC scale at a 1% significance level indicating concurrent validity. According to confirmatory factor analysis, the UUIACS had an acceptable goodness of fit. Given these findings, the UUIACS was judged to have satisfied the criteria for use in a clinical setting, although further investigation was required.

Keywords

Unruptured Intracranial Aneurysms, Endovascular Coiling, Uncertainty Scale

1. Introduction

Given the increased use of brain scans, cranial MRA/3D-CTA, and other minimally-invasive diagnostic imaging techniques, there has been a sharp increase in patients unexpectedly diagnosed with unruptured intracranial aneurysms (UIA) [1]. In Japan, more than 10,000 individuals a year receive this diagnosis. A UIA can lead to a subarachnoid hemorrhage, for which the fatality rate is extremely high; therefore, it has been recommended that patients meeting the accepted criteria for medical treatment, receive preventative surgery (neurosurgical clipping or cerebral endovascular coiling treatment), with the aim of preventing a rupture [2] [3].

When a UIA is detected, people face an uncertain situation. Beginning from the time before the development of symptoms, an individual is aware of the potential dangers of this illness. People who are asymptomatic and have been diagnosed with a UIA unexpectedly, become aware of its existence with inadequate psychological preparation, and consequently start to show an increase in uncertainty [4] [5], a decline in their quality of life (QOL) [6], and a deterioration in their mental health [7]. Furthermore, people who are currently healthy have difficulty making decisions about treatment for a UIA, such as choosing whether to undergo preventative medical care and choosing among the options of neurosurgical clipping, neurosurgical endovascular coiling, and active observation. A fairly large number of endovascular surgery patients have problems with imperfect closure and recanalization, requiring surgical correction [8] [9]. The results of prior studies [10] suggest that from their first diagnosis until their recovery from treatment, patients undergoing endovascular surgery to correct a UIA may experience emotional distress, such as anxiety and conflict linked to their recognition of uncertainties, such as the ambiguity of late-stage impairment and inadequate dissemination of information about new treatments. Therefore, it is important to assess in detail and with accuracy, the degree of uncertainty that patients with a UIA are aware of over the course of their treatment and recuperation, and to offer assistance aimed at mitigating or removing this uncertainty.

Despite the development of a Japanese version [11] of the Mishel Uncertainty in Illness Scale-Community Form (MUIS-C) [12], which measures uncertainty in illness, and the Universal Uncertainty in Illness Scale to be used for Inpatients and Outpatients (UUIS) [13], a similar measure that can be used regardless of the treatment setting. These linear scales do not reflect this illness's particular discomfort or specific conditions.

Therefore, this study focuses on the general idea of uncertainty concerning the subjective interpretations of responses to illness and medical treatment. A scale is also developed to measure the uncertainty that affects patients who have undergone endovascular surgery to treat a UIA, and to assess the scale's validity and reliability.

Definition of Uncertainty

The definition of uncertainty in this study is based on Mishel's definition as "the inability to determine the meaning of illness-related events…, the cognitive state created when the person cannot adequately structure or categorize an event because of the lack of sufficient cues" [14].

2. Methodology

The name of the measure being developed and evaluated is the Uncertainty in Unruptured Intracranial Aneurysm Patients Undergoing Endovascular Coiling Scale (henceforth referred to as the UUIACS).

2.1. Initial Development of the UUIACS

An item pool was compiled with passages describing uncertainty, which had been excerpted from interview data of 31 patients diagnosed with UIA at the Department of Neurosurgery at Metropolitan A University Hospital. The interviewed patients had no previous experience of surgery related to intracranial aneurysms, and were undergoing endovascular coiling for the first time. Questions were developed using existing scales that measure uncertainty: the Mishel Uncertainty in Illness Scale-Community Form (MUIS-A) [15], the MUIS-C Japanese edition [11], and the UUIS [13].

Next, similar and overlapping content were clustered, and 52 questions were developed. The questions were classified based on their meaning and organized into 6 categories: 1) Nature of the disease; 2) The treatment characteristics; 3) Information; 4) Decision making; 5) Course of the future; and 6) Living with UIA [16].

The 52 questions were checked by another researcher, two doctors, two nurses, and four patients who previously underwent endovascular coiling to ensure that the expressions used were appropriate; some revisions were made. The questionnaire consisted of 52 items each with five response options (strongly disagree, disagree, undecided, agree, strongly agree) rated on a scale of 1 - 5 points. Pilot tests were conducted with 50 UIA patients. The analysis found that two questions had a ceiling effect (percentage of patients who scored at the ceiling level—that corresponded to 10% best results on the scale), and one had a floor effect (percentage of patients who scored at floor level—equivalent to the 10% worst results on the scale); these items were eliminated, leaving the questionnaire with 49 questions. Additionally, a final analysis was performed to confirm the internal consistency and wording of the scale. In the end, the original draft of the UUIACS had 6 categories and 49 questions.

2.2. Developing the UUIAS-C and Analyzing Its Validity and Reliability

The survey portion of the UUIACS was distributed to develop it and analyze its validity and reliability. Exploratory factor analysis, internal consistency, validity testing, and confirmatory factor analysis were performed on the survey.

2.3. Participants

2.3.1. Target Group

The survey was administered at two different institutions to convenience samples of UIA patients who underwent neurosurgery and endovascular coiling as part of their treatment. The candidates in the target group were patients who were undergoing endovascular coiling for the first time and had consented to participate in the study.

2.3.2. Participants' Characteristics

Patients' gender, age, smoking behavior, family composition, medical history, and other patient attributes were surveyed via medical examination and patient interviews. The first author performed structured interviews. The content of the question included smoking behavior, family composition, medical history, and circumstances of discovery.

2.4. Measures

2.4.1. Uncertainty

The original draft of the UUIACS consisted of 6 categories and 49 questions, with responses on a 5-point scale (strongly disagree, disagree, undecided, agree, strongly agree) ranging from 1 - 5 respectively. The total and subscale scores were calculated by simply summing the scores, a higher score indicated a higher degree of uncertainty experienced.

2.4.2. Scales Used for Assessing Criterion-Related Validity

1) Universal Uncertainty in Illness Scale (UUIS)

The UUIS, developed by [13] to measure uncertainty, is a linear scale composed of 26 items and 6 subscales. The scale can be used regardless of whether the medical treatment is administered on an inpatient or outpatient basis, and it better reflects how Japanese patients experience uncertainty in relation to their illness. A higher score indicates a higher level of uncertainty.

2) Health Locus of Control Scale (HLC Scale)

The HLC scale [17] measures subjective feelings of control over one's health. Health Locus of Control focuses on whether or not one believes that there is a cause associated with an event resulting from one's own behavior related to health and illness, and whether one believes that one had control over its cause. Questions 26-30 clearly relate to uncertainty [18] [19]. The scores for the HLC Scale range from 11 to 33 points, with a higher score indicating stronger subjective feelings of control over one's health.

3) Short Form-36v2® Health Survey-Japanese Version (SF-36v2®)

The SF-36v2® survey [20] [21], which measures health-related quality of life, SF-36v2®, consists of items related to physical functioning, everyday role functioning (physical), bodily pain, overall health, vitality, social functioning, everyday role functioning (mental), and eight subscales measuring mental health. The score is converted to a 0-100-point scale, and a higher score indicates a higher quality of life.

2.5. Survey Method

A questionnaire survey method was used. The researchers explained the intent of the survey and any ethical considerations to the patients. After obtaining informed consent, the questionnaires were distributed and the participants' responses were requested. The responses were collected on the same day, or they were returned by mail. The data collection was conducted from July 2013 to March 2014.

2.6. Data Analyses Methods

The following analyses were performed using statistics software SPSS 21.0J and Amos 22.0J. Item analysis was used to examine ceiling and floor effects and item-total correlations. Construct validity was tested by comparing the 6 categories that were developed when composing the original draft with the factors that were extracted from exploratory factor analysis. Criterion-related validity was tested by analyzing the correlation coefficients using UUIS, the HLC scale, and the Japanese version of the SF36v2®. Internal consistency was assessed by calculating Cronbach's alpha coefficients for the entire scale and each subscale. The model's degree of conformance was examined using confirmatory factor analysis, which was performed on the latent variables that included the items of the UUIACS that were selected as factors as a result of exploratory factor analysis. The UUIACS model's degree of conformance was tested using the goodness of fit index (GFI), degree-of-freedom adjusted goodness of fit index (AGFI), comparative fit indicator (CFI), and root mean square error of approximation (RMSEA).

2.7. Ethical Considerations

This study was conducted with the approval of the medical ethics committees of the institutions that implemented the survey in June 2013. The participants gave their consent after the study's intent was explained to them. At that time, the freedom of the participants to withdraw from the study and the protection of their anonymity were explained verbally and in writing, after which signatures were obtained indicating their consent. Their responses to the questionnaire were collected on the same day, and when this was not possible, the questionnaire was taken home and returned by mail.

3. Results

3.1. Clinical Research Settings and Data Collection Procedures

A request for cooperation was made to two institutions, both of which agreed. Questionnaires were distributed to 201 participants and 173 were retrieved (68.1% return rate); 10 of the returned questionnaires had missing responses; 9 of them were missing fewer than 10% of the total responses. Therefore, the total score was adjusted to reflect the average of the UUIACS, UUIS, HLC scale, and SF-36v2® (Japanese version). One of the returned questionnaires was missing more than 10% of the total responses and was eliminated from the study. Valid responses from 172 patients were used in the analysis of the data (response rate: 99.4%).

3.2. Participants

As shown in **Table 1**, the participants consisted of 54 men and 118 women, with an average age of 62.3 (SD = 10.9); 44 participants had a family history of subarachnoid haemorrhage and 128 did not; 55 were smokers, and 117 were not.

3.3. Item Analysis

The item-total correlations ranged from 0.22 to 0.64; none of the questions had a correlation coefficient below 0.2; therefore, none of them were trimmed. Descriptive statistics were calculated and 15 questions were eliminated: 8 questions had ceiling effects (e.g. "I do not know the cause of my intracranial aneurysm") and 7 questions had floor effects (e.g. "I have not decided whether to continue medical examination going forward").

3.4. Factors Selected through Exploratory Factor Analysis

Exploratory factor analysis using promax rotation, was conducted on 34 questions (after eliminating 15 questions) (**Table 2**). A scree plot using principal component analysis showed that there were 4 factors, and after

Table 1. Demographic characteristics of participants (n = 172).

		Number	Proportion (%)
Age	Mean ± SD	62.3 ± 10.9	
Sex	Male	54	31.4
	Female	118	68.6
Employed	Yes	99	57.6
	No	73	42.4
High blood pressure	Yes	82	47.7
	No	90	52.3
Smoker	Yes	55	32.0
	No	117	68.0
Drinks alcohol	Yes	62	36.0
	No	110	64.0
Family history	Yes	44	25.6
	No	128	74.4
Circumstances of discovery	Screening for UIA	123	71.5
	Symptoms	49	28.5
Size[a]	Mean ± SD	4.9 ± 2.1	
	5 mm or more	69	40.1
	Less than 5 mm	103	59.9

[a]Alternate option for UIA size was >5 mm.

eliminating questions with a factor loading of less than 0.4, as shown in **Table 2**, 4 factors and 17 questions achieved a valid factor structure and were extracted for use in the UUIACS. The cumulative contribution ratio before rotation was 45.85%, and the Spearman's correlations between the four factors ranged from 0.36 - 0.60, all of them having significant positive correlations.

3.5. Subscale Naming

The contents of the items selected for each of the four extracted factors were interpreted. The first factor (6 items) pertained to uncertainty concerning the complexity of decision making (e.g. "I do not know which to choose, endovascular surgery or craniotomy" and "I do not know whether it is good that the unruptured intracranial aneurysm was detected"). This factor was named "Lack of decision-making cues". The second factor (5 items) pertained to uncertainty about the lack of information and the interpretation of information (e.g. "I feel like the more I learn about my illness and treatment, the less I understand and the more questions mount up" and "I do not know what other people with the same illness may be experiencing"). This factor was named "Lack of information, complexity of information interpretation". The third factor (3 items) pertained to uncertainty about the inability to specify the nature of the illness, as it was discovered at an asymptomatic stage before a rupture (e.g. "I do not know whether or not an unruptured intracranial aneurysm is an illness"). This factor was named "The ambiguous nature of the disease". The fourth factor (3 items) pertained to uncertainty about living with a UIA because it is a relatively recent illness (e.g. "Unruptured intracranial aneurysm is an illness with which I am not very familiar"). This factor was named "The unpredictable living with UIA".

3.6. Assessment of Reliability (Internal Consistency)

Cronbach's alpha for the overall UUIACS (17 questions) was 0.84, and for each of the four factors, it ranged from 0.61 - 0.82 (**Table 2**).

3.7. Assessment of Validity

3.7.1. Assessment of Construct Validity

The items that fell under the four factors extracted through exploratory factor analysis (1) "Lack of decision-

Table 2. Major factor analysis of UUIACS.

Factor[a] <Naming of subscale>	New No	Items of UUIACS	Factor loadings: 1st factor	2nd factor	3rd factor	4th factor	Communality	Cronbach's alpha coefficient
1st factor	A1	26 I don't know which to choose, endovascular surgery or craniotomy	0.80	0.11	0.06	-0.10	0.7	
<Luck of decision-making cues>	A2	24 I don't understand the degree of the risk of UIA	0.75	0.00	-0.04	0.06	0.58	
	A3	25 If I take the treatment, I may not be cured completely	0.65	0.12	-0.09	-0.04	0.44	0.82
	A4	12 If I don't choose the treatment, I will continue to take the angiography and MRA	0.64	−0.12	0.03	0.01	0.37	
	A5	29 I don't know whether it's good that the UIA was detected	0.51	−0.10	−0.07	0.31	0.37	
	A6	27 I'm not sure if a preventive craniotomy is necessary	0.45	0.00	0.19	0.10	0.35	
2nd factor	A7	33 I don't know the angiography is necessary	0.03	0.78	−0.07	0.11	0.68	
<Luck of information and complexity of information interpretation>	A8	18 The more I know about UIA and the treatment the more questions I have	0.00	0.64	−0.16	−0.12	0.28	
	A9	15 The explanation of medical professionals don't go down with me	−0.02	0.58	0.01	0.07	0.39	0.70
	A10	34 I don't know whether I should continue to take the angiography and MRA	0.04	0.52	0.17	−0.40	0.28	
	A11	20 I don't know the experience of others	−0.07	0.44	0.04	0.36	0.49	
3rd factor	A12	9 I don't know wheter it's good or not that I don't have any subjective symptoms	−0.05	−0.60	0.99	−0.09	0.84	
<The ambiguous nature of the disease>	A13	8 I don't understand what exactly UIA is	0.03	−0.15	0.73	0.12	0.52	0.74
	A14	10 I don't know if UIA is even a disease	0.07	0.24	0.40	−0.07	0.32	
4th factor	A15	21 UIA is an unfamiliar disease	0.05	0.00	0.16	0.62	0.53	
<The unpredictabiliy living with UIA>	A16	22 I don't know what my actions might be increasing the risk of rupture	−0.09	0.27	0.09	0.57	0.60	0.61
	A17	16 I don't know how interprete the explanation of madical professionals	0.10	−0.18	−0.12	0.52	0.21	
		Loading sum of square after rotation	3.52	2.16	2.42	2.68		0.84[c]
		Correlation between factors[b] 1st factor	1					
		2nd factor	0.32	1				
		3rd factor	0.42	0.54	1			
		4th factor	0.58	0.26	0.4	1		

[¥]: see materials and methods, Table 1. [dw]: values were calculated on dry weight basis, [a,b,c,...]: Means with the same letter in the same raw into each parameter are not significantly different ($p > 0.05$), [A,B,C,...]: Means with the same letter in the same column are not significantly different ($p > 0.05$).

making cues"; 2) "Lack of information, complexity of information interpretation"; 3) "The ambiguous nature of the disease"; and 4) "The unpredictable living with UIA") were compared with the items that were classified under the six categories derived from the content analysis when creating the original draft of the questionnaire 1) "Nature of the disease"; 2) "The treatment characteristics"; 3) "Information"; 4) "Decision making"; 5) "Course of disease"; and 6) "Living with a UIA"). The results showed that the factor, "Lack of decision-making cues" consisted of the same items as categories 2) and 4). "Lack of information, complexity of information interpretation" consisted of the same items as category 3). "The ambiguous nature of the disease" consisted of the same items as category 1) and "The unpredictable living with UIA" consisted of the same items as categories 5) and 6).

3.7.2. Assessment of Criterion-Related Validity

To assess criterion-related validity, Spearman's correlations were calculated between the total UUIACS score, and the scores on the UUIS, HLC scale, and the SF-36c2® Japanese edition. As shown in **Table 3**, the analyses yielded a positive correlation of $r = 0.65$ with UUIS, and a negative correlation of $r = -0.25$ with the HLC scale, that was significant at the 0.01 level. A problem remained with the SF-36v2® (Japanese version), which had a negligible correlation of $r = -0.14$.

3.8. Examination of the Model's Goodness of Fit

The goodness of fit of the hypothetical model obtained through exploratory factor analysis was assessed through confirmatory factor analysis. If the four factors are treated as latent variables, this should result in a GFI of 0.90 and an AGFI of 0.85, satisfying the goodness of fit criteria of a GFI of 0.9 or above, an AGFI of 0.85 or above, with the GFI greater than the AGFI. The GFI of 0.92 in this study, satisfied the criterion that the GFI should be above 0.9, and the RMSEA of 0.07 satisfied the criterion of 0.08. Between the latent variables and the observed variables, as shown in **Figure 1**, all of the items achieved a valid path coefficient of 0.50 or above.

4. Discussion

This study attempted to develop a scale to measure the uncertainty that affects patients undergoing endovascular surgery for a UIA, focusing on uncertainty as a general concept concerning the subjective interpretation of illness and treatment. The result was the creation of the UUIACS, composed of 17 items and 4 subscales.

4.1. The Reliability and Validity of the UUIACS

Regarding the reliability of the UUIACS, Cronbach's alpha for the overall scale (17 questions) was 0.84, and ranged from 0.61 to 0.82 for each of the four subscales. Factors 1-3 exceeded 0.7. Only the fourth factor, at 0.61, fell below the criterion of 0.7. This finding could be caused by fewer questions. However, the Cronbach's alpha of 0.84 for the overall scale exceeded the criterion; therefore, it can be considered a generally reliable measure.

The scale's content validity was conducted the experts panel, criterion-related validity was tested by analyzing the correlation coefficients using UUIS, the HLC scale, and the Japanese version of the SF36v2®, and construct validity were examined by comparing 6 categories of the original draft from exploratory factor analysis. Content validity was examined during the creation of the original UUIACS draft, with consideration of whether or not the instrument had been adequately conceptualized to encompass the entire field, as understood from the literature review conducted as part of a qualitative study. The items of the UUIACS inquire about the uncertain-

Table 3. Criterion-related validity (n = 172).

Scale	Spearman's correlation coefficients			
	UUIACS total score	UUIS	HLC scale	SF-36v2®
UUIACS total score	-			
UUIS	0.65**	-		
HLC scale	−0.25**	−0.15*	-	
SF-36v2®	−0.14	−0.06	0.17*	-

**$p < 0.01$, *$p < 0.05$.

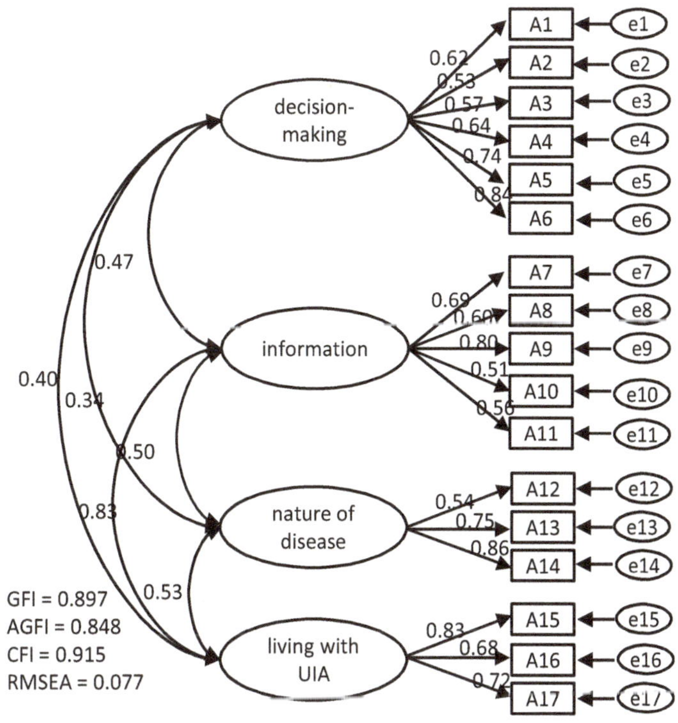

Figure 1. Test of goodness of fit.

ty of patients who undergo endovascular coiling for an UIA. The scale is not only for specialists who have received university degrees and are conversant in the development of linear scales; it also is of practical value for obtaining opinions from doctors and nurses who examine and treat large numbers of UIA patients, as well as the UIA patients who experience this type of uncertainty.

Regarding the scale's criterion-related validity, a strong positive correlation was observed between the total UUIACS score and the UUIS score. A significant negative correlation, although weak, was observed with the HLC scale score, confirming a degree of concurrent validity. However, there remains the issue of revising the scale because of the lack of a correlation with the SF-36v2® (Japanese version) and this issue will influence the future studies that are conducted.

In terms of the scale's construct validity, the 6 categories that were extracted through content analysis by the researchers during the original drafting stage of the UUIACS had an almost identical structure to the four factors that were extracted through exploratory factor analysis. Before rotation, the four factors' cumulative contribution ratio was 45.85%. Consequently, the UUIACS can be considered to have construct-related validity. Based on this finding, we can that the UUIACS is a scale with adequate validity and reliability, and may be used in clinical settings because it satisfied the criteria for the model's goodness of fit through confirmatory factor analysis.

4.2. Significance of the UUIACS's Characteristics and Development

The UUIACS, a linear scale measuring uncertainty, consists of 17 items in 4 subscales. The significance and characteristics of this scale can be discussed in comparison with the MUIS, which has been used around the world and with the UUIS, which was developed in Japan.

Mishel's scale was developed using American patient data (Mishel 1981) [15]. However, the UUIACS was based on Japanese patient data, so it might be a more accurate measure of how uncertainty is recognized by patients with a Japanese cultural background. Furthermore, the UUIS, has overcome problems with mis-translations and word nuances that affected the use of Mishel's scale [15] with Japanese people. It can be used regardless of treatment site, whether a patient is hospitalized or recuperating at home on an outpatient basis, so it is particularly useful for measuring uncertainty on an ongoing basis. The UUIACS was developed based on a longitudinal qualitative study, and reflects the specific phenomenon of UIA patients undergoing endovascular coiling; therefore, it can be used continuously, as a measure that is highly relevant to this medical specialty. For this reason, there is a greater chance of acquiring a better understanding of the characteristics and changes of patients with this illness.

Moreover, the MUIS and UUIS measure the uncertainty recognized by patients while they are ill. However, UIA patients often express that "it is unclear whether an unruptured intracranial aneurysm is an illness", as the UIA is discovered at an asymptomatic stage; hence, this creates a key discrepancy between the MUIS and UUIS, which assume that the respondent must be experiencing the illness. Furthermore, UIA is a relatively new illness, and endovascular surgery is a relatively new treatment. Although making decisions regarding medical treatment is extremely difficult, the MUIS and UUIS do not include the concept of complex decision-making. Further, the UUIACS better reflects the nature and source of the uncertainties characteristic of UIA patients, and may help in the development of policies that remove the uncertainty faced by patients undergoing endovascular coiling to treat a UIA, or mitigate its effects.

4.3. Potential Use of the UUIACS to Evaluate Nursing Support

The UUIACS may be used to assess the uncertainty that UIA patients experience during recovery. For this reason, it can be used as an assessment tool for nurses. Furthermore, it is useful for examining how nurses might set goals and provide concrete support to patients by understanding their source, nature, and degree of uncertainty. For instance, when dealing with the lack of information or ambiguous subjective symptoms due to uncertainty over disease characteristics, uncertainty can eased and transformed into certainty by providing information, explaining whether subjective symptoms are due to UIA or not. On the other hand, with regard to decision making, uncertainty will not necessarily be transformed into certainty, most helpful information. In such cases, teaching probabilistic thinking skills helps patients to at least partially accept this certainty. Using the UUIACS, together with the HLC scale and a depression scale, may enable nurses to evaluate the results of their nursing support.

5. Study Limitations and Recommendations for Future Research

The UUIACS was developed through a region-based study that experienced difficulty guaranteeing an adequate number of participants. More than half of the scale's questions had to be eliminated during the item and factor analysis stages of its development; yet, problems with the expression of items remained. There was almost no correlation between the scale and the Japanese version of the SF-36v2®, and this finding will determine future plans for the scale's further development.

6. Conclusion

The development of a scale that can reflect the uncertainty experienced by patients undergoing endovascular surgery due to UIA is attempted. The result of this endeavor is a scale consisting of 17 items in 4 factors named, "Lack of decision-making cues", "Lack of information and complexity of information interpretation", "The ambiguous nature of the disease", and "The unpredictable living with UIA". The validity and reliability of the UUIACS are verified by assessing the scale's criterion-related validity and internal consistency.

Acknowledgements

The authors acknowledge that this study received funding assistance from JSPS KAKENHI Grant Number 24890253.

The authors are grateful to the subjects of this study who provided us with invaluable information. They would also like to thank the outpatient nurses, senior staff, doctors, and nurses of the hospital ward.

Conflict of Interest

The authors have no financial conflicts of interest to disclose concerning the research.

References

[1] Jung, Y.J., Ahn, J.S., Park, E.S., Kwon, D.H., Kwun, B.D. and Kim, C.J. (2011) Surgical Results of Unruptured Intracranial Aneurysms in the Elderly: Single Center Experience in the Past Ten Years. *Journal of Korean Neurosurgical*

Society, **49**, 329-333. http://dx.doi.org/10.3340/jkns.2011.49.6.329

[2] Sonobe, M., Yamazaki, T., Yonekura, M. and Kikuchi, H. (2010) Small Unruptured Intracranial Aneurysm Verification Study: SUAVe Study, Japan. *Stroke*, **41**, 1969-1977. http://dx.doi.org/10.1161/STROKEAHA.110.585059

[3] UCAS Japan Investigators (2012) The Natural Course of Unruptured Cerebral Aneurysms in a Japanese Cohort. *New England Journal of Medicine*, **366**, 2474-2482. http://dx.doi.org/10.1056/NEJMoa1113260

[4] Otawara, Y., Ogasawara, K., Kubo, Y., Tomitsuka, N., Watanabe, M., Ogawa, A., Yamadate, K., *et al.* (2004) Anxiety before and after Surgical Repair in Patients with Asymptomatic Unruptured Intracranial Aneurysm. *Surgical Neurology*, **62**, 28-31. http://dx.doi.org/10.1016/j.surneu.2003.07.012

[5] van der Schaaf, I.C., Brilstra, E.H., Rinkel, G.J.E., Bossuyt, P.M. and van Gijn, J. (2002) Quality of Life, Anxiety, and Depression in Patients with an Untreated Intracranial Aneurysm or Arteriovenous Malformation. *Stroke*, **33**, 440-443. http://dx.doi.org/10.1161/hs0202.102335

[6] Yamashiro, S., Nishi, T., Koga, K., Goto, T., Kaji, M., Muta, D., Fujioka, S., *et al.* (2007) Improvement of Quality of Life in Patients Surgically Treated for Asymptomatic Unruptured Intracranial Aneurysms. *Journal of Neurology, Neurosurgery & Psychiatry*, **78**, 497-500. http://dx.doi.org/10.1136/jnnp.2006.098871

[7] Brilstra, E.H., Rinkel, G.J.E., van der Graaf, Y., Sluzewski, M., Groen, R.J., Lo, R.T.H. and Tulleken, C.A.F. (2004) Quality of Life after Treatment of Unruptured Intracranial Aneurysms by Neurosurgical Clipping or by Embolisation with Coils. *Cerebrovascular Diseases*, **17**, 44-52. http://dx.doi.org/10.1159/000073897

[8] Cheong, J.J., Ghinea, N. and van Gelder, J.M. (2004) Estimating the Annual Rate of de Novo Multiple Aneurysms: Three Statistical Approaches. *Neurosurg Focus*, **17**, 1-8. http://dx.doi.org/10.3171/foc.2004.17.5.8

[9] Tsutsumi, K., Ueki, K., Morita, A. and Kirino, T. (2008) Risk of Aneurysm Recurrence in Patients with Clipped Cerebral Aneurysms: Results of Long-Term Follow-Up Angiography. *Stroke*, **39**, 1276-1285.

[10] Masuda, M. and Inoue, T. (2010) Experience of Uncertainty in Patients with Unruptured Intracranial Aneurysms Treated with Endovascular Coiling and Their Nursing Care. *Journal of Japan Academy of Critical Care Nursing*, **6**, 16-25. http://dx.doi.org/10.11153/jaccn.6.3_16

[11] Nogawa, M. (2004) Study on the Reliability and Validity of the Japanese-Language Version of the Mishel Uncertainty in Illness Scale-Community Form. *Japan Journal of Nursing Science*, **24**, 39-48. http://dx.doi.org/10.5630/jans1981.24.3_39

[12] Mishel, M.H. and Epstein, D. (1997) Uncertainty in Illness Scales Manual. University of North Carolina, Chapel Hill.

[13] Nogawa, M. (2012) Development of a Universal Uncertainty in Illness Scale to Be Used for Inpatients and Outpatients. *Japan Journal of Nursing Science*, **32**, 3-11. http://dx.doi.org/10.5630/jans.32.1_3

[14] Mishel, M.H. (1988) Uncertainty in Illness. *Journal of Nursing Scholarship*, **20**, 225-232. http://dx.doi.org/10.1111/j.1547-5069.1988.tb00082.x

[15] Mishel, M.H. (1981) The Measurement of Uncertainty in Illness. *Nursing Research*, **30**, 258-263. http://dx.doi.org/10.1097/00006199-198109000-00002

[16] Masuda, M., Ohishi, H. and Yamamoto, M. (2014) Uncertainty in Patients with Unruptured Intracranial Aneurysms Undergoing Endovascular Surgery: A Qualitative and Inductive Study. *Nursing Research*, **63**, 366-374. http://dx.doi.org/10.1097/NNR.0000000000000050

[17] Wallston, K.A. and Wallston, B.S. (1981) Health Locus of Control Scale. In: Lefcourt, H.M., Ed., *Research with the Locus of Control Construct*, Academic Press, New York, 15-63. http://dx.doi.org/10.1016/b978-0-12-443201-7.50010-5

[18] Edwards, J.A. and Weary, G. (1996) Antecedents of Causal Uncertainty and Perceived Control—A Prospective Study. *European Journal of Personality*, **12**, 135-148. http://dx.doi.org/10.1002/(SICI)1099-0984(199803/04)12:2<135::AID-PER301>3.0.CO;2-Y

[19] Mast, M.E. (1995) Adult Uncertainty in Illness—A Critical Review of Research. *Scholarly Inquiry for Nursing Practice: An International Journal*, **9**, 3-24.

[20] SF-36v2® Health Survey © 1992, 2000, 2003 Quality Metric Incorporated, Medical Outcomes Trust and Shunichi Fukuhara.

[21] Fukuhara, S. and Suzukamo, Y. (2004) Manual of SF-36v2 Japanese Version. Institute for Health Outcomes & Process Evaluation Research, Kyoto.

11

Pain Assessment as a Tool in Back-to-Work Rehabilitation

Aud Moe*, Aud Evensen, Karin Torvik, Hildfrid V. Brataas

Faculty of Health Science, Nord-Trøndelag University College, Steinkjer, Norway
Email: *aud.moe@hint.no, AudEmelie.Evensen@hint.no, Karin.Torvik@hint.no, hildfrid.brataas@hint.no

Abstract

The purpose of this study was to elucidate participant experiences with a way to use pain assessment as a tool in vocational rehabilitation and see if the process is perceived to be important for the rehabilitation process in a four-week lasting rehabilitation back to work program for people with chronic pain, mental illness and fatigue symptoms. Design: A qualitative study. Purposeful typical case sampling. Semi-structured qualitative interviews with rehabilitation back to work participants were thematic content analyzed. Setting: Interviews at the end of the 4th week of rehabilitation took place at a Rehabilitation Center in Central Norway. Subjects: Six women and four men aged 23 to 57 years, suffering from chronic pain and mild mental illness symptoms. Main outcome measure: This paper describes the participants' experiences with pain mapping in back-to-work rehabilitation, used as a tool in a rehabilitation model for people suffering from chronic pain and mild mental illness. Results: The main topic was "empowered to insights". The results illustrate a process where mapping tools were experienced relevant in the process of growing discovery of pain and ways of pain management. Pain assessment as a joint aid for both themselves and the staff provided a clearer pain understanding. Conclusion: Mapping as own activity, and co-operation with supportive personnel showing respect for patients' own experiences, may promote empowerment, and further motivate own efforts and progress of the rehabilitation process.

Keywords

Pain Assessment, Rehabilitation to Work, Empowerment, Qualitative Research

1. Introduction

The article deals with a study of participants' experiences when using pain assessment as a tool in back-to-work

*Corresponding author.

rehabilitation called Responsibility for Self-Mastery (AFEM) [1] for people on sick leave who have compound problems, such as chronic pain, musculoskeletal disorders, psychological distress, and signs of fatigue. AFEM is a comprehensive four-week lasting psychosocial and psycho-educative rehabilitation back to work program in Central Norway [2]. The model includes pain assessment and total appraisements based on the International Classification of Functioning, Disability and Health model (ICF) [3]. Based on this health understanding, participants' pain experiences can be understood as complex, with links between biological, psychological, and social aspects of the experience [4] [5]. According to an agreement with The Central Norway Regional Health Authority, the AFEM rehabilitation model from 2007 is used as a specialist health measure for people on sick leave in Mid-Norway [6].

A comprehensive pain assessment can be used in biomedical and psychosocial domains [7]. In the assessment of chronic musculoskeletal pain, quantitative tools [8] and health-related quality of life instruments [9] can be used, since pain may affect quality of life [10]. The pain phenomenon can be understood as personal experience, and consequently only the person experiencing pain may fully assess the pain character and intensity. Therefore, self-reporting is seen as valid pain assessment [11].

Rehabilitation for workers with musculoskeletal pain have shown improvement in participants' employability and job performance through their development of pain self-efficacy [12]. From an empowerment perspective [13], self-reporting and pain assessment instruments may both strengthen the patient involvement and his/her pain self-efficacy. The patient's perception of involvement and control are key components of empowerment in rehabilitation [14]. Wikman and Fältholm [15] studied patient empowerment and found that support from health professionals was of significance for the patients' involvement in their rehabilitation.

Experience creates expectations, and our expectations are important for what we perceive [16]. Lillrank [17] found that women with chronic pain had the experience that some doctors did not take subjective pain seriously when diagnosing chronic pain. Other studies, however, have shown the positive and supportive attitudes of health professionals [15] [18] [19]. A study conducted by Coutu *et al.* [20] showed that being met with positive attitudes led to a changed way of thinking about pain [20]. This may show that professionals' communication of attitudes may have an impact on how patients perceive the world [16] [21] and own pain. Expectations and thoughts concerning pain appear to have an impact on perception of pain. In anticipation of pain, one can easily perceive something painful. For the chronically ill, the perspectives "illness-in-foreground" and "wellness-in-foreground" may have specific functions in the person's world [22] [23]. A life with chronic ailments can be an ongoing and changing process, where the focus is mainly on pain rather than on well-being. Is it, in that case, possible to turn over the perspective? Does the pain assessment further pain focus, or vice versa—does it put painful focus in the background, and focus on what brings well-being in life? How pain is focused, and how are the pain assessment activities experienced in the context of AFEM back-to-work rehabilitation?

Little has been studied about participant experiences of the pain assessment in vocational rehabilitation; nothing has been studied in the AFEM rehabilitation arena. Experience-based knowledge about pain assessment may be important for further development and use of assessment in rehabilitation for individuals with chronic pain. The purpose of this study was to elucidate participant experiences with a way to use pain assessment as a tool in vocational rehabilitation and see if the process is perceived to be important for the rehabilitation process.

2. Method

The study had a qualitative descriptive and interpretive design, with individual interviews about the informants' experiences of pain assessment in the rehabilitation process. Analyses of interview data were done by content analysis in order to integrate narrative information in relation to key concepts and themes [24]. The research team had experience as researchers and as nurses in various areas of health care, including rehabilitation, chronic pain, and mental health care.

Pain Assessment used in AFEM rehabilitation

Pain assessment was carried out at three different times: before the person came to rehabilitation, in the first week, and in the last week (week 4) of the rehabilitation program. Assessment of pain was carried out using the SF-36 Health Survey (two questions of pain) [10], and the Brief Pain Inventory [25].

The SF-36 Health Survey, SF-36 [10] [26] [27] is a health and quality of life assessment tool with indexes of physical functioning, bodily pain, general health, physical vitality, social and emotional functioning, and mental health. One question was about bodily pain and one about how bodily pain affect every day work and activities. Responses are based on a Likert scale.

Brief Pain Intervention [25] identifies pain, pain intensity, daily variation, and how pain affects the patient's functioning in relation to daily life. The form has one input issue that maps whether or not the patient has pain. The form includes a body map where the participant marks the pain areas on the body. Questions concerning daily variation and impact of pain on the patient's functional level is relative to the last 24 hours. All variables scored are by means of an 11-point numeric scale. Participants may fill out these forms without any help from the staff.

Sample and sampling

Purposeful sampling focuses on selecting information-rich cases that will shed light on the question under study [28]. Among the population that had chronic pain in Mid-Norway, the sample represented a selected group admitted as patients in the AFEM rehabilitation program. Approximately 40 people have attended AFEM rehabilitation annually since 2007. The inclusion criteria for the study were persons on sick leave with pain who participated in the AFEM rehabilitation. The informants reported idiopathic unexplained pain. Selection of informants for the study was carried out as "Typical case sampling" [24] [28] of persons holding key information about typical assessment experiences at this rehabilitation. Twelve rehabilitation participants were requested. Ten agreed to participate in the study, of which six were women and four were men, aged 23 years to 57 years. Before the stay at the rehabilitation institution the informants had been on sick leave from one month to several years.

Data Collection

Data was collected during 2013. Interviews were carried out by the first, second, and fourth authors and took place at the rehabilitation institution the last week of the rehabilitation program (week 4). To talk undisturbed, the interviewer and the interviewee withdrew from the arena where the rehabilitation activities took place. The interviewer asked open-ended questions, and the interviewees spoke about their experiences of pain assessment and the importance of the use of assessment tools in the rehabilitation process. A semi-structured interview guide began with questions related to pain assessment before admission. Then, the informants were encouraged to talk about the meaning of pain assessment as they experienced this at the end of the rehabilitation program. Finally, the interviewer opened the conversation for suggestions about the improvement of pain assessment practices at the clinic. The duration of the interviews was 20 - 30 minutes. The interviews were recorded on a digital recorder and thereafter transcribed to text.

Data analysis

Transcribed texts were analyzed by content analysis to determine the content and meaning of the stories; this method was inspired by Graneheim and Lundman [29]. The analysis started with reading the entire text several times to obtain an overall impression. The next step was to identify meaning units that were relevant for the study's purpose. Next, the units of meaning were condensed into condensed text, which were subsequently coded. "Labelling a condensed meaning unit with a code allows the data to be thought about in new and different ways" [29]. The codes were compared for similarities and differences, and sorted into six sub-categories under three categories that emerged from the manifest content. Two researchers performed independently analysis of subcategories, categories and development of theme. In order to validate the subcategories, categories and themes independently, the findings were compared. Thereafter, all four researchers participated in meetings where the analysis of meaning unit, categories, and theme discussed were until there was agreement on a common result formulation. The researchers reflected on the latent underlying meaning at an interpretative level based on the relationship or "thread" in the manifest content, expressed as sub-categories and categories [29]. From this analysis, a theme emerged as an overarching pattern in the material ref. **Table 1**.

Table 1. Subcategories, categories, and theme.

Subcategory	Category	Theme
Relevance of the pain assessment tools User-friendliness of the pain assessment tools	Charting of pain	
Participation through collaboration Complicity through involvement	Discovery through participation	Empowerment to own insights
Awareness through notes making and reflection Increased understanding of own pain	Pain clarification and development of own insights	

Ethical considerations

Permission to conduct the study was given from the Regional Committee for Medical and Health Research Ethics, Region Central (2013/534). The Head of Administration for the rehabilitation institution was informed about the project. He informed the participants verbally, gave them written information from the researchers, and requested participation in the study. Participants were informed of the possibility to withdraw from the study at anytime; they were also informed the study would have anonymity, confidentiality, and the use of de-identification of the information gathered through interviews. Participants gave written informed consent to participate before the interviews started.

A request communicated by the Head of Administration could be perceived as pressure to participate in the study, although the manager was not responsible for the rehabilitation program. To ensure voluntary participation, the researcher repeated the information about the request and the opportunity to withdraw from participation before the interviews started. Ten of the twelve subjects requested agreed to participate. The Head of Administration was not aware of who did not wish to participate.

3. Findings

From the interviews with the ten AFEM rehabilitation participants, the following categories emerged: Charting of pain, Discovery through participation, and Pain clarification due to assessment experiences. From further interpretation the theme "Empowered to own insights" emerged.

Charting of pain

Charting of pain was described as mapping headaches; neck pain; pain in the arms, shoulders, legs, pelvis, lower back, and knees; and stomach pains. Some also reported to have a deep inner pain of grief and despair. It could be difficult to distinguish between physical and psychological pain.

One of the forms used offsets, whereas the second additionally provided an opportunity for marking on a bodymap. The ability to visualize the pain was relevant to establish the location of the physical pain. One of the participants filled out the survey tool far in advance of their stay at the institution, and thought it was not very relevant. Another participant felt he really did not have much pain and there was little to chart. Still another had a lot of pain when they charted before the rehabilitation started.

Most participants had not thought of the importance of the assessment, but on reflection argued that the assessment was well done this way. Mapping tools encompassed the ability to identify the pain as it was experienced, and the tools were considered accurate and detailed. The tools provided an opportunity to see the logic in using them; they were relevant as part of the overall rehabilitation program. There was no one who proposed amendments to this charting of pain.

Charting pain meant that participants appreciated the ease of use of the tools. User-friendliness was about the design of the questionnaires. Shading pain areas on a drawing was especially appreciated and motivated participation in mapping:

> "I could see on the drawing where I crossed and scribbled. It was really just thinking about it – and then I knew it. This was the smartest way to show the pain, rather than just describe the pain"

Through illustrations and grading the questions, they received options to answers that they could relate to. User-friendliness also was strengthened by the fact that the mapping went quickly with little expenditure of time.

Participants who experienced much pain thought the charting tools were relevant, because they made their experiences and reflections of pain location specific and highlighted the complexity of the pain.

Discovery through participation

Discovery through participation in the charting process revolved around the patient; they had the opportunity to do the charting by self-report. The fact that the rehabilitation nurses wanted information and that the participants could fill it out on their own was a motivating experience, even before rehabilitation. This gave them a sense of positive and helpful attitudes among the staff.

In the pain assessment, done at the start of rehabilitation, their own participation and involvement varied. Some had not filled out the form, but conversed about pain assessment with employees. Others had filled out the form in collaboration with the staff, and some had been independent in filling out charting forms. At that time, participants regarded pain mapping as a tool for employees in their work.

All participants experienced equality among the staff, and they showed confidence in them. Such confidence strengthened informants' trust in the employees and the overall rehabilitation program. Pain assessment was marked by the respect that boosted participants' confidence and self-respect.

When participants were shown that an interest in the knowledge of their own pain experience was in demand, they did not feel left to themselves. Doing pain assessments during their stay in the institution actualized the relationship with the rehabilitation nurse as an active helper. Thus, the assessment was an activity of importance in cooperation with the recovery process:

> "We collaborate. I can fill out, and then I am in the process itself. You are not 'overrun' at a single point. You are constantly a part of the process."

Personalized complicity built on mutual trust and support from competent helpers helped participants realize they were participants in the rehabilitation process.

At first, they had looked at mapping as a tool for employees. Eventually, they considered pain assessment as an aid in collaboration between the participant and staff. Participants went from passive participation to active participation through collaboration and "good relations".

Pain clarification and development of own insights

For one participant this experience was about raising awareness through the recording and reflection of writing and drawing on paper, which led to an awareness of the situation as it was. Records could even provide insight, and as a result, some of the informants had "laid down" exhausting thoughts that influenced pain. Regarding what one had experienced "at a distance", this provided a fresh start by going back to what made sense before the pain experiences.

Pain clarification also meant raising awareness through the experience of change, which appeared to some at the beginning of the stay:

> "Good to see if one thinks of that pain map when coming to rehabilitation, I see how it has changed. One becomes conscious of that. Because I did not think about that anymore and I did not have that kind of pain to map any longer."

Another talked about awareness through repeated assessments:

> "It was quite funny, really—because I saw the difference, but I did not think of it until a few days after I had filled it out. At that time the pain had begun to quit-then I thought about it—when I was going to fill it out and look over it again—then I saw it—I had no more pain."

Some felt that raising awareness through mapping experiences could be utilized for even more active participation in the use of the forms under the rehabilitation process. To be aware of one's own pain was all about "raising awareness of body and mind", as expressed. Pain assessment could also be helpful in placing their responsibility on suffering, accountability, and self-awareness. This could in turn, result in a feeling of greater control over the situation.

The general theme for the three categories was "Empowered to own insights".

4. Discussion

The purpose of this study was to elucidate participant experiences with a way to use pain assessment as a tool in vocational rehabilitation and see if the process is perceived to be important for the rehabilitation process. The result illustrates a process through the participants' pain mapping and their use of relevant tools. The active participation led to an emerging discovery that the assessment could be a common aid for both patient and staff. Through these experiences a new awareness emerged and led to a deeper and more holistic understanding of their own pain situation. The topic "Empowered to own insights" demonstrated relationships between categories.

Charting of pain may be useful in routine assessments that can relate to other problems, such as physical functioning, emotional functioning, and the different experiences of satisfaction and quality of life [9]. Standardized self-report instruments to assess patients' pain [7] were experienced as relevant tools for the way they were used in AFEM rehabilitation. Personalized involvement built on mutual trust was, in this study, a support from the rehabilitation nurse that helped patients discover themselves as participants with their own responsibilities in the rehabilitation process.

Several studies [15] [18] [30] [31] point out that the process meetings for people with chronic pain are important for the experience of being respected and taken seriously. In this study participants discovered thorough participation. Empowered thinking requires that personnel have basic confidence in the individual's ability to make decisions and act in their best interest. Individually oriented empowerment is all about to initiation processes in order to boost confidence, knowledge, and skills [32]. Doas [21] found that actively listening can improve personal relationships and foster trust, mutual respect, and patient compliance. The trust that the participants were shown through repeated self-reports and conversations about pain assessment seemed to support a gradual build-up of more self-confidence and self-respect. The mapping tools used in communication with the rehabilitation nurse appear to be both trustworthy and lead to the development of insight. Communication and the nurse's behavior seem to be central to the participants' sense making processes [16]. Personnel appear to signal basic confidence that patients themselves can take responsibility and be active in the acquisition of knowledge about themselves, their pain, and perspectives on life. Mutual trust and respect are essential in the relationship between patient and health professionals [16] [19]. To be confirmed as a whole person, and not identified with a disorder, can be a force for patient participation [16] and for raising awareness of their own thinking. It is through the development to find individual strength and confidence that the individual realizes their resources and acquires more power and control over their lives [13].

The participants in this study experienced pain clarification and development of own insights through the rehabilitation process. Lillrank [17] found that when patients who previously had not been taken seriously for their subjective experience of pain, met health professionals who took their pain seriously, it was a turning point that could lead to "solve the puzzle" of the troublesome pain. Suffering can be enhanced and extended in duration by the stigma of pain, but troublesome pain can be changed if the person with pain is taken seriously [15] [17] [19].

Experiences of chronic pain appear to be shaped by biomedical and psychosocial factors [3] [7] [33]. The two assessment tools used in the study reflect these factors [10] [25]. When participants map their pain experiences, what proceeds comes from their individual background and understanding and shapes their interpretation in the context of their understanding of an ongoing order in life [16]. They do not deal with the world event by event, but rather frame events in larger meaning structures that provide them with an interpretive template within which they can make sense of relevant aspects of the events they experience [34]. During the assessment process a reflection process occurs; during this they make sense of their pain experiences, and a new, expanded self-knowledge seems to develop. A new way of thinking can be constructed through the experience of control [20]. A "turning point" is when the meaning of the experiences of the past and the individual's identity lead to new insights [17]. Research shows that workers on sick leave who returned to work after a rehabilitation program underwent an "illness-transformation", where their illness identity was abandoned because they experienced control of symptoms through pain management [20]. By spending time and attention to pain mapping, awareness of pain character and intensity may appear [11]. Positive results through a work rehabilitation program are shown as a reduction in pain intensity by developing a new way of thinking that changes the perception of pain [20]. This study's results show a new way of thinking in the sense of being more aware of both detail and comprehensiveness in their own pain experience by being empowered to own insights.

On the one hand, individual-oriented empowerment-thinking is criticized; health is seen as an "instrument" to get patients to act differently by adopting established knowledge (*i.e.*, knowledge that the nurse holds) [13]. On the other hand, Anderson and Funell [35] argue that the empowerment to own insights represents a health promotion of thinking that has led to a paradigm shift among health care workers. Our findings about the raising of awareness through the experience, education, and empowerment that the participants in the rehabilitation experience supports the assumption of a paradigm shift-a shift that includes and values the patient's thinking.

Method discussion

The study provided information about how persons within a selected group participating at a specific rehabilitation program perceived use and usefulness of pain assessment scheme employed. Transferability consideration should be in light of the sample character, the rehabilitation arena, and the Central Norwegian context. The mapping tools do not specifically relate to the rehabilitation model. Therefore, the assessment experiences may be of relevance when considering mapping in other arenas.

To protect participants' anonymity, omitted are diagnoses, occupations and personal information. The study included a small sample and short stories, but the material was rich enough to get data about categories creating coherence within the main theme. More informants and redundant conversations could possibly provide more and detailed information about the topic. In the analysis of meaning units, the researchers were aware that interviews swung between experiences with mapping and experiences with the overall AFEM rehabilitation program. Through joint reflection among scientists, consensus emerged on relevant units of meaning. Credibility handled was through a detailed description. The analysis process, in which four researchers participated, strengthens the study reliability.

5. Conclusions

Pain assessment tools mapped physical pain, while notes, reflections, and collaboration with the rehabilitation nurse helped participants to reflect more holistic on pain experiences, this seemingly influencing a change in pain understanding and focus. Awareness and self-knowledge seemed promoted through an individually managed mapping, assessment, and through collaboration with the rehabilitation staff, this taking place in an empowerment process. Trust and respect led to the experience of involvement in the individual's rehabilitation process.

The participants had no suggestions for changes to the mapping practice. On the other hand, assessment possibly to greater extent could be used. There is a need for more knowledge about the importance of individual pain assessment as a tool for raising awareness, increasing control, and changes that may promote rehabilitation back to work.

Author Contributions

Study design: Aud Moe and Hildfrid V. Brataas. Data collection: Aud Moe, Aud Evensen and Hildfrid V. Brataas. Analyses and manuscript preparation: All four authors; Aud Moe, Aud Evensen, Karin Torvik, Hildfrid V. Brataas.

Sources of Support

The study was supported by Central Norway Regional Health Authority; Smednestrivselsgåd as, N 6590 Tustna, Norway.

References

[1] Indergaard, E. (2002) AFEM Model 2002. http://www.smednes-trivselsgard.no/afem-rehabilitering/afem-modellen

[2] Evensen, A., Brataas, H.V. and Landstad, B. (2010) Individuell læring i psykoedukativkognitiv rehabilitering. *Nordisk Tidsskrift for Helseforskning*, **6**, 70-83.

[3] World Health Organization (2001) International Classification of Functioning, Disability and Health. WHO, Genova.

[4] Butler, D. and Moseley, L. (2008) Explain Pain. NOI Group. http://www.noigroup.com/en/Product/EPBII

[5] Garguilo, H., McCaffrey, R. and Frock, T.L. (2003) Understanding Chronic Pain and the Mindbody Connection. *Holistic Nursing Practice*, **6**, 281-289.

[6] Norway. Helse Midt-Norge. Raskere tilbake (Fasterreturn). (2014). http://www.helse-midt.no/no/Pasient/Behandlingstilbud/Raskere-tilbake/84352/

[7] Dansie, E.J. and Turk, D.C. (2013) Assessment of Patients with Chronic Pain. *British Journal of Anaesthesia*, **111**, 19-25.

[8] Chapman, J.R., Norvell, D.C., Hermsmeyer, J.T., Bransford, R.J., DeVine, J., McGirt, M.J. and Lee, M.J. (2011) Evaluating Common Outcomes for Measuring Treatment Success for Chronic Low Back Pain. *SPINE*, **36**, S54-S68.

[9] Salaffi, F., Ciapetta, A. and Carotti, M. (2012) Pain Assessment Strategies in Patients with Musculoskeletal Conditions. *Reumatismo*, **64**, 216-229. http://dx.doi.org/10.4081/reumatismo.2012.216

[10] Ware, J.E. and Sherbourne, C.D. (1992) The MOS 36-Item Short-Form Health Survey (SF-36). *Medical Care*, **30**, 473-483. http://dx.doi.org/10.1097/00005650-199206000-00002

[11] International Association for the Study of Pain (2013) http://www.iasp-pain.org

[12] de Vries, H.J., Reneman, M.F., Groothoff, J.W., Geertzen, J.H.B. and Brouwer, S. (2013) Self-Reported Work Ability and Work Performance in Workers with Chronic Nonspecific Musculoskeletal Pain. *Journal of Occupational Rehabilitation*, **23**, 1-10. http://dx.doi.org/10.1007/s10926-012-9373-1

[13] Askheim, O.P. (2012) Empowerment i helse-og sosialfaglig arbeid: Floskel, styringsverktøy eller frigjøringsstrategi (Empowermentin Healthand Social Work: cliché, managementorreleasestrategy)? Gyldendal Akademiske, Oslo.

[14] Zimmerman, M.A., Israel, B.A., Schulz, A. and Checkoway, B. (1992) Further Explorations in Empowerment Theory: An Empirical Analysis of Psychological Empowerment. *American Journal of Community Psychology*, **20**, 707-727. http://dx.doi.org/10.1007/BF01312604

[15] Wikman, A.M. and Fältholm, Y. (2006) Patient Empowerment in Rehabilitation: Somebody Told Me to Get Rehabilitated. *Advances in Physiotherapy*, **8**, 23-32. http://dx.doi.org/10.1080/14038190500494774

[16] Hargie, O., Brataas, H.V. and Thorsnes, S.L. (2009) Cancer Patients' Sensemaking of Conversations with Cancer Nurses in Outpatient Clinics. *Australian Journal of Advanced Nursing*, **26**, 70-78.

[17] Lillrank, A. (2003) Back Pain and the Resolution of Diagnostic Uncertainty in Illness Narratives. *Social Science & Medicine*, **57**, 1045-1054. http://dx.doi.org/10.1016/S0277-9536(02)00479-3

[18] Rørtveit, K., Hansen, B.S., Leiknes, I., Joa, I., Testad, I. and Severinsson, E. (2015) Patients' Experiences of Trust in the Patient-Nurse Relationship A Systematic Review of Qualitative Studies. *Open Journal of Nursing*, **5**, 195-209. http://www.scirp.org/journal/ojn http://dx.doi.org/10.4236/ojn.2015.53024

[19] Nordin, C., Gard, G. and Fjellman-Wiklund, A. (2013) Being in an Exchange Process: Experiences of Patient Participation in Multimodal Pain Rehabilitation. *Journal of Rehabilitation Medicine*, **45**, 580-586. http://dx.doi.org/10.2340/16501977-1136

[20] Coutu, M.-F., Baril, R., Durand, M.-J., Cote, D., Rouleau, A. and Cadieux, G. (2010) Transforming the Meaning of Pain: An Important Step for the Return to Work. **35**, 209-219.

[21] Doas, M. (2015) Are We Losing the Art of Actively Listening to Our Patients? Connecting the Art of Active Listening with Emotionally Competent Behaviors. *Open Journal of Nursing*, **5**, 566-570. http://www.scirp.org/journal/ojn http://dx.doi.org/10.4236/ojn.2015.56060

[22] Moe, A., Enmarker, I. and Hellzén, O. (2012) Daily Life for Chronically Ill Oldest Old Persons. *Nursing Reports*, **2**, e8.

[23] Paterson, B.L. (2001) The Shifting Perspectives Model of Chronic Illness. *Journal of Nursing Scholarship*, **33**, 21-26. http://dx.doi.org/10.1111/j.1547-5069.2001.00021.x

[24] Polit, D.F. and Beck, C.T. (2012) Nursing Research: Generating and Assessing Evidence Fornursing Practice. 9th Edition, Wolters Klüwer, Phladelphia.

[25] Klepstad, P., Loge, J.H., Borchgrevink, P.C., Mendoza, T.R., Cleeland, C.S. and Kaasa, S. (2002) The Norwegian Brief Pain Inventory Questionnaire: Translation and Validation in Cancer Pain Patients. *Journal of Pain and Symptom Management*, **24**, 517-25. http://dx.doi.org/10.1016/S0885-3924(02)00526-2

[26] Ware Jr., J.E., Kosinski, M. and Keller, S.K. (1994) SF-36 Physical and Mental Health Summary Scales: A User's Manual. The Health Institute, Boston.

[27] Ware Jr., J.E. (2011) SF-36 Health Survey Update. http://www.sf-36.org/tools/SF36.shtml

[28] Patton, M.C. (2002) Qualitive Research & Evaluation Methods. 3th Edition. http://onlinelibrary.wiley.com/cochranelibrary/search.

[29] Graneheim, U.H. and Lundman, B. (2004) Qualitative Content Analysis in Nursing Research: Concepts, Procedures and Measures to Achieve Trustworthiness. *Nurse Education Today*, **24**, 105-112. http://dx.doi.org/10.1016/j.nedt.2003.10.001

[30] Andersson, S., Sundberg, T., Johansson, E. and Falkenberg, T. (2012) Patients' Experiencesand Participations of Integrative Care for Back and Neck Pain. *Alternative Therapies*, **18**, 25-32.

[31] Drachler, M.L., Leite, J.C., Hooper, L., Hong, C.S., Pheby, D., Nacul, L., Lacerda, E., Campion, P., *et al.* (2009) The Expressed Needs of People with Chronic Fatigue Syndrome/Myalgic Encephalomyelitis: A Systematic Review. *BMC Public Health*, **11**, 458. http://dx.doi.org/10.1186/1471-2458-9-458

[32] Askheim, O.P. (2011) Pasientopplæring og empowerment (Patient educationandempowerment). In: Brataas, H.V., Ed., *Sykepleiepedagogisk praksis* (*NursingEducationalPractice*), Gyldendal Akademiske forlag, Oslo, 71-100.

[33] Fagermoen, M.S. and Lerdal, A. (2011) Teoretiske modeller for læring og mestring (Theoreticalmodelsfor Learning Andmastering). In: Lerdal og Fagermoen, ed., Læring og mestring—et helsefremmende perspektiv i praksisog-forskning (Learning and Mastering—A Health Promotion Perspective in Practice and Research). Gyldendalakademisk, Oslo, 17-37.

[34] Mills, C. (2009) A Case of Making Sense of Organisational Communication. In: Hargie, O. and Tourish, D., Ed., *Auditing Organisational Communication*: *A Handbook of Research*, *Theory and Practice*, Routlede, London, 370-390.

[35] Anderson, R.M. and Funell, M.M. (2010) Patient Empowerment: Myths and Misconceptions. *Patient Education and Counseling*, **79**, 277-282. http://dx.doi.org/10.1016/j.pec.2009.07.025

12

Emergency Preparedness Nursing Education: Learner and Faculty Perspectives

Geraldine Jody Macdonald

Associate Professor, Teaching Stream, Bloomberg Faculty of Nursing, University of Toronto, Toronto, Canada
Email: g.macdonald@utoronto.ca

Abstract

Over the past decade, entry-to-practice emergency preparedness competencies have been identified as an essential component of nursing education. In this paper the author reports upon a small Canadian study which explores the perspective of undergraduate learners and faculty members who participated in and/or facilitated an Emergency Preparedness Simulation (EPS) module during a primary health care praxis course. The central purpose of this study was to explore the related experiences of learners and faculty who participated in or facilitated an Emergency Preparedness Simulation (EPS) module academic year and their perspectives on the effectiveness of the simulation in preparing learners to respond to emergencies in the future. The EPS module included a seminar followed by a mass-casualty simulation experience. The mass-casualty simulation experience included a "Teddy Bear" triage and an "Explosion" triage. The constructivist data analysis identified four related patterns for both the learner and faculty participants: Strengths (S), Objections (O), Suggestions (S), and Feelings (!) [SOS!]. Three themes were identified in each pattern: relevance, design, and engagement. In comparing the learner and faculty perspectives, there is a clear congruence between the strengths identified, the objections identified, and the power of feelings for both learners and faculty who participate in the emergency preparedness scenarios. Learners and faculty had different suggestions. Learners suggested more time on developing skills, particularly around first aid of individual clients, and recommended all students begin with the "Teddy Bear" triage. Faculty suggested a re-thinking of the "Explosion" triage simulation to emphasize community based emergency preparedness and responsiveness. Such re-focusing would support the integration of key primary health care principles and values including equity, social justice, and social determinants of health. Learners and faculty valued the EPS module and recommended it continue to be a learning component of the primary health care course.

Keywords

Emergency, Mass-Casualty, Simulation, Learners, Faculty

1. Introduction

The increasing number of emergencies in the community related to natural, manmade, and technological disasters has prompted new standards in emergency preparedness nursing education locally and globally [1] [2].

Since September, 2007 all undergraduate nursing programs in Ontario, Canada have been directed by the College of Nurses of Ontario (CNO) to incorporate emergency preparedness within the undergraduate nursing curriculum [3]. The College of Nurses of Ontario sets the competencies for entry-level Registered Nurse practice in Ontario. By definition, a nursing competency identifies "the knowledge, skill, ability and judgment required for safe and ethical nursing practice" [3]. An entry-level Registered Nurse must be prepared to demonstrate knowledge of emergency preparedness and to participate in emergency preparedness and disaster planning [3]. The Canadian Association of Schools of Nursing (CASN) identifies applying public health sciences in nursing practice as an expected competency, including "health emergency preparedness and disaster response" [4].

Globally, many nursing education programs are incorporating some aspects of emergency preparedness in their nursing education programs and in their accreditation standards. The American Association of Colleges of Nursing (AACN) incorporates emergency preparedness in their competency standards. American accreditation requirements include "disaster and mass-casualty education" [5]. The AACN standards state graduates are expected to be able to "prepare for and minimize health consequences of emergencies" [6].

The addition of emergency preparedness has created new challenges for faculty. Community nursing faculty members have, unexpectedly, become responsible for implementing effective educational opportunities that meet the new accreditation standards for emergency preparedness. In particular, they have needed to ensure nursing curricula incorporate "...mass-casualty education" [5].

In this paper the author reports upon a small Canadian study which explores the perspective of undergraduate nursing learners and faculty members who participated in and/or facilitated an emergency preparedness simulation (EPS) module.

2. Background, EPS Module, & Study Introduction

Senior year nursing students have developed health assessment skills, communication skills, and leadership skills that are valuable during an emergency situation whether it is a pandemic, bio-terrorism, violence, or natural disaster such as ice/wind storms. Nevertheless, most nursing students have little experience or preparation to respond to an emergency.

To meet the challenge of embedding emergency preparedness skills into the curriculum faculty designed a pilot emergency preparedness simulation module for all senior year students in a second entry undergraduate nursing program. All senior year students were expected to participate in this emergency preparedness simulation module in their primary health care praxis course, with their seminar peers. There were approximately 150 students in the senior year of the BScN program. Half completed the EPS module in the fall term, and half in the winter term. There were five sections of the primary health care course in the fall term, and five in the winter term. Each section was facilitated by a faculty member and normally fifteen students. All five seminar groups completed the EPS module in the same week. Half of the students in each course section started with the "Teddy Bear" triage, and half with the "Explosion" triage.

The learning objective for the EPS module was outcomes based, stating that by the completion of the EPS module learners would be prepared to demonstrate the Ontario College of Nurses expectations of new graduates in terms of emergency preparedness. As previously stated, this meant having the required knowledge and preparation needed to participate in emergency preparedness and disaster planning [3].

The first component of the EPS module was a three hour Monday morning seminar. The seminar began by reflecting upon local and global disasters prompted by images on power point slides. This led to a rich discussion. The faculty then facilitated a discussion of the seminar readings that investigated the role of nurses in planning for and responding to emergencies and disasters. More specifically, the readings considered emergency preparedness [7], mass casualty [8], ability and willingness to report to duty [9], and debriefing [10]. Faculty highlighted ethical standards for emergency response during the seminar [11]. At the end of the seminar students were reminded of the time of their simulation experience later in the week, and advised that the simulation would relate to the seminar theme of preparing to participate in emergency preparedness and disaster planning.

The second component of the EPS module was participation in a mass-casualty simulation experience. Each section of the course was booked into a specific two hour simulation lab time, on a clinical practice day. Students had to travel to the university prior to or after their clinical practice that day and were given credit for a half day of clinical practice. The simulation experience included a welcome and briefing prior to both the "Teddy Bear" mass casualty triage and the "Explosion" mass casualty triage. After each simulation exercise that the students completed, the faculty facilitated a thorough and thoughtful debriefing. Students completed evaluations of the simulation experience in the final ten minutes. The simulation experience was guided by the National League for nursing theoretical framework for simulation design [12]. This theoretical framework was further developed by Jeffries & Rogers [13]. It is now referred to as the NLN/Jeffries Simulation Framework [14]. The NLN/Jeffries Simulation Framework identifies effective educational practices, simulation design characteristics, and participant outcomes [14].

An internally funded, descriptive educational research study was designed to provide needed feedback from learners and faculty on the educational effectiveness of the 2007/2008 emergency preparedness simulation module (EPS). Ethics approval was obtained from the University of Toronto, Office of Research Ethics. Completion of the Survey Monkey questionnaire provided informed consent for the learner participants and ensured participant anonymity. Faculty participants signed a consent form prior to the start of their focus group.

2.1. Purpose

The central purpose of this study was to explore the related experiences of learners and faculty who participated in or facilitated an Emergency Preparedness Simulation (EPS) module in the 2007/08 academic year and their perspectives on the effectiveness of the simulation in preparing learners to respond to emergencies in the future. As well, the study identified learner perspectives on the simulation design, educational practices, and learner satisfaction and confidence. This study was a descriptive educational study, including the collection and analysis of quantitative and qualitative data from learner participants and qualitative data from faculty participants.

This study was anticipated to provide valuable insight into the related experiences and perspectives of the learners and the faculty members involved in the EPS module. It was anticipated that the study findings would guide planning for the EPS module in future years, enhance the educational experience of future BScN learners, and contribute to the safety of Canadians during emergencies.

2.2. Review of Literature

The focus of simulation research in nursing education in Canada, and internationally, has been primarily in undergraduate nursing education [15]-[17] with interest in simulation in the practice environment growing, particularly in relation to emergency preparedness [17] [18]. Emergency preparedness is a particular concern because of the increasing number of emergencies being faced in the community related to violence/terrorism [18], natural disasters [19], pandemic preparedness [20] and technological disasters [21].

Simulation research suggests that key learner outcomes of simulations relate to knowledge development, skill performance, learner satisfaction, critical thinking, and self-confidence [22]. Active learning, high fidelity simulations that closely mimic real practice, and immediate constructive feedback, are proposed to result in more positive student outcomes [22]. Faculty involvement in the simulation is encouraged with faculty taking on roles in the simulation [23], guiding simulation debriefing [24] [25], and taking responsibility to assess the ongoing impact of participating in the simulation on the students and faculty members, as participation may be anxiety provoking and/or exhausting [23].

Prior to the research proposal development, no published studies were located that specifically described faculty perspectives related to the design and/or implementation of simulated learning or the related experiences/perspectives of learners and faculty involved in an emergency preparedness simulation. Subsequently, Jose & Dufrene [25] completed an integrative review of disaster preparedness in undergraduate nursing education globally. They found that all disaster preparedness nursing education studies incorporated simulations within their design, typically engaging students actively in responding to a disaster scenario [25]. Faculty-facilitated debriefing was an integral component of these studies with a focus on facilitating reflection upon the simulation experiences of the students [25]. Adams, Canclini, and Frable [21] argue that nursing programs must ensure that there are appropriate learning experiences that facilitate students learning about emergency preparedness nursing, including imagining how they will participate in future emergencies as a Registered Nurse. Simulation based learning

(SBL) has been confirmed as an appropriate clinical learning approach in pre-licensure nursing programs, one that leads to effective learning and successful passing of the NCLEX-RN registration exam [26].

3. Study Methodology

3.1. Guiding Research Questions

The guiding research questions for the study were:

1) What is the nature of the related experiences of learners who participated in the Emergency Preparedness Simulation (EPS) module and the faculty who facilitated the EPS module?

2) What are the learner and faculty perspectives on the effectiveness of the EPS module as a learning approach to prepare learners to respond to emergencies in the future?

3) What are the learner perspectives on the simulation module design, educational practices, and learner satisfaction and self-confidence?

3.2. Participants

All senior students/learners in the BScN program at the researcher's university who participated in an Emergency Preparedness Simulation module during their Primary Health Care course (N = 150), in the 2007/2008 academic year, were invited to participate. Learners were invited to participate via an e-mail from the faculty registrar as the faculty research protocol did not permit the principle investigator (PI) to contact students directly. Learners then had to initiate a direct e-mail to the PI and state that they would like to participate in the study. Following this, the learners' contact data (e-mail) was uploaded into Survey Monkey by the research assistant (RA).

Nine learners volunteered to participate in the study. This was a disappointing response rate of 6%. Barriers to participation were thought to be the fact that data collection occurred during the final two week of the BScN program, when students were completing a clinical practicum off campus, and the requirement to read the registrar's e-mail and take the initiative to respond directly to the PI.

All faculty (n = 6) who facilitated a simulation during an EPS module, in the 2007/08 academic year, were invited to participate in the study. They were invited to attend a two hour focus group in July, 2008. Three faculty participated in the study (n = 3) for a response rate of 50%. Two of these faculty also attended an optional focus group to review the preliminary data findings and thus provided face validity for the findings. Focus group tapes and notes were transcribed into a word document creating paper transcripts for qualitative analysis. A constructivist analysis was used to identify patterns in the qualitative data and then themes within each of the patterns.

3.3. Learner Methods

Learners (n = 9) in their final year of a second-entry BScN program completed survey questions using the secure, on-line survey tool, Survey Monkey. Survey questions for the learner participants included one demographic question which asked if they completed the EPS in the fall or winter term of the 2007/08 academic year, two open-ended qualitative survey questions, and fixed-choice questions from three tested and reliable NLN/Laerdal instruments that have established their value in educational research, specifically, "... all three measures are both reliable and valid" [27]. The three instruments are: The Simulation Design Scale (SDS), the Educational Practices Questionnaire (EPQ), and the Student Satisfaction and Self-Confidence in Learning (SCLS) instrument [27]. Data collection was completed in June, 2008. Learner participants were not invited to attend the optional focus group to review the preliminary data analysis and as they had graduated and ethical approval had not included contacting these alumni.

Survey Monkey was set to ensure all responses remained anonymous. Learner participants had a two week window to complete the survey questions after access to the survey questions in Survey Monkey was opened. One reminder was sent to learner participants via Survey Monkey to highlight the deadline date. Once the deadline date was reached, the survey questions on Survey Monkey were removed. Data was stored initially on Survey Monkey, in a secure, password-protected account, accessible only to the research team. Data was then transferred into word documents stored in the research team members' secure, password-protected computers. Hard copies were stored in secure, locked cupboards.

3.4. Faculty Methods

Faculty were initially contacted by the PI via e-mail with an attached letter providing a description of the study and an invitation to participate in one focus group. Faculty were also advised that they would have the option to participate in a second focus group to respond to preliminary data analysis, but this was not required to be eligible to participate in the study. Faculty indicated their willingness to participate in the research study by responding to the PI via e-mail. The focus group was held in July 2008, on the university campus, at a time which was convenient for faculty participants.

The PI and the RA attended the focus group along with the faculty participants. It was anticipated that from 3 - 6 faculty participants would attend the focus group and three attended (n = 3), two in person and one via telephone conference call. The two hour focus group was moderated by the PI. Faculty participants were invited to respond to six open-ended questions. During the focus group the RA audio-recorded the discussion, using a tape recorder and a digital voice recorder, and recorded highlights in writing and on a computer. Following the focus group the recorded dialogue and notes were cleaned and transcribed into a word document available for qualitative analysis. In May, 2009 the faculty participants were invited to meet for an additional, optional, focus group discussion to validate the preliminary findings. Two faculty participants attended this optional focus group. Feedback from this additional focus group was recorded via notes taken by the PI and was included in the final data analysis to support faculty face validity for the findings.

4. Data Analysis

Overall, a constructivist analysis guided the data analysis. As Pickard and Dixon [28] confirm, the individual is central in a constructivist analysis and the challenge of the researcher is to offer an analysis of the individual's lived experience. The researcher seeks to explicate the meaning of the individual's experience, necessitating a holistic approach that attends to the broad context of the experience, including an ecological analysis that identifies the multiple realities experienced by the individual, attending to their complexities and interconnections, and thus identifying the multiple realities and finally the meaning of the individual's experience [28]. It is essential to collect data that will provide the rich text needed for a trustworthy analysis [29] [30].

Lincoln [31] argues that constructivist is consistently relativist. Analysis in constructivist inquiry is responsive to the data, in contrast to much positivist, post positivist, and critical theory research which begins the analysis by choosing to examine the data through the lens of a predetermined theoretical model [31] [32]. The patterns that emerge from a constructivist analysis may demand a deeper critical analysis that acknowledges concerning contradictions and, if so, the analysis may include a balance of constructivist and deconstructivist inquiry [32]. What is clear is the importance of attending to the data to inform the analysis, and to attend to the multiple realities of the participants' experiences. Constructivist researchers value a subjective perspective, researcher and subject form interdependent relationships, and the subjective experiences of the researcher are made explicit and valued [30]. To judge the quality of an interpretive, constructivist inquiry, soundness of the inquiry is judged by the trustworthiness, meaning the establishment of credibility through measures such as triangulation, peer debriefing, and most importantly, member checks; transferability of the findings; dependability established by the inquiry audit, and confirmability that the "...subjective knowledge of the researcher can be traced back to the raw data..." [30]. The PI and RA kept detailed field notes throughout the research process, including recording their own responses to the faculty focus group questions prior to interviewing the faculty participants to ensure that they have processed their lived/heuristic experiences. By expressing their own experience prior to inviting the faculty participants to express their experience, the researchers are prepared to be able to open and listen to the experience of the faculty participants and learner participants.

Qualitative data for learners and faculty were analyzed separately and then results were compared as reported in this paper.

4.1. Learner Quantitative Data Analysis

Pickard & Dixon [28] suggest that tensions remain among qualitative researchers about collecting qualitative and quantitative data within a study, and thus mixing paradigms, leading to limitations, but argue this may be needed to answer central questions in the research study. In this study, the researcher included three valid questionnaires, composed of fixed-response questions, for the learners, along with one demographic question and a number of open-ended questions. This would require integration during data analysis but was considered the best data collection methodology to provide a response to the final research question "What are the learner perspectives on the simulation module design, educational practices, and learner satisfaction and self-confidence?" As well, the results were to establish a baseline that future research might be compared to and to create an opportunity to examine the relationship between the quantitative and qualitative responses. And so the overall constructivist analysis was intended to include the statistical analysis of the quantitative questions.

Due to the low learner response rate (6%, n = 9) the quantitative data was not considered to be representative of the experience of learners in the class. Guided by the advice of a statistician, the raw data was reviewed, using the following numeric values: strongly disagree (−2), disagree (−1), undecided (0), agree (1), strongly agree (2). A positive average confirms learner agreement with the simulation tool statements while a negative average indicates disagreement with the simulation tool statements. A positive average indicates strengths of the simulation from the learners' perspectives. The demographic question asked learners to identify which term they had completed the simulation but due to the low response rate this data was not included in the analysis. The two open-ended qualitative survey questions were analyzed using a constructivist analysis and are reported under the qualitative findings.

Each of the three instruments used drew upon a 5-point scale that rated student participants' attitudes or beliefs: 1-strongly disagree, 2-disagree, 3-undecided, 4-agree, and 5-strongly agree [27]. *The Simulation Design Scale* (SDS) (20 items) uses a 5-point scale to assess the quality of simulations relating to objectives/information, learner support, problem-solving component, feedback/debriefing, and fidelity/realism [22]. The tool has established content validity and reliability [27]. *The Student Satisfaction and Self-Confidence in Learning* (SCLS) (13 items) uses a 5-point scale to assess learner satisfaction with simulation learning and self-confidence in learning during the simulation. The tool has established content validity and reliability [27]. *The Education Practices Questionnaire* (EPQ) (16 items) uses a 5-point scale to assess the quality of simulations related to educational practices including active learning opportunities, collaboration with peers, diverse ways of learning, and clarity of expectations. The tool has established validity and reliability [27].

4.2. Learner Quantitative Findings

Overall, all three simulation tools report positive averages indicating that the simulation was of high quality from the perspective of the nine participants in the study. The categories reviewed included objective and information, support, problem solving, feedback/guided reflection, fidelity (realism) from the SDD; active learning, collaboration, diverse ways of learning, and high expectations from the EPSS; and from the SSLS satisfaction with current learning and self-confidence in learning. Of the 49 subcategories, 44 reported positive averages and 5 reported negative averages. The five subcategories reporting negative averages were: the chance to discuss the simulation objectives with my teacher, availability of the instructor to discuss individual learning needs, the opportunity to goal set during the simulation, and the scenario resembled a real-life situation.

The researcher acknowledges that the timing of the data collection, from four to eight months following the emergency simulation, and the fact that learners may have discussed their experience with their peers, may impact the validity of the responses of the learner participants to the NLN/Laerdal Instruments. Learner participants were advised that if they had trouble responding to any of the questions they did not have to complete them.

Overall, all three simulation tools report positive averages indicating that the simulation was of high quality from the perspective of the nine participants in the study. The learner quantitative data findings provided limited but valued guidance to local faculty planning future emergency preparedness simulations in the study institution. The low response rate limited further data analysis.

4.3. Learner Qualitative Data Analysis

Qualitative data from the two open-ended learner survey questions were reviewed, and a constructivist analysis was used to identify patterns emerging from the data. Open-ended survey questions data stored in word documents were line numbered and printed in hard copy. Qualitative data analysis included reviewing the data from the open-ended learner questions and identifying emerging broad patterns related to the experiences and perspectives of the learners. Coloured highlighters were used to mark connections/emerging patterns within the data. Once the broad patterns were identified/coded, data was organized within these patterns, by identifying themes. Each pattern was explored in depth to establish the meaning of the learner experience.

4.4. Learner Qualitative Results

This qualitative analysis of the learner open ended questions led to four patterns: Strengths, Objections, Suggestions, and Feelings (SOS!). The pattern of Strengths identified the learners' perspectives of the positive components of participating in the EPS module. Objections identified the concerns learners shared about participating in the EPS. Learners did have a number of Suggestions for improving the learning experience of students in the EPS. And finally, students shared strong Feelings about participating in the EPS, both positive and concerning. Within each of these four patterns was evidence of three themes: relevance, design, and engagement. Relevance spoke to the valuing of the EPS module by learners, design spoke to the organization of the lab and flow of the triage simulations, and engagement reflected the learners' ability to pay attention and create meaning from their experience in the EPS module. The four patterns and three themes are integrated in this SOS! analysis.

In the strengths pattern, learners identified relevance "*the idea of having an EPS is very essential*" and design features "*The teddy bear triage was effective*"... "*The debriefing was helpful and when we repeated our* [explosion] *scenario*". Engagement was also a strength "*I now know that during an emergency it is not feasible to perform CPR*"... "*I recognize my potential role as a leader in such a situation because of my knowledge base and experience.*"

In the objections pattern, learners identified relevance by their concerns that their learning was not optimal—"*I still feel under qualified to provide first aid for trauma, bleeds, burns, breaks, dislocations etc.*" The design was not optimal either—"*During the simulation our group really wasn't sure what to do so it seemed awkward*"... "*The set-up was very unrealistic*". And one learner objected to the "Teddy Bear" triage simulation, directly stating that engagement was a concern—"... *the scenario itself was not engaging.*"

Learner suggestions were focused on the simulation design, identifying changing the order of the simulations and requesting faculty provide demonstrations: "*If I had seen the bears first* [before the Explosion simulation]" and "*time ... for actual teaching/demonstrations by the facilitators ... what a response should look like given our lack of experience and knowledge ...*"

And learners identified strong feelings associated with the simulation including feeling engaged prior to the simulations and feeling upset about the [Explosion] simulation design: "*I was pretty eager to do this module prior to the day of ...*" *but* ... "*during ... I was feeling very ill-prepared ... helpless ...*"

4.5. Learner Discussion

It was clear from the strengths learners identified, that the EPS module was a valued and relevant learning experience for most of the learner participants. Emergency preparedness is an engaging topic and learners were engaged in the EPS module. Learner responses did not mention the seminar. Responses related to the two simulations which they anticipated with excitement. The "Teddy Bear" triage worked well for most students. It was safe, challenging, and the design flowed well.

Objections addressed the design of the "Explosion" triage simulation. Learners were uncertain, felt unable to take charge of the situation, and didn't feel confident in their first aid skills. They also wished their teachers had been more supportive and had given them more guidance. This scenario didn't work as well particularly for learners who started with this simulation first.

Learners suggested that the "Teddy Bear" triage be the first simulation for all students. They also suggested faculty be more involved in the "Explosion" triage as faculty are in the "Teddy Bear" triage.

And finally, learners experience a range of powerful emotions while completing this EPS module. Learners didn't like feeling powerless. They wanted more support from faculty, more role modelling, more direction.

5. Faculty Perspectives

5.1. Results

The constructivist data analysis revealed four patterns in the faculty perspectives, aligning closely with the learner qualitative patterns: Strengths (S), Objections (O), Suggestions (S), and Feelings (!) or SOS!. Within each of these four patterns were three themes: relevance, design, and engagement. The patterns and themes are integrated into the discussion following the direct faculty quotes.

5.1.1. Strengths

Faculty identified a number of strengths related to the topic and the enhancement of the course by using the simulation lab which the learners valued:

"*Okay, prior to it I, I was quite excited because it's quite close to my heart as you know I am in public health and we are also going through a similar experience and I was really happy to hear that* [*the university*] *was a taking it on.*"

"*I was actually intrigued about how we would use the lab to do something in community. To me that was quite novel and so from that perspective I was really quite excited to see how that would play out.*"

5.1.2. Objections

Faculty objections were related to feelings about their own competency to teach the EPS module, their role in the simulations, and how they would support students.

"*I didn't know what my role was until the day before, a couple of days before the actual class. So it was that part that I was a little bit apprehensive.*"

"*... really not knowing what to expect and having really no trauma experience or experience in this field I was probably anxious about what I would be expected to know and how I would be expected to support the students and that was that was before we actually started...*"

"*And then when we came to the actual* [explosion] *mass casualty I was, I thought it was, I thought it left a lot open for the students to feel powerless... partly because the activity was structured around one person who got to be in charge and they held all the information.*"

5.1.3. Suggestions

Faculty had suggestions to share which would incorporate values and principles of primary health care, including focusing on community level analysis:

"*... I would say that this curriculum needs to be expanded to include other forms of disasters like—you know it was a bomb at that time but it could be—other kinds of disasters like a train derailment, that kind of thing.*"

"*... in the fall I remember, putting in a couple of articles around like the critical analysis using race, gender, class and disaster management. Things that lead to disaster, social determinants and I don't think in the winter term there was an opportunity to do this. I mean I thought that that was an element that was missing and it was not necessarily going to be encompassed by the way this was set up. So I think there has to be or it would be useful for the students in linking that more clearly to okay so what kinds of analysis is also important here. It is more that a how to understanding okay, so who is it that are more vulnerable etc.*"

5.1.4. Feelings

Faculty experienced a range of feelings during the lead up to and during the facilitation of the "Teddy Bear" and "Explosion" simulations.

"*...but I don't really feel as if I have all the knowledge, skills and confidence to do this.*"

"*Yeah, casualty. It was a bit of feeling that scattered kind of feeling and I was trying to put myself in the real situation when that happens and that was a bit traumatic and the students when they were in that situation they were sort of very disorganized and they were kind of scattered and they took on the attitude of laissez faire... I was a little unsure of what to do as a faculty member and I was asked not to say anything.*"

"*Now, I seem to recall teddy bear triage going about the same in the fall and the winter. A very positive experience. The* [Explosion] *casualty experience was a bit different in the fall than the winter. Seems to me in the winter, there was a second chance and so that changed the outcome for the students, and because I was made aware of that before things started, I think I felt a bit different.*"

5.2. Discussion

The faculty experience identified strengths relating to relevance of the emergency preparedness module, design of the "Teddy Bear" triage, and personal engagement with learning new skills and developing a new competency. Faculty suggested that in future the design of the simulations would have all students complete the "Teddy Bear" triage prior to the "Explosion" triage as students had recommended.

Faculty objections related to the design of the "Explosion" triage which limited feedback to students and was not considered safe for students; limited relevance to the course learning objectives as the design focused on responses to individual clients rather than taking the broad community perspective of the course including critical analysis of PHC principles and values and key SDOH such as race, gender, class issues. Concerns about confidence, competence, and preparation for the EPS were also voiced as objections.

Faculty participants contributed suggestions for future EPS modules that were invaluable including making the critical analysis a central part of the modules, so that in keeping with the course objectives faculty do consider issues of vulnerability/social justice. As well, the faculty suggested that the design of the "Explosion" triage needed to be clearer and proposed that a setting such as MSF (Doctors without Borders) or Red Cross might be a more viable simulated setting in which to conduct the triage.

Faculty reported a range of feelings including liking the simulation, feeling excited, and happy to more problematic feelings such as feeling disempowered because of the lack of control over the design of the "Explosion" triage, a design some felt was not safe for the students.

6. Learner and Faculty Interpretations

6.1. Learner Interpretations

Learners identified key strengths of the "Teddy Bear" Triage, objections to the design of the "Explosion" triage, valuing of including the emergency preparedness simulation in the course, and the emergence of powerful feelings associated with the two simulations, including feeling that faculty should be demonstrating emergency preparedness skills for the learners. They suggested specific changes to improve the learner experience including starting all students in the "Teddy Bear" triage, and then proceeding to an "Explosion" triage that was more realistic, that focused more on first aid, one that included active participation of the faculty who would then provide role modelling and offer support and guidance to the learners.

6.2. Faculty Interpretations

Overall, faculty were engaged with the EPS module and became far more engaged with the topic of emergency preparedness, a new competency for a number of the faculty. Faculty identified the design of the "Teddy Bear" triage as one that worked well—it was safe, structured, clear, and non-threatening. The design and facilitation of the "Explosion" triage was problematic. Faculty were concerned about students and the lack of supports outside of the faculty to support students. Faculty also acknowledge that planning and leading the "Explosion" triage stimulated a range of powerful feelings, some positive but predominantly feeling concerned for the safety of students and missing congruency between the simulations based learning (SBL) and the primary health care principles and values guiding the course.

Faculty suggestions focused on continuing to incorporate the EPS module in the Primary Health Care course but shifting the focus of the "Explosion" triage to one that is more community oriented, away from a first aid approach, to look at community level responses. This confirmed that faculty felt there was value in preparing students for emergency preparedness in their future practice. Faculty proposed new readings to be integrated into the seminar, to ensure a positive link between the EPS learning and the course expectations. As well, faculty recommended considering how to identify the impact of emergencies on our most vulnerable clients such as our homeless population, within the context of a community response to emergency preparedness. The SOS! analysis was an effective one to interpret both the learner and the faculty perspectives on the emergency preparedness simulation.

7. Study Conclusion: Comparing the SOS! Findings for Learners and Faculty

In comparing the learner and faculty perspectives, there is a clear congruence between the strengths identified, the objections identified, and the power of feelings for both learners and faculty who participate in the emergency preparedness scenarios. However, while the learners asked for more demonstration of emergency preparedness skills, particularly around first aid of individual clients, the faculty offered another perspective when identifying suggestions.

Faculty advocated for a re-thinking of the Explosion triage to shift the focus of the learning away from individual to community based preparedness and responsiveness. Such re-focusing would tap into the strengths of the faculty teaching the course, would reduce the tension students felt about being prepared to provide care to critically injured clients in an unpredictable environment, and would support the integration of key course themes around equity, accessibility, social justice, social determinants of health, race, gender and class.

The SOS! analysis effectively supports the interpretation of both learners and faculty participants in this study. While the sample size was limiting, the study was able to inform future emergency preparedness simulations in the local context. It is less clear that the study will be of benefit for other nurse educators and students in other nursing programs. However, this study may provide some guidance for nurse educators who are just beginning to integrate emergency preparedness into their curriculum. There was a clear support by both faculty and learners for the value of including emergency preparedness into the BScN curriculum.

Future research studies are needed to confirm the value of emergency preparedness simulations for BScN curriculum, to explore learner perspectives and to continue to develop our understanding of nurse educator perspectives.

8. Limitation

The study response rate was low related to timing and university student recruitment policies. This negatively impacted the value of the quantitative data collected. While few learners participated in the study (n = 9), their qualitative data remains of value. The participation of faculty was small (n = 3) but it represents a RR of 50%, which is acceptable. The study data was collected seven years ago. However, as the outcomes of the study continue to guide the current EPS module, and as students and faculty continue to evaluate this EPS very positively, the study is considered to be of current value to nurse educators.

Acknowledgements

In memory of Ms. Betty Burcher, a Lecturer at the Bloomberg Faculty of Nursing, University of Toronto who was the second author for the study proposal. Funding support was provided from the Bloomberg Faculty of Nursing, University of Toronto, NERF Fund ($6810.00).

References

[1] Adams, L.M., Canclini, S.B. and Frable, P.J. (2015) Skip the Infection, Get the Injection: A Case Study in Emergency Preparedness Education. *Nurse Education in Practice*, **15**, 58-62. http://dx.doi.org/10.1016/j.nepr.2013.12.004

[2] Weiner, E. (2006a) Preparing Nurses Internationally for Emergency Planning and Response. *OJIN: The Online Journal of Issues in Nursing*, **11**, Manuscript 3. http://www.nursingworld.org/MainMenuCategories/ANAMarketplace/ANAPeriodicals/OJIN/FunctionalMenu/AboutOJIN

[3] College of Nurses of Ontario (2007, 2014) Competencies for Entry-Level Registered Nurse Practice, Toronto: Author. http://www.cno.org/docs/reg/41037_EntryToPracitic_final.pdf

[4] Canadian Association of Schools of Nursing (CASN) (2014) Entry-to-Practice Public Health Nursing Competencies for Undergraduate Nursing Education. http://www.casn.ca/2014/12/entry-practice-public-health-nursing-competencies-undergraduate-nursing-education-2/

[5] Austin, E.N., Bastepe-Gray, S.E., Nelson, H.W., Breitenbach, J., Ogle, K.T., Durry, A., Green, S.D., Crabtree, L.A., and Haluska, M. (2014) Pediatric Mass-Casualty Education: Experiential Learning through University-Sponsored Disaster Simulation. *Journal of Emergency Nursing*, **40**, 428-434. http://dx.doi.org/10.1016/j.jen.2014.05.015

[6] American Association of Colleges of Nurses (AACN) (2008) The Essentials of Baccalaureate Education for Professional Nursing Practice. 1-62. http://www.aacn.nche.edu/education-resources/BaccEssentials08.pdf

[7] Rodriquez, D. and Long, C.O. (2006) Emergency Preparedness for the Home Healthcare Nurse. *Home Healthcare Nurse*, **24**, 20-27. http://dx.doi.org/10.1097/00004045-200601000-00006

[8] Riba, S. and Reches, H. (2002) When Terror Is Routine: How Israeli Nurses Cope with Multi-Casualty Terror. *Online Journal of Issues in Nursing*, **7**, 1-14. http://www.nursingworld.org/MainMenuCategories/ANAMarketplace/ANAPeriodicals/OJIN/FunctionalMenu/FAQs.aspx

[9] Qureshi, K., Gershon, R.M., Sherman, M.F., Straub, T., Gebbie, E., McCollum, M., Erwin, M.J. and Morse, S.S. (2005)

Health Care Workers' Ability and Willingness to Report to Duty during Catastrophic Disasters. *Journal of Urban Health*, **82**, 378-388. http://dx.doi.org/10.1093/jurban/jti086

[10] Hollister, R. (1996) Critical Incident Stress Debriefing and the Community Health Nurse. *Journal of Community Health Nursing*, **13**, 43-49. http://dx.doi.org/10.1207/s15327655jchn1301_4

[11] Canadian Nurses Association (2008) Ethics in Practice: Nurses' Ethical Considerations in a Pandemic or Other Emergency. CNA, Ottawa. http://cna-aiic.ca/~/media/cna/page-content/pdf-en/ethics_in_practice_august_2008_e.pdf?la=en

[12] Jeffries, P.R. and Rodgers, K. (2007) Theoretical Framework for Simulation Design. In: Jeffries, P.R. and National League for Nursing, Eds., *Simulation in Nursing Education*: *From Conceptualization to Evaluation*, National League for Nursing, New York, 21-33.

[13] Jeffries, P.R. and Rogers, K.J. (2012) Theoretical Framework for Simulation Design. In: Jeffries, P.R. and National League for Nursing, Eds., *Simulation in Nursing Education*: *From Conceptualization to Evaluation*, 2nd Edition, National League for Nursing, New York, 25-41.

[14] Ravert, P. and McAfones, J. (2014) NLN/Jeffries Simulation Framework: State of the Science Summary. *Clinical Simulation in Nursing*, **10**, 335-336. http://dx.doi.org/10.1016/j.ecns.2013.06.002

[15] Canadian Association of Schools of Nursing (CASN) (2007) CASN/ACESI Clinical Placements Projects, Project 3: Inventory of the Use of Simulated Clinical Learning Experiences and Evaluation of Their Effectiveness. www.cihc.ca/files/complementary/CASN Inventory of Simulation.pdf

[16] Miller, J.L., Rambeck, J.H. and Synder, A. (2014) Improving Emergency Preparedness System Readiness through Simulation and Inter Professional Education. Public Health Reports, Supplement 4, 129-135.

[17] Weiner, E. (2006) Addressing Emergency Preparedness and Response Competencies for Nurses through Simulation Experiences. *Clinical Simulation in Nursing Education*, **2**, 10-14. http://dx.doi.org/10.1016/j.ecns.2009.05.017

[18] Albores, P. and Shaw, D. (2007) Government Preparedness: Using Simulation to Prepare for a Terrorist Attack. *Computers & Operations Research*, **35**, 1924-1943. http://dx.doi.org/10.1016/j.cor.2006.09.021

[19] Qureshi, K.A. and Merrill, J.A. (2002) Emergency Preparedness Training for Public Health Nurses: A Pilot Study. *Journal of Urban Health*: *Bulletin of the New York Academy of Medicine*, **79**, 413-416. http://dx.doi.org/10.1093/jurban/79.3.413

[20] Maunder, R.G., Leszcz, M., Savage, D., Adam, M.A., Peladeau, N., Romano, D., Rose, M. and Schulman, R.B. (2008) Applying the Lessons of SARS to Pandemic Influenza. *Canadian Journal of Public Health*, **99**, 486-488.

[21] Adams, L.M., Canclini, S.B. and Frable, P.J. (2015) "Skip the Infection, Get the Injection": A Case Study in Emergency Preparedness Education. *Nurse Education in Practice*, **15**, 58-62. http://dx.doi.org/10.1016/j.nepr.2013.12.004

[22] Jeffries, P.R. and Rizzolo, M.A. (2006) Designing and Implementing Models for the Innovative Use of Simulation to Teach Nursing Care of Ill Adults and Children: A National, Multi-Site, Multi-Method Study. National League for Nursing and Laerdal Medical, New York.

[23] Austin, E.N., Bastepe-Gray, S.E., Nelson, H.W., Breitenbach, J., Ogle, K.T., Durry, A., Green, S.D., Crabtree, L.A., and Haluska, M. (2014) Pediatric Mass-Casualty Education: Experiential Learning through University-Sponsored Disaster Simulation. *Journal of Emergency Nursing*, **40**, 428-434. http://dx.doi.org/10.1016/j.jen.2014.05.015

[24] Dreifuerst, K.T. and Decker, S.I. (2012) Debriefing: An Essential Component for Learning in Simulation Pedagogy. In: Jeffries, P.R. and National League for Nursing, Eds., *Simulation in Nursing Education*: *From Conceptualization to Evaluation*, 2nd Edition, National League for Nursing, New York, 105-130.

[25] Jose, M.M. and Dufrene, C. (2014) Educational Competencies and Technologies for Disaster Preparedness in Undergraduate Nursing Education: An Integrative Review. *Nurse Education Today*, **34**, 543-551. http://dx.doi.org/10.1016/j.nedt.2013.07.021

[26] Jeffries, P.R. (2015) Reflections on Clinical Simulation: The Past, Present and Future. *Nursing Education Perspectives*, **36**, 278-279. http://dx.doi.org/10.5480/1536-5026-36.5.278

[27] Franklin, A.E., Burns, P. and Lee, C.S. (2014) Psychometric Testing on the NLN Student Satisfaction and Self-Confidence in Learning, Simulation Design Scale, and Educational Practices Questionnaire Using a Sample of Pre-Licensure Novice Nurses. *Nurse Education Today*, **34**, 1298-1304. http://dx.doi.org/10.1016/j.nedt.2014.06.011

[28] Pickard, A. and Dixon, P. (2004) The Applicability of Constructivist User Studies: How Can Constructivist Inquiry Inform Service Providers and Systems Designers? *Information Research*, **9**, Paper 175. http://InformationR.net/ir/9-3/paper175.html

[29] Freeman, M., deMarrais, K., Preissle, J., Roulston, K. and St. Pierre, E.A. (2007) Standards of Evidence in Qualitative Research: An Incitement to Discourse. *Educational Researcher*, **36**, 25-32. http://dx.doi.org/10.3102/0013189X06298009

[30] Lincoln, Y.S. (1995) Emerging Criteria for Quality in Qualitative and Interpretive Research. *Qualitative Inquiry*, **1**,

275-289. http://dx.doi.org/10.1177/107780049500100301

[31] Lincoln, Y.S. (1990) The Making of a Constructivist: A Remembrance of Transformations Past. In: Guba, E.G., Ed., *The Paradigm Dialog*, SAGE Publications, Newbury Park, 67-87.

[32] Macdonald, G. (1996) Sustaining Energy for Caring: The Experience of Mothers Who Are Nurses. Ed.D. Dissertation, Ontario Institute for Studies in Education, University of Toronto, Toronto.

13

Perceptions of Couples Who Use Jadelle Implant in Blantyre District, Malawi

Brima Osaio Kamara*, Rachel Rodriguez, Genesis Chorwe-Sungani, Angela Chimwaza

Kamuzu College of Nursing, University of Malawi, Blantyre, Malawi

Email: *brimaosaiokamara@gmail.com

Abstract

Malawi has a high total fertility rate of 5.7 per woman and Jadelle implant may be an ideal option for couples who want to practice family planning. Jadelle is a long term contraceptive which is inserted just under the skin of a woman's upper, inner arm by a nurse or midwife and prevents a woman from getting pregnant for a period of five years. But the use of Jadelle for family planning depends on perceptions of couples. The purpose of this study was to explore the perceptions of couples who choose Jadelle as their family planning method at a Central Hospital in Blantyre district. This study used a descriptive qualitative design. A purposive sample of 5 couples was used. Ethical clearance was granted by relevant authorities. Data was analysed through content analysis. The findings showed that the following nine themes emerged from the qualitative data: 1) men and women perspectives about mode of action of Jadelle; 2) knowledge about effectiveness and efficacy of Jadelle among men and women; 3) sources of information about Jadelle; 4) information given to Jadelle users by providers; 5) benefits of Jadelle; 6) challenges associated with Jadelle; 7) myths associated with Jadelle; 8) attitudes of providers of Jadelle and 9) role played by men regarding use of Jadelle. In conclusion, this study found that both men and women generally lacked knowledge of Jadelle. Men play a vital role when couples are choosing contraceptives. Every opportunity should be utilised at antenatal, postnatal and family planning clinics to teach individuals about family planning. This may allow women and men to make informed choices about the use of Jadelle.

Keywords

Perception, Jadelle, Couples, Family Planning

1. Introduction

Malawi has a high total fertility rate of 5.7 per woman [1] and Jadelle implant may be an ideal option for

*Corresponding author.

couples who want to practice family planning. Jadelle is a long term contraceptive which is inserted just under the skin of a woman's upper, inner arm by a nurse or midwife [2] and prevents a woman from getting pregnant for a period of five years. The use of Jadelle for family planning depends on perceptions of couples. Some men and women perceive that using contraceptive methods helps them to live a healthy life and participate in development activities. Others perceive that a man becomes weak (impotent) if he sleeps with a woman who is using contraceptives such as Jadelle [3]. Similarly, men and women may also perceive that women who use modern family planning methods to reduce the number of children God intended for them and they will be punished with infertility on reincarnation [4]. This shows that perceptions may encourage or discourage couples from using Jadelle and other family planning methods. The misperceptions about contraceptive use and little perceived risk of pregnancy are some of the reasons for unplanned pregnancy [5]. This may be true for Malawi where unplanned pregnancies are common. These unplanned pregnancies mostly end up in unsafe abortions which lead to increased deaths of women.

It is evident that 17% of maternal deaths are due to unsafe abortion globally [6]. Nonetheless, the effective use of contraceptives saves women's lives and preserves their health by protecting them from the health risks of frequent childbirth and unsafe abortion [7]. Most maternal deaths in Malawi are due to complications of unsafe abortions from unwanted pregnancies that can have been prevented through effective use of contraceptive methods. The rate of abortions in Malawi is high at 38 per 1000 women of reproductive age [8]. Besides that, maternal mortality rate for the country (675/100,000 live births) is amongst the highest in the world [1]. This was corroborated by Khunga and Lupickwho asserted that 807 women per 100,000 died in child birth in Malawi in 2010 [8]. These high levels of maternal mortality may be reduced by encouraging couples to use Jadelle which effectively prevents unplanned pregnancies. However, Jadelle is the least used contraceptive method at 0.3% [1] and most women use short term contraceptive methods which may sometimes be out of stock in the country [9]. Couples may not use Jadelle because they may have fear of perceived complications. There is evidence that women have concerns about family planning methods, including fear of side effects from hormonal methods [7]. Furthermore, a woman may feel that she has or lacks control over her own fertility due to social constructs of gender roles and expectations in her society [10].

Gender inequality, for example, may determine who has access to family planning information, which holds the power to negotiate contraceptive use or to withhold sex, who decides on family size, and who controls economic resources to obtain family planning related health services. These hurdles vary from culture to culture, yet they exist throughout the world and can often lead to negative family planning health outcomes. These problems are partly dealt with in Malawi by the Sexual Reproductive Health and Rights Policy for Malawi which proposes that individuals and couples have a right to decide freely and responsibly the number, spacing and timing of children and shall be provided with the means to do so without coercion [11]. The policy also provides for the availability of long lasting and permanent methods of contraceptives such as Jadelle at all levels of health care services in the country. This is vital for Malawi where stock-outs of short-term contraceptives are common and Jadelle offers a vital option for couples who want to delay or space child-bearing [9]. Nonetheless, the perceptions of men and women towards the use of Jadelle as a family planning method are not well documented in Malawi. Therefore, this study was conducted to explore the perceptions of couples who choose Jadelle as their family planning method at Queen Elizabeth Central Hospital in Blantyre district.

2. Methodology

2.1. Design

This study used descriptive design employing a qualitative method to explore perceptions of couples who choose Jadelle implant as their family planning method.

2.2. Setting

Setting for this study was a family planning clinic at Queen Elizabeth Central Hospital in Blantyre district.

2.3. Sample and Sampling

Target population was all couples who were using Jadelle implant. The sample comprised of 5 couples (5 men and 5 women) who were purposively sampled because participants were required to be experientially fit for the study. Qualitative inquiry is deliberately biased hence selection was based on the participants' experience that fits the research questions [12]. The decision to interview 5 couples only was based on the fact that the data became saturated. In this study, the researcher identified the participants at the Family Planning Clinic when they were attending check-up visits. The inclusion criteria were as follows: 1) being a married couple in which a woman is on Jadelle implant or had used it before; 2) expressing willingness to participate in the study and 3) being able to communicate in Chichewa. Couples who accepted to participate in the study were asked to sign a written consent.

2.4. Data Collection

An interview guide was used to collect data from the participants through in-depth interviews. Female participants were interviewed by a female research assistant while males were interviewed by a male research assistant considering the sensitivity of some issues that may come up during interviews. The length of each interview was between 30 and 45 minutes. Participants were interviewed in Chichewa because it is the most widely spoken language in Malawi. The individual interviews were conducted face to face in a private room at the family planning clinic. Couples were allowed to receive the services from the service provider before they were interviewed. Interviews were audio recorded and later transcribed and typed verbatim. Transcripts were assigned code numbers for identification.

2.5. Data Analysis

The collected data were analysed through content analysis. Themes were derived by analysis of words so that word repetitions, key indigenous terms, and key words in the contexts were identified. In addition themes were identified through a careful reading of larger blocks of texts, comparing and contrasting information and searching for missing information. Themes were also developed by conducting a comparative analysis of concepts coded in different participants group or setting codes. Demographic data was analysed manually using descriptive statistics.

2.6. Ethical Considerations

Ethical approval was granted by College of Medicine Research and Ethics Committee (COMREC) and institutional clearance was obtained from Director of Queen Elizabeth Central Hospital prior to data collection to ensure participants' protection. Participants volunteered to take part in the study and they gave a written consent. They were also assured that they would not be denied health care services because of their withdrawal or refusal to participate in the study.

2.7. Limitations of This Study

The limitation of this study is that a small sample size was used which might have limited the depth of information which was gathered in this study.

3. Findings

Demographic characteristics of participants of this study are presented in **Table 1**. The following nine themes emerged from the qualitative data: 1) men and women perspectives about mode of action of Jadelle; 2) knowledge about effectiveness and efficacy of Jadelle among men and women; 3) sources of information about Jadelle; 4) information given to Jadelle users by providers; 5) benefits of Jadelle; 6) challenges associated with Jadelle; 7) myths associated with Jadelle; 8) attitudes of providers of Jadelle and 9) role played by men regarding use of Jadelle.

3.1. Theme 1: Men and Women Perspectives about Mode of Action of Jadelle

The findings of this study revealed that men and women have various perspectives about the mode of action of Jadelle. Some participants linked the mode of action to their personal care or various perspectives. Other participants linked it to their personal agreement with the kind of care or knowledge given to them by providers. One participant said that Jadelle *makes semen to be weak, so that no fertilization takes place*. Similar views were

Table 1. Demographic characteristics of participants.

Demographic characteristics	Male	Female	Total
	n	n	n
Age group			
25 - 30	1	3	4
31 - 35	2	2	4
36 - 40	2	0	2
Education level			
PSLC	2	1	3
JCE	1	1	2
MSCE	2	3	5
Occupation			
Business	1	4	5
Intelligence officer	1	0	1
Cleaner	1	0	1
Hospital attendant	0	1	1
Cook	1	0	1
Welder	1	0	1
Religion			
Seventh day Adventist	1	1	2
CCAP	0	1	1
Catholic	2	3	5
Assemblies of God	1	0	1
Mbawa first Christian church	1	0	1
Tribe			
Lomwe	2	1	3
Ngoni	2	0	2
Chewa	1	1	2
Yao	1	0	1
Sena	0	1	1
Tonga	1	0	1

shared by another participant who reported that *it kills… do we say the uterus? So that when men's power come, should not have effect in the women's body*. Participants also connected the mode of action of Jadelle to the ovulation. Two participants said that *Jadelle helps women not to become pregnant by stopping ovulation*. One participant also emphasized on the men and women perspectives about the mode of action of Jadelle. She said that it *prevents women from getting pregnant when they have sexual intercourse with their husbands*.

3.2. Theme 2: Knowledge about Effectiveness and Efficacy of Jadelle among Men and Women

The study findings showed that men and women decide to use Jadelle as family planning method because of its effectiveness and efficacy. One male participant said that *they just say it is good and it can stay for 5 years while using it*. This was supported by a female participant who said that *it is best because you do not think of coming to the hospital now and then, once inserted for 5 years to come again to the hospital.* Male participants also emphasized the effectiveness and efficacy of Jadelle as family planning method when compared to other contraceptives. They said that *the method is effective because you can have sex with your wife any how without her getting pregnant unlike the injection.* A female participant who had similar views reported that *Jadelle is a good method; you can stay for 5 years without any problem.* Couples are choosing Jadelle in place of the other contraceptives because it is a long-lasting and reversible. A male participant reported that *Jadelle is long acting rather than pills and injection. Pills are used daily and sometimes you forget going to the hospital for injection.*

3.3. Theme 3: Sources of Information about Jadelle

The findings of the study indicated that participants get information about Jadelle implant from different sources. A male participant reported that he got information about Jadelle from his wife. He said that *I came to know Jadelle through my wife who explained the method.* On the contrary two female participants said that they got the information from different sources. One said that *I heard about Jadelle from a certain staff, one of the sisters from the family planning clinic* while the other one said *I knew of Jadelle when I came to the hospital for check-up of my baby after 6 weeks of delivery. That was the time they taught us of family planning methods and I choose Jadelle.*

Two male participants reported that they heard about Jadelle from the radio. One participant said that *the radios and televisions advertised Jadelle as one of the best methods of family planning. We listen to those messages and use them.* Another male participant got the information from different source said that *I heard about Jadelle from my friends because men share ideas on issues affecting the country when interacting. Ihave heard that there are several family planning methods from my wife and other people.*

3.4. Theme 4: Information Given to Jadelle Users by Providers

This study showed that participants generally got the information about Jadelle from a health facility especially postnatal and family planning clinics. However, it was also clear from the findings that the information which is given to them is usually inadequate. One male participant said that *I would have loved that those health workers were educating people about side effects caused by Jadelle if you do not go along with it and other options which are there.* This was supported by a female participant who felt that *most women do not know the benefit of Jadelle, if they are taught well and understand they might choose this method.* The little information Jadelle users receive from providers give them few options in using the method. This is clearly noticed in statements made by a male participant who said that *health workers should have enough time when doing different activities to share this information wherever they are working. People should be helped to understand what they are supposed to do because there are some who look like they know but they do not know and they rely upon this information to reach them.*

Some of the responses from participants showed the level of information given to users by providers was confusing. For instance a female participant who was experiencing a problem with Jadelle went to the clinic for advice and the information she was given was very misleading. She reported that *I came to complain so that they can remove the implants but I was told that they do not remove before 5 years and even if it is removed I would not stop bleeding.* Participants requested that providers should be reaching users in their communities by educating them on the effectiveness of Jadelle, its side effects and its benefits for the individual and the country. This was clear in sentiments made by a male participant who suggested that *if they have enough time, they can be moving around in areas educating people because there are some people who have transport problems cannot come to hospitals that are usually far away.*

3.5. Theme 5: Benefits of Jadelle

In Malawi participants are reportedly testifying that Jadelle has benefits for the individual and the country since its introduction as a family planning method. One male participant narrated that *you can have enough space for a mother to care for a child to grow up well, you can have a good time for 5 years. It gives you enough time to do what you want with regard to development of family and the country.* Another male participant also said that *this family planning method can be one way of reducing deaths of women due to giving birth frequently.* A female participant who shared similar sentiments said that *if women are not giving birth now and again there are going to be enough drugs in the hospitals and women will have time to participate in development project in the country*. Participants acknowledged that there are increased dangers associated with having too many children or having children too closely together. One male participant narrated that *using Jadelle helps a person to be able to achieve his plans and the woman will be healthy. Because if the woman is giving birth frequently, her body becomes unhealthy*. The findings are unique in demonstrating male and female reasons for using the implant Jadelle as a long-lasting contraceptive. This is supported by one male participant who narrated that *a person can easily forget to take Oral pills while as for Jadelle once inserted it is done and you just wait for its removal.*

3.6. Theme 6: Challenges Associated with Jadelle

The findings of this study revealed that there are challenges associated with Jadelle which influence couples' use of Jadelle. One male participant said that *his* **spouse** *had a problem of continuous menstruation week in week out without stopping*. Another male participant with a different experience reported that *the cessation of menstruation causes problems in his spouse such as noise from abdomen, her body becomes weak without strength and she suffers from other sicknesses*. Participants emphasized on the challenges they faced when using Jadelle. The following is a summary of views of two female participants: *Sometimes I miss my monthly periods for a month then the following month I could have it normally. A woman may have monthly period normally whilst to others they have continuous monthly period.*

3.7. Theme 7: Myths Associated with Jadelle

There are lots of myths associated with the use of implant Jadelle. There are misconceptions associated with insertion procedure or how Jadelle works in the body. Some women believe that the insertion of implants requires major surgery or that insertion is very painful and causes infection. Some male participants commented that *the things that they inserted have gone much deeper and after* 5 *years those things slowly come to the surface but at the moment it's impossible and if they remove it its effect will be there for* 5 *years because the contraception have already taken its root*. Some women believed that implants reduce a woman's libido or affect a couple's sexual life in some way. A female participant said that *the husband does not have desire*; *the woman has no desire because of Jadelle*. This view was supported by a male participant who said that *since my wife started using Jadelle I can go for a week without having any sexual desires and deep in my heart I have been thinking that this maybe happening because of the method of family planning we are practicing now*.

3.8. Theme 8: Attitudes of Providers of Jadelle

The findings of this study revealed that some Jadelle users linked their choice to the attitudes of providers. One participant said that *I came here telling them that I want the Jadelle removed and they told me that it was impossible*. The attitudes of providers can influence a couple decide to use Jadelle or reject it. A male participant also connected attitude of providers to the choice of Jadelle. He said that *they did not assess her what they did was just insertion of Jadelle*. Some female participants emphasized that attitude of providers also play a decisive role in the choice of Jadelle. There is no pre-insertion counseling and potential disadvantages should be discussed. One female participant said that *women are not being taught well and most of them do not know the benefits of Jadelle*.

3.9. Theme 9: Role Played by Men Regarding Use of Jadelle

The findings of the study also looked at the role played by men regarding the use of Jadelle as a family planning method, in a society which is male dominated. The role of the male is very crucial in the use of contraceptive or the size of the family. A female participant who envisaged that said that *had it been that my husband is a trouble maker as of now the marriage could have not been still there. I considered the* 5 *years as a long period*. Men feel positive and wish to be involved in issues about contraceptive used by their partners, discussing contraceptive problems together and resolving the problems. One male participant supported this by saying that *most of the times a man is not realistic because he might use a condom when happy and the next day he changes and does not use a condom. This means that he has not followed properly the method of family planning*. He even went on to say that they should continue with the same method of family planning, Jadelle, until the time they make up their minds to have another child in future. Since women in the developing countries are either under collective decision making with their partners or completely rely on the male partners' decision on issues that affect their reproductive lives. A male participant said that *it is good that as a family we made a decision to choose this method of family planning which can go along with her body system and also people should have a right to decide the number of children to bear according to how they see their own family.*

4. Discussion

This study provided us with valuable information that couples have some knowledge about Jadelle although it is sometimes inadequate and at times inaccurate. They generally knew that Jadelle prevents pregnancy but they did not know its correct mode of action except for one woman. There is evidence that non-barrier method users are generally less knowledgeable about how their current contraceptive method works [13]. This is corroborated by Bogale and colleagues who found that many rural residents lacked knowledge of contraception's mode of action apart from knowing that it prevents pregnancy [14]. The lack of knowledge about mode of action of Jadelle may influence choices of family planning methods among men and women. It is evident that knowledge transfer about the mode of action of the chosen method improves efficiency and compliance to contraceptive method use [13]. As such it is important that family planning providers equip users of Jadelle with correct knowledge about its mode of action to promote effective use of Jadelle and consequently preventing unplanned and unwanted pregnancies.

Participants of this study appreciated the effectiveness of Jadelle as a family planning method in preventing pregnancy. This result is similar to Power *et al.* [15] who found that women accepted Jadelle as a very effective contraceptive in the prevention of pregnancy when compared to other methods of contraception. This may be attributed to their knowledge about Jadelle. Having better knowledge about family planning methods is associated with decision making power of women to use contraceptives [14]. In this study, couples revealed that they get information about family planning methods from significant others, media and health talks. Nevertheless, men reported that they usually get information about Jadelle from their spouses. Dissimilar results were found in Korea where husbands were the major source of information regarding contraceptive issues [16]. This may be due to differences in culture and levels of male involvement in maternal and child health issues. In Malawi, most men do not attend antenatal and post natal clinics with their spouses where health talks on family planning are given [17]. This is in line with one of the findings of this study whereby unlike men, women mentioned health education at clinics as a source of information. For this reason, it is proper to encourage men to accompany their wives to antenatal, postnatal and family planning clinics so that they can both get correct information about Jadelle. It is evident that many women remembered education they received during antenatal and postnatal health talk and this promoted their utilization of family planning services [18]. Nonetheless, men find it difficult to attend antenatal clinic because it is feminine in nature [17]. Consequently, men do not have access to relevant information about Jadelle from professionals. There is need to de-feminise maternal health services and maternal health education must be given to men and women [17]. Therefore, every opportunity should be utilised at antenatal, postnatal and family planning clinics to teach individuals about family planning because if people accept the advice, they are likely to apply it to their own family [19].

This study also suggests the use of media to complement the dissemination of information about Jadelle to men and women. Radio was reported as one of the main sources of information among participants. There is evidence that media is the most common source of information about contraceptives [20]. Nurses and other health professionals are the least source of family planning information [21]. This is a great concern because nurses are the major contact persons for family planning clients. In this study it was clear that couples were not given adequate information during Pre-insertion and Post-insertion counselling of Jadelle. In addition participants felt that they were not adequately informed by health workers about side effects of Jadelle which caused some women to request removal of the implant. The low and poor contraceptive usage results from ineffective conveyance of relevant information to clients by health care workers [7]. Nurses are well placed to provide relevant information about family planning to people [20] they should intensify one-on-one counselling to all clients so that even illiterate individuals can have adequate information about Jadelle. Counselling is an important aspect in family planning because it allows women to make informed choices about contraceptive methods and ultimately influences their compliance [22].

Some women who participated in this study felt that use of Jadelle allowed them freedom and removed the burden of frequent hospital visits to obtain contraceptives. They were able to continue with their business freely because it has long lasting effectiveness. It is evident that women perceive that using contraceptives allows them to take better care of themselves and their family [23] because implants are long acting contraceptives with a high efficacy rate over a 5 years period after insertion [24]. The use of Jadelle has a potential to decrease maternal mortality [25] and its use must be promoted in Malawi where the maternal mortality rate is very high. However, it was clear that some men who participated in this study were not comfortable with the side effects of Jadelle such as menstrual irregularities experienced by their spouses. These men advised their wives to change the method because they felt that the wife was losing too much blood. On the contrary other men perceived that Jadelle did not cause any side effects which were caused by other contraceptives in their wives. This implies that past experiences influence their choice of Jadelle. People do not consider other contraceptives because they have tried them before [26]. Furthermore, myths and misinformation discouraged use of Jadelle among couples in this study. For instance, one female participant reported that if a man sleeps with a woman who is on contraceptives, the power of the contraceptive makes the man weak and loses his sexual power. This is consistent with Okanlawon and colleagues who found that respondents in their study believed that contraceptives are harmful, dangerous and can cause damage to the reproductive system [27]. It is worrisome because Jadelle is not commonly chosen due to inadequate information, possible misinformation and side effects [21]. As such, it is important that couples are provided with correct information if they are going to choose Jadelle.

Participants indicated that the most common side effect of Jadelle that affects them is the disruption of the menstrual cycle such as prolonged menses. Some women are unwilling to use contraceptives due to fear of side effects [28]. It is evident that excessive vaginal bleeding and weight gain are some of the reasons for discontinuation of Jadelle use [26] [29]. Couples should be given adequate information about side effects and benefits of Jadelle so that they are motivated to utilise it. In addition, family planning providers should effectively assist women who are experiencing side effects so that they can continue using Jadelle. Men usually get irritated with prolonged menstruation which occurs in women using Jadelle because in Malawi culture does allow a man to have sex with a woman who is menstruating [3]. Apart from the side effects, this study also revealed that poverty influences the couples' choices on the use of Jadelle because many people in the rural areas cannot afford to pay for transport to attend family planning clinics. Lack of money is a barrier to contraceptive access and use [30]. In a similar study that was conducted by Okanlawon *et al.* respondents indicated that they experienced difficulties in gaining access to the family planning clinics due to transportation cost and distance [27]. As such efforts must be made to bring family planning services closer to poor communities so that there is improved accessibility of Jadelle. It is clear that women cannot always access Jadelle in many rural health centres in Malawi and this limits the couples' options to choose from.

Participants in the study revealed that the attitudes of individuals towards contraceptives influence their choices. For instance, men demonstrated positive attitudes towards Jadelle as a family planning method. It is evident that men's general attitudes concerning the ideal family size influence women's preferences and opinions [31]. The attitudes of men towards Jadelle may stem from their cultural beliefs. For example, male partners would not want to stop having children if their wives were having only girl children because of the cultural value placed on male offspring and patrilineal heritage [32]. The attitudes of family planning providers also matter because they can serve as motivators or barriers to use of contraceptives among couples. In this study, a participant complained that she was denied the removal of Jadelle when she wanted it removed and this nearly put her marriage in jeopardy. It is necessary that family planning providers should demonstrate positive attitudes because their negative attitudes maybe a barrier to contraceptives utilization [33].

This study provided vital information about participants' decision making regarding contraceptive use. It was clear from the findings that both men and women make decisions on the use of Jadelle as a family planning method. Nonetheless it is evident that men are main decision makers in most African countries such as Malawi and should be involved in prevention of unplanned and unwanted pregnancies [20] [34]. Male involvement in family planning increases uptake of contraceptives [34]. Conversely, men are usually left out when decisions about reproductive health issues are discussed [19]. This may have a negative impact on women's decision to use contraceptives. Sometimes women fail to use contraceptives because of rejection by their spouses [19]. It is important that women in Malawi are empowered to make their own decisions on use of contraceptives. Women who have adequate knowledge about contraceptives have better decision making power about family planning [14]. Thus women should be empowered by providing them with accurate information about contraceptive methods so that they are able to make informed choices. It is encouraging that some men who participated in this study were involved in making decisions about family planning issues. It is evident that men want to be involved in open discussion about types of contraceptives used by their partners, their side effects and playing a role in resolving problems arising from contraceptive failures [20].

5. Conclusion

In conclusion, this study found that both men and women generally lacked knowledge about the mode of action of Jadelle as a family planning method. They reported that their main sources of information about family planning methods were significant others, media and health talks. Nonetheless, every opportunity should be utilised at antenatal, postnatal and family planning clinics to teach individuals about family planning. Further to that they must be given adequate information during pre-insertion and post-insertion counselling which might in turn increase utilisation of the implant Jadelle. As such family planning providers should intensify one-on-one counselling to all the family planning clients to ensure that even the women and men can have clear and adequate information about Jadelle. This may allow women and men to make informed choices about the use of Jadelle.

Acknowledgements

We are grateful to all couples who took part in this study.

References

[1] National Statistical Office (NSO) and ICF Macro (2011) Malawi Demographic Health Survey 2010. NSO, Zomba, ICF Macro, Calverton.

[2] Quinn, H. and Le May, A. (2008) Introducing the Contraceptive Sino Implant II (Zarin) in Sierra Leone. Marie Stopes International, London.
https://www.k4health.org/sites/default/files/Introducing%20the%20Contraceptive%20Impant%20to%20Sierra%20Leone%20finalDraft%20HQ.pdf

[3] Chipetal, E.K., Chimwaza, W. and Kalilani-Phiri, L. (2010) Contraceptive Knowledge, Beliefs and Attitudes in Rural Malawi: Misinformation, Misbeliefs and Misperceptions. *Malawi Medical Journal*, **22**, 38-41.
http://dx.doi.org/10.4314/mmj.v22i2.58790

[4] Nyanzi, S., Nyanzi, B. and Kalina, B. (2005) Contemporary Myths, Sexuality Misconceptions, Information Sources, and Risk Perceptions of *Bodabodamen* in Southwest Uganda. *Sex Roles*, **52**, 111-119.
http://dx.doi.org/10.1007/s11199-005-1198-3

[5] Wang, X., Chen, C., Wang, L., Chen, D., Guang, W. and French, J. (2003) Conception, Early Pregnancy Loss, and Time to Clinical Pregnancy: A Population-Based Prospective Study. *Fertility and Sterility*, **79**, 577-584.
http://dx.doi.org/10.1016/S0015-0282(02)04694-0

[6] World Health Organization (2007) Unsafe Abortion: Global and Regional Estimates of Incidence of Unsafe Abortion and Associated Mortality in 2003. 5th Edition, World Health Organization, Geneva.

[7] Omo-Aghoja, L.O., Omo-Aghoja, V.W., Aghoja, C.O., Okonofua, F.E., Aghedo, O., Umueri, C., Otayohwo, R., Feyi-Waboso, P., Onowhakpor, E.A. and Inikori, K.A. (2009) Factors Associated with the Knowledge, Practice and Perceptions of Contraception in Rural Southern Nigeria. *African Journal of Reproductive Health*, **15**, 135.

[8] Khunga, S. and Lupick, T. (2011) Malawi: Unsafe Abortions Lead Cause of Maternal Death. *Daily Times*, **5**, 12.

[9] Futures, C. (2008) Analysis of the Operational Policy Barriers to Financing and Procuring Contraceptives in Malawi. Health Policy Initiative, USAID.

[10] Levy, J. (2008) Reaching the Goals of Cairo: Male-Involvement in Family Planning (Carolina Papers on International Health No. 28). Center for Global Initiatives, NC: UNC Global.

[11] Ministry of Health (MOH) (2009) National Sexual and Reproductive Health and Rights Policy. Ministry of Health, Lilongwe.

[12] Munhall, P.L. (2007) Nursing Research: A Qualitative Perspective. 4th Edition, Jones & Bartlett Publishers, Boston.

[13] Topsever, P., Alvur, T.M., Aladağ, N., Topall, R., Ciğerli, O. and Görpelioğlu, S. (2006) Counselling and Knowledge about Contraceptive Mode of Action among Married Women; A Cross-Sectional Study. *BMC Women's Health*, **6**, 1-6.
http://dx.doi.org/10.1186/1472-6874-6-12

[14] Bogale, B., Wondafrash, M., Tilahum, T. and Girma, E. (2011) Married Women'S Decision Making Power on Modern Contraceptive Use in Urban and Rural Southern Ethiopia. *BioMed Central Public Health*, **11**, 42.
http://dx.doi.org/10.1186/1471-2458-11-342

[15] Power, J., French, R. and Cowan, F.M. (2012) Subdermal Implantable Contraceptives versus other Forms of Reversi-

ble Contraceptives or other Implants as Effective Methods for Preventing Pregnancy (Review). http://onlinelibrary.wiley.com/doi/10.1002/14651858.CD001326.pub2/pdf

[16] Wiebe, E.R., Henderson, A., Joyce Choic, J. and Trouton, K. (2006) Ethnic Korean Women'S Perceptions about Birth Control. *Contraception*, **73**, 623-627. http://dx.doi.org/10.1016/j.contraception.2006.02.001

[17] Kululanga, L.I., Sundby, J., Malata, A. and Chirwa, E. (2012) Male Involvement in Maternity Health Care in Malawi. *African Journal of Reproductive Health*, **16**, 145-157.

[18] Duong, D.V., Lee, A.H. and Binns, C.W. (2005) Contraception within Six Month Postpartum in Rural Vietnam: Implications on Family Planning and Maternity Services. *European Journal of Contraception and Reproductive Health Care*, **10**, 111-118. http://dx.doi.org/10.1080/13625180500131527

[19] Ikechebelu, J.I., Joe-Ikechebelu, N.N. and Obiajulu, F.N. (2005) Knowledge, Attitude and Practice of Family Planning among Igbo Women of South-Eastern Nigeria. *Journal of Obstetrics and Gynaecology*, **25**, 792-795. http://dx.doi.org/10.1080/01443610500328231

[20] Maja, T.M. (2007) Involvement of Males in Promoting Reproductive Health. *Curationis*, **30**, 71-76. http://dx.doi.org/10.4102/curationis.v30i1.1054

[21] Monjok, E.E., Smesny, A., Ekabua, J.E. and Essien, E.J. (2010) Contraceptive Practices in Nigeria: Literature Review and Recommendation for Future Policy Decisions. *Open Access Journal of Contraception*, **1**, 9-22. http://dx.doi.org/10.2147/OAJC.S9281

[22] Cremer, M., Ditzian, L., April, A., Peralta, B., Klausner, D., Podolsky, R. and Dierking, E. (2011) Depot-Medroxyprogesterone Acetate Contraception Use among Salvadoran Women: An In-Depth Analysis of Attitudes and Experiences. *Journal of Women's Health*, **20**, 1751-1756. http://dx.doi.org/10.1089/jwh.2010.2264

[23] Frost, J.J. and Lindberg, L.D. (2012) Reasons for Using Contraception: Perspectives of US Women Seeking Care at Specialized Family Planning Clinics. *Contraception*, **87**, 465-472. http://dx.doi.org/10.1016/j.contraception.2012.08.012

[24] Ladipo, O.A. and Akinso, S.A. (2005) Contraceptive Implants. *African Journal of Reproductive Health*, **9**, 16-23. http://dx.doi.org/10.2307/3583156

[25] Stover, J. and Ross, J. (2010) How Increased Contraceptive Use Has Reduced Maternal Mortality. *Maternal Child Health Journal*, **14**, 687-695. http://dx.doi.org/10.1007/s10995-009-0505-y

[26] Kane, R., Brown, S., Parkes, N., Walling, M. and Kallick, S. (2009) Long Acting, Reversible and Permanent Methods of Contraception: Insight into Women's Choice of Method. *Quality in Primary Care*, **17**, 107-14.

[27] Okanlawon, K., Reeves, M. and Agbaje, O.F. (2010) Contraceptive Use: Knowledge, Perceptions and Attitudes of Refugee Youths in Oru Refugee Camp, Nigeria. *African Journal of Reproductive Health*, **14**, 17.

[28] Krakowiak-Redd, D., Ansong, D., Otupiri, D., Tran, S., Klanderud, D., Boakye, I., Dickerson, T. and Crookston, B. (2011) Family Planning in a Sub-District Near Kumasi, Ghana: Side Effect Fears, Unintended Pregnancies and Misuse of a Medication as Emergency Contraception. *African Journal of Reproductive Health*, **15**, 135

[29] French, K. (2009) Long-Acting Reversible Contraceptive. *Primary Health Care*, **19**, 40-46. http://dx.doi.org/10.7748/phc2009.05.19.4.40.c7029

[30] Haider, S., Todd, C., Ahmadzai, M., Rahimi, S., Azfar. P., Morris, J.L. and Miller, S. (2009) Childbearing and Contraceptive Decision Making amongst Afghan Men and Women: A Qualitative Analysis. *Health Care for Women International*, **30**, 935-953. http://dx.doi.org/10.1080/07399330903052129

[31] Ijadunola, M.Y., Abiona, T.C., Ijadunola, K.T., Afolabi, O.T., Esimai, O.A. and OlaOlorun, F.M. (2010) Male Involvement in Family Planning Decision Making in Ile-Ife, Osun State, Nigeria African. *Journal of Reproductive Health*, **14**, 45

[32] Imbuki, K., Todd, C.S., Stibich, M.A., Shaffer, D.N. and Sinei, S.K. (2010) Factors Influencing Contraceptive Choice and Discontinuation among HIV-Positive Women in Kericho, Kenya. *African Journal of Reproductive Health*, **14**, 98-109.

[33] Tilahun, M., Mengistie, B., Egata, G. and Reda, A.A. (2012) Health Workers' Attitudes toward Sexual and Reproductive Health Services for Unmarried Adolescents in Ethiopia. *Reproductive Health*, **9**, 19. http://dx.doi.org/10.1186/1742-4755-9-19

[34] Shattuck, D., Kemer, B., Gilles, K., Hartmann, M., Ng'ombe, T. and Guest, G. (2011) Encouraging Contraceptive Uptake by Motivating Men to Communicate about Family Planning: The Malawi Male Motivator Project. *American Journal of public health*, **101**, 12-18. http://dx.doi.org/10.2105/ajph.2010.300091

14

Patients' Perspectives on Pre-Operative Education for Total Hip Replacement

Yi-Li Ko[1], Wei-En Chu[2], Pi-Chu Lin[3*]

[1]Department of Nursing, College of Medicine, Fu Jen Catholic University, Taiwan
[2]Nurse, Kaohsiung Veterans General Hospital, Taiwan
[3]School of Nursing and Master Program in Long-Term Care, College of Nursing, Taipei Medical University, Taiwan
Email: *pclin02@gmail.com

Abstract

The purpose of this qualitative research was to explore subjective experiences related to pre-operative patient education experience with total hip replacement (THR). Semi-structured, in depth interviews were used to collect data. Eleven participants aged 44 to 76 were recruited. Data were analyzed using a constant comparative method. Three categories emerged from interview data. 1) Obedience professions' knowledge: trust professions' authority, synchronization with instruction and satisfy information; 2) Worries restrict mobility and lose job: post-op activities changes and impact on daily work; 3) Information wanted by personal preference: motivation differently. Hopefully insights on pre-operative education to THR patients experience will provide valuable references for application in teaching materials for orthotics' nurse to improve THR care.

Keywords

Total Hip Replacement, Patient Education, Qualitative Study

1. Introduction

In parallel with the increasing number of older people in Taiwan, the proportion of individuals with osteoarthritis is increasing. Severed osteoarthritis caused pain and disability posing a heavy burden on the patient. Total Hip Replacement (THR) is an effective way to solve severe osteoarthritis [1] [2]. As a THR patient hospitalized 5 - 7 days and has paid by Taiwan National Health Insurance according to the Diagnosis related groups (DRG) system. Most of the patients are in hospital at the day before the operation. Only half a day limit time have to implement the whole pre-operative preparation, including the patient education. This is a big challenge to nurse staff through Taiwan surgical ward workload which is rapidly and routinely patient education. Little is known

*Corresponding author.

about patients' real preference of THR patient education under this urgent rhythm. Especially late middle age group/young elderly group, who face to this surgery risk often worry disability postoperatively. Therefore, the purpose of this study is to realize THR patients' views about subjective experience, education content and process. Through this study, we hope that we can realize patients' feelings to education, and then distinguish patients' education needs; moreover, become reference of patient-centered education intervention in the future.

1.1. THR Patient's Physiological and Psychological Distress

THR patient is defined as one who is admitted for received an elective surgery hospitalized 5 - 7 days but requires several months' rehabilitation for recovery. Under this surgical treatment and then is the main purpose is to decrease joint pain and improve joint function [3]. Patients' diagnosis with hip osteoarthritis, rheumatoid arthritis and femoral head osteonecrosis will receive THR. Following new analgesics developed and arthritis patients' pain could get more relieved. However, THR surgery is still the terminal step to solve their pain. Although the successful rate of operation is more than 90%, patients still need to face problem including operative risk, complications, post-operative care and rehabilitation. Therefore, patients need to know more about the operation and its influence to the future [4].

Studies showed patients who just hospitalized will feel stress because of the change of living environment, threated by uncertainty of the disease, unknown to medical terminology, endured pain from examination and treatment, and worried about family or friends' response. They were even high anxiety before the operation [5] [6]. Scholar indicated that patients' fear of pre-operation and disease could induce high anxiety. Lue, Chang, Liu, Chen and Lu [7] investigated knee and hip replacement patients' anxiety degree and found that 31.33% of the patients have mild anxiety; 10.81% of the patients have moderate to high anxiety. Patients worried about including safety of anesthesia, success rate of the operation, complications, mortality, how long can awake after operation, wound pain, discomfort, post-operation physical function, rehabilitation time, when can walk and independent self-care, and recover level etc. If they adjusted inadequately, it will cause negative impact on their health [8].

Meanwhile, every patient had different anxiety level. Peoples' anxiety level will influence by their past experience and preconceptions experience. Non-experienced and negative-previous experience patients had higher pre-operative anxiety. Younger, female and lower education level had higher anxiety [9]. Female patients worry about postanesthesia can not awake, and male patients worry about pain [6]. Every patient has its individuality and different afraid item. Therefore, individual assessment is necessary before operation. As what is concluded from the above, nurses need to face many challenges when provide emotional care for pre-operative patients.

Not only based on the medical treatment but also humanity caring, nurses hope to help patient recovered from operation fast and safe. Joint replacement patients need to actively participate in pain control, rehabilitation and daily care [10]. The pre-operative education is an important part of operation; it can enhance patient's knowledge about operation and their compliance. Pre-operative patients with psychologically distress will have more pain complaint and lower satisfaction level [9]. So be careful to manage patients' psychological distress is very important.

1.2. Education for THR Patient

Recently, inform pre-operative patient that they have the right to know is taken seriously. Under the pressure of hospital administrator, nurses explain the purpose and risk of the operation, routine process, the situation they may face and future management at a day before operation or the operation day. Let patient receive huge information in one time [11]. According to American Association of Orthopedic Surgeons (AAOS), patients' education should include knowledge about operation and rehabilitation, sign of pulmonary embolism (such as shorten breath, tachycardia, anxiety, chest pain, hemoptysis, hypotension and dizziness) and deep vein thrombosis [4]. Taiwan scholars suggested hip replacement education should include operating leg correct positioning, turning, ambulation, rehabilitation, walker or crutches using, self-care and home care [12] [13].

2. Methodology

The study consisted of 11 qualitative interviews of THR preoperative hospitalized patients at one medical center in northern Taiwan. All patients were informed about the study verbally by the researcher. After giving their written consent, the patients were guided to the meeting room of the ward. Exclusion criteria were difficulties in speaking and understanding the Mandarin Chinese and obvious dementia.

Based on the authors' clinical experience and previous study, a semi-structured interview guide was constructed before the study [14]. The guide was tested on one THR patient and then revised slightly. The guide was then reviewed by a group of researchers with interviewing experience (**Table 1**). Eleven of the interviews were done by the third author who has been working as an orthopedics nursing clinical supervisor for about 20 years. Each interview took about 30 - 40 min. Interviews were tape-recoded. Demographic data and diseases information and past operative experience were collected from the patient records.

2.1. Analysis

Data were analyzed using qualitative content analysis as described by scholars [15]. First, the recorded tapes were repeatedly listened to and all the interview records were read through in order to get an overall sense of the patients' views. Next, the verbatim data were read line-by-line in order to identify statements related to THR. These statements were marked, and tentative codes were written in the margin for the detection of emerging patterns. Differences and similarities among codes were compared, and codes that were similar in content were subsequently grouped and classified into various categories.

2.2. Trustworthiness

To validate the results, responses to questions were further probed several times during the interview, to gain deeper understanding. Coding and development of the categories were done by the first author. The third author read all the condensed units of meaning and also questioned the preliminary analysis. After 11 interviews, no new categories or subcategories were developed, and then stop collected. The third author has been working as an orthopedics nursing clinical supervisor for about 20 years and the first author is a senior researcher in nursing.

2.3. Ethical Considerations

Ethical considerations were observed according to the recommendations of Helsinki declaration, as suggested by Wilkie [16]. This study has been approved by the Institutional Review Board of the hospital where the study was conducted (IRB No: 93-11-08A).

3. Findings

A total of 11 THR patients were interviewed in the ward. The patients were between 44 and 66 years of age. The average age was 58.5 years; most of their marital status was married; most of their education level was elementary school. All patients had operation experience before. More demographic data can be found in **Table 2**.

Three major categories emerged from the participants' experience with THR patient education. First category is "Obedience professions' knowledge". This category comprised three subcategories: believe in physicians' authoritative, passive learning and accept the fate. Second category is "Worries to mobilized and lose the job". This category comprised two subcategories: post-op activities changes and impact on daily work. Third category is "Information wanted by personal preference". This category comprised one subcategory: Learning motivation individual differently. The following are the findings of the categories and subcategories (**Table 3**):

Table 1. Interview guide.

After welcome and introduction of researcher:
Have you had surgery experience before?
Do you feel anxiety about the THR surgery? If do, what strategy have you done to adjust this anxiety?
Please describe what kind of the THR education nurse gave to you in the ward and THR education means to you?
Did you feel current THR patient education is effective?
Did you satisfy current THR patient education arranged? Did it (THR patient education) reach your individual needs?

Table 2. Demographic data.

Patient no.	Age	Gender	Marital status	Educational level	Primary Diagnosis	Past operative experience
C1	47	Male	Married	College	R't THR Loosening	Yes
C2	53	Male	Married	College	P't FNF s/p pinning loss of reduction	Yes
C3	63	Female	Married	Elementary school	L't THA Loosening	Yes
C4	51	Female	Married	Elementary school	L't OA hip	Yes
C5	60	Female	Married	Elementary school	L't OA hip	Yes
C6	49	Female	Married	Senior high school	R't INFH	Yes
C7	76	Male	Married	Elementary school	R't INFH	Yes
C8	74	Female	Married	Senior high school	L't OA hip	Yes
C9	50	Male	Divorced		L't AS hip	Yes
C10	76	Female	Widowed	Elementary school	Bil OA hip	Yes
C11	44	Male	Married		Bil INFH	Yes

Table 3. The category and subcategory of nursing education for pre-op THR patient.

Category	Subcategory
Obedience professions' knowledge	1. trust professions' authority 2. synchronization with instruction 3. felt satisfy information
Worries restrict mobility and lose job	1. post-op activities changes 2. impact on daily work
Information wanted by personal preference	1. motivation differently

3.1. Obedience Professions' Knowledge

3.1.1. Trust Professions' Authority

Ask around who is the best/famous doctor, wandering on the hospitals searching for second opinion, ask physicians with different treatment strategies, and feel secure more to be educated by physicians. As a case (C5) said: "*I have a friend had a same problem. She told me which doctor is the best. Well, we are business people, so we had heard much information related to the plans to solve THR.*" Other case (C2) said: "*I prefer doctor do the THR education for me or let me participate my education process. If so, I feel it is more effective and give me confidence.* Another case (C7) said: "*I trust on Director Chen, I felt proud that he did the operation for me.*"

3.1.2. Synchronization with Instruction

Patients' education needs were just part of patient role obligation in Taiwan. Generally, patients didn't want to get more information and not used to questioning. They expressed lower desire to get more THR information from their physicians or nurses. On the other side, because of heavy working load (average take care of 8 patients/dayshift), nurses just want to finish THR education in the admission as soon as possible. Thus, patients' THR individual education needs are easy to be neglected consequently. If the doctor as a case (C10) said: "*What is THR education? Oh, I know! It is just a piece of paper that a physician (or a nurse) gave me at outpatient clinic.*"

3.1.3. Felt Satisfy Information

Influence by Confucianism and Moderation thinking, Taiwanese adapt themselves to circumstances. This view also reflects on their disease experience. Patients pleased with the information which enables them to understand the disease, as patients, not to ask questions too much. As (C4) said: "*I have seen the education pamphlet. I de-*

liver my body and disease to the institution (hospital and doctors). It is a nature thing; I didn't understand the disease, though I didn't dare to ask."

3.2. Worries Restrict Mobility and Lose Job

Patients afraid that physical activity will be affected after operation. In addition, they worry about lose job and not qualified the job requirement they used to be.

3.2.1. Post-Op Activities Changes

Some cases mentioned about activities changes after THR surgery. A case (C2) asked some questions about activity, sex life and diet: "*What kind of position should I avoid? Should I avoid moving heavy objects? How long should I stop intercourse?*" "*What nourishment, as calcium, should I intake?*" "*Like my case, put bone nail into the leg will it take more time to recover?*" Another case (C4) said: "*Crutch is necessary for months after joint replacement. After that, can I walk without assistive devices?*"

3.2.2. Impact on Occupation

After THR operation, patients need to take sick leave for a period of time. Thus, some patients worked in private company worry about their job can't maintain. As a case (C1) work in service industry said: "*I work at a private company, they don't allow me to take sick leave too long. Everybody has different work content. If I took three month off, others have to cover my works. Although they didn't mind it, I will still feel embarrassed.*" Another case (C7) worry that taken too many days off will affect their career "*The rehabilitation took too long, that was very inconvenient*". An advertising company employee (C7) said: "*I got laid off, so I came here had time do the THR. I will find a new job after THR recovery.*"

3.3. Information Wanted by Personal Preference

Motivation Differently

The depth of educational content depends on personal demand. Somebody felt scared if the image was too realistic; somebody wanted to know more, but somebody thought they won't understand so just asked their children to be educated. As a case said (C7): "*Handout is better because I forget the contents soon after I watched the education video.*" Another said (C9): "*I have an operation before and the THR educational content is similar.*" Despite repeat THR information provided, patients confirmed and accepted the education. As a case (C6) said: "*I knew more about it after I watched the video. I won't know it if I didn't watch it. This video can help me to be well prepared.*" Another said (C5): "*I think the education was clearly with that video. My family would also know how to take care of me if they watched it together.*" The other said (C8): "*Could you tell us whether the operation have some risks? Is it dangerous? What should I do before the operation? Could you please tell me more details after the operation?*" And case C8 said *he refuse to watch the video because he scared blooded and realistic images.* "*I thought I would see some operative images in the video.*"

4. Discussion

4.1. Obedience Professions' Knowledge

We found that the patients admire the hospital workers' authority with which it was not possible to argue or disagree. The patients believe the superior knowledge of health care professionals especially the doctor is a health team leader, which enhances patients' confidence. Edwards, Davies and Edwards [17] used meta-study approach to synthesis 7 studies. There were three themes of information exchange were found including non-empowered who non-user of information relies on doctor as ultimate information source; disempowered who healthcare practitioner regulated information, and empowered who patient-regulated information. Patients' motivation to seek information, the management of that information and its risks and information exchange in consultations can lead to empowerment. Our results are not quite the same with Edwards *et al.* [17] study. In present study, we found that patients only passively accept authoritative advice, they did not feel participation—but did not want to either. It may be patient with older age and the traditional Chinese character with more docile. However, patient empowerment is still the future direction to improve information exchange between patients with professionals.

4.2. Worries Restrict Mobility and Lose Job

After THR surgery, patients worry about mobility changed, similar as Japanese Scholar's study osteoarthritis patients after THR experience. In their study found that participants' anxiety was heightened around the time of discharge because of worries about dislocation and living at home with prosthesis [18]. The result of this study was similar with the previous results [19] [20]. Gustafsson, Ekman, Ponzer and Heikkilä [21] use phenomenology to interview 16 knee or hip replacement elderly people (above 65 years old). One of them said: "When I was young, I had been in hospital for a long time because of hip fracture. Maybe that's why now I feel more afraid of this hip replacement operation." Another also questioned about post-op life type: "Will I have more quality of life after THR? Can I do everything just like before?" It told that they worried whether they could have a regular life like before.

4.3. Information Wanted by Personal Preference

Most of the participants of this study were middle age and early elderly; this age group generation had lower learning motivation than younger. Thus, it seems possible that the preference of patients belongs to non-participant in THR education learning process. Little of patients can express preference of THR education. The study has investigated THR patients' perspectives of pre-operation THR education. It showed they did not clearly express their THR education needs. They want to be informed and listened to; they wanted to enjoy top-down communication with their health education providers. The result is similar with the previous study. Loft, Mc William, and Ward-Griffin [22] found five themes emerged centering on a strong desire to maintain independence through data analogist. Overall, participants experienced disempowered relationships with professional in-home care providers and a more equitable empowered relationship with nonprofessional care providers.

Limitation

This generalizability of these findings is limited by the small sample of subjects from only one medical centre in Taipei.

Further Research Suggestion

In future need to consideration the elderly THR education preference for participation in their hospital care. More research is needed to realize the elderly THR patients' needs. Hopefully to find a way that can take into both efficient and satisfy patients' individual needs.

Clinics should provide valuable THR information that fit the speed of orthopedic wards via pamphlet and/or audio-visual materials to increase THR knowledge and increase awareness of the THR education demands. And encourage patients to share THR successful experience and strengthen out-patient clinic THR education.

References

[1] Walker, J. (2012) Care of Patients Undergoing Joint Replacement. *Nursing Older People*, **24**, 14-20. http://dx.doi.org/10.7748/nop2012.02.24.1.14.c8898

[2] Yeh, M.L., Chen, X.X. and Liu, B.X. (2004) Hip Joint Replacement Nursing: Research and Test of Multimedia CD and Manual. *The Journal of Health Science*, **6**, 141-152.

[3] National Joint Registry (2009) NJR StatsOnline. http://www.njrcentre.org.uk/njrcentre/Healthcareproviders/Access-ingthedata/StatsOnline/NJRStatsOnline/tabid/179/Default.aspx

[4] Johansson, K., Katajisto, J. and Salanterä, S. (2010) Pre-Admission Education in Surgical Rheumatology Nursing: Towards Greater Patient Empowerment. *Journal of Clinical Nursing*, **19**, 2980-2988. http://dx.doi.org/10.1111/j.1365-2702.2010.03347.x

[5] Chang, J.P., Tsai, Y.F., Chen, Y.C. and Huang, S.L. (2002) Anxiety and Its Related Factors in Burn Patients. *Formosan Journal of Medicine*, **6**, 661-671.

[6] Walker, J.A. (2002) Emotional and Psychological Preoperative Preparation in Adults. *British Journal of Nursing*, **11**, 567-575. http://dx.doi.org/10.12968/bjon.2002.11.8.10166

[7] Lue, Y.J., Chang, J.K., Liu, M.F., Chen, S.M. and Lu, Y.M. (2003) Anxiety in Patients with Lower Extremity Arthroplasty. *Formosan Journal of Physical Therapy*, **28**, 317-323.

[8] Lam, E., Lee, M. Brull, R. and Wong, D.T. (2007) Effect of Anesthesia Consultation on Patients' Preoperative Concerns. *Canadian Journal of Anesthesia*, **54**, 852-853. http://dx.doi.org/10.1007/BF03021718

[9] Hossain, M., Parfitt, D.J., Beard, D.J., Darrah, C., Nolan, J., Murray, D.W. and Andrew, G. (2011) Does Pre-Operative Psychological Distress Affect Patient Satisfaction after Primary Total Hip Arthroplasty? *BMC Musculoskeletal Disorders*, **12**, 122. http://dx.doi.org/10.1186/1471-2474-12-122

[10] Parker, R.J. (2011) Evidence-Based Practice Caring for a Patient Undergoing Total Knee Arthroplasty. *Orthopaedic Nursing*, **30**, 4-8. http://dx.doi.org/10.1097/NOR.0b013e3182057451

[11] Weiner, B.K. and Essis, F.M. (2006) Patient Preferences Regarding Spine Surgical Decision Making. *Spine*, **31**, 2857-2860. http://dx.doi.org/10.1097/01.brs.0000245840.42669.f1

[12] Ding, Z.F., Zhou, X.L. and Chen, M.M. (2006) A Project to Provide Instruction in the Nursing of Elderly Patients with Total Hip Replacement. *The Journal of Nursing*, **53**, 36-45.

[13] Wu, H.F. and Lin, Q.Z. (2007) Nursing Experience in Caring a Systemic Lupus Erythematosus (SLE) Patient Undergoing Total Hip Replacement. *VGH Nursing*, **24**, 236-243.

[14] Chiang, H.M., Jou, H.J., Kao, C.H. and Tsao, L.I. (2009) Disturbance Experiences and Vaginal Symptom Self-Management among Menopausal Women. *The Journal of Nursing*, **56**, 43-51.

[15] Polit, D.F. and Beck, C.T. (2012) Nursing Research: Generating and Assessing Evidence for Nursing Practice. 9th Edition, Lippincott Williams & Wilkins, Philadelphia.

[16] Wilkie, P. (1997) Ethical Issues in Qualitative Research in Palliative Care. *Palliative Medicine*, **11**, 321-324. http://dx.doi.org/10.1177/026921639701100411

[17] Edwards, M., Davies, M. and Edwards, A. (2009) What Are the External Influences on Information Exchange and Shared Decision-Making in Healthcare Consultations: A Meta-Synthesis of the Literature. *Patient Education and Counseling*, **75**, 37-52. http://dx.doi.org/10.1016/j.pec.2008.09.025

[18] Fujita, K., Makimoto, K. and Hotokebuchi, T. (2006) Qualitative Study of Osteoarthritis Patients' Experience before and after Total Hip Arthroplasty in Japan. *Nursing & Health Sciences*, **8**, 81-87. http://dx.doi.org/10.1111/j.1442-2018.2006.00253.x

[19] Huang, G.J., Wu, X.C., Liang, J. and Tsai, G.Z. (2005) The Relation between Pre- and Postoperative Anxiety and Uncertainty in Orthopaedic Surgical Patients. *Taiwan Journal of Physical Medicine and Rehabilitation*, **33**, 1-10.

[20] Wei, Q.G., Qui, X.J., Yang, X.T., Chen, S.Z. and Ye, H.Y. (2006) The Effects Analysis of Intervention Programs for the Patient of Artificial Hip Joint Replacement. *Journal of Oriental Institute of Technology*, **26**, 241-250.

[21] Gustafsson, B.Å., Ekman, S.L., Ponzer, S. and Heikkilä, K. (2010) The Hip and Knee Replacement Operation: An Extensive Life Event. *Scandinavian Journal of Caring Sciences*, **24**, 663-670.

[22] Loft, M., McWilliam, C. and Ward-Griffin, C. (2003) Patient Empowerment after Total Hip and Knee Replacement. *Orthopaedic Nursing*, **22**, 42-47. http://dx.doi.org/10.1097/00006416-200301000-00012

15

The Impact of an eLearning Course on Nurses' Attitudes towards Mental Illness

Anneli Pitkänen[1], Raija Kontio[2,3], Mari Lahti[4,5], Jouko Katajisto[6], Maritta Välimäki[5,7]

[1]Tampere University Hospital, Tampere, Finland
[2]Helsinki University, Helsinki, Finland
[3]Department of Psychiatry, Helsinki University Hospital, Helsinki, Finland
[4]Turku University of Applied Science, Turku, Finland
[5]Department of Nursing Science, University of Turku, Turku, Finland
[6]Department of Statistics, University of Turku, Turku, Finland
[7]Turku University Hospital, Turku, Finland
Email: anneli.pitkanen@pshp.fi

Abstract

Patients with mental illness are stigmatized. Health care professionals may even perpetuate stigma towards mental illness. Thus it is important to ensure that health care professionals have positive attitudes towards patients with mental illness. The aim of this study was to estimate the impact of an eLearning course on psychiatric nurses' attitudes towards mental illness. A cluster-randomized trial (ISRCTN32869544) design was used. Twelve wards were randomly assigned to the eLearning course (ePsychNurse.Net) group or the education as a usual group. The participants (N = 228) were allocated to the intervention (n = 115) or control group (n = 113) according their baseline ward affiliation. Attitudes were rated according to the Community Attitude towards the Mentally Ill scale. Both groups were found to have positive, not stigmatized attitudes towards mental illness. No statistically significant changes were found at three-month or nine-month follow-up. It may be that by developing the ePsychNurse.Net course to include more material related to nurses' attitudes and as nurses become more familiar with eLearning, the course may be effective in shaping nurses' attitudes towards mental illness. On the other hand, our study's nine-month time span may have been too short to change nurses' attitudes.

Keywords

eLearning, Psychiatric Nursing, Cluster-Randomized Intervention Trial, Stigma

1. Introduction

In recent years, mental health has been recognized as a priority area in most European countries [1]. One key challenge on the political agenda is tackling stigma [2] [3]. Stigma of mental illness is a global problem which may lead to negative discrimination [4] [5] affects in many areas of life [1], such as health care services, housing, education, employment and social relationships [6]. It may also lead to poor quality of life for these people [5]. Moreover, stigma and discrimination against people with mental illness is the main obstacle to the development of mental health care [7]. It is important to ensure that mental health professionals have positive, not stigmatized attitudes towards patients with mental illness [8]. Nurses' positive attitudes may be defined as holding sympathetic and compassionate views towards people with mental illness and disagreeing with the view that those people are inferior or a threat to society and thus need to be excluded or coercively handed [9].

Nurses' positive attitudes are crucial since stigmatized attitudes can have serious implications for patients' recovery [8]. Earlier studies have shown that mental health nurses' attitudes towards mental illness differ across countries [9]. In general, nurses who work in mental health settings have largely positive attitudes towards mental illness [9] and more positive attitudes than general medical nurses [10]. However, stigmatized attitudes are not unknown among mental health professionals [8]. Some research findings indicate that nurses have more stigmatized attitudes towards mental illness than do psychiatrists or the general population [4]. Moreover they may even contribute to perpetuating stigma regarding mental illness [10].

Stigma may not only be seen in nurses' negative attitudes but can contribute to the abuse of human rights in institutions [3]. It is noteworthy that nurses' positive attitudes may reduce coercive interventions [11] since negative experience of discrimination may be related to prior coercive mental health service intervention [5]. Thus it is important to ensure that nurses have positive attitudes towards patients with mental illness. Vocational education may have a positive effect on nurses' attitudes and values in clinical work [12] [13].

This study is based on a large project conducted in six European countries and funded by the European Commission of Leonardo da Vinci (FI-06-B-F-PP-160701). The overall goal of the collaborative project was to ensure high quality, ethically appropriate and therapeutically effective interventions to enable nurses to manage distressed and disturbed patients on psychiatric wards. Based on this goal, an eLearning course (ePsychNurse.Net) was developed [14] since e-learning has been dramatically increased as a promising new method of delivering courses [15].

We have earlier reported findings from Finnish data related to how the ePsychNurse.Net course impacts on knowledge, attitudes towards seclusion and restraint, job satisfaction and general self-efficacy [16] [17], how nurses are able to transfer knowledge from e-learning course to their clinical practice [18] and how the course impacts on the rates and duration of seclusion and mechanical restraint [19]. The aim of this study was to explore the impact of the ePsychNurse.Net course on nurses' attitudes towards mental illness. The hypothesis was that nurses completing the ePsychNurse.Net course would have more positive attitudes towards mental illness.

2. Materials and Methods

2.1. Design

A multicentre randomized controlled open label design was used and the study protocol has been registered (ISRCTN32869544). The study was conducted according to CONSORT guidelines [20].

2.2. Study Setting, Recruitment and Participants

The study was conducted from January to November 2009 on twelve closed acute psychiatric wards in three hospitals in Southern Finland. There were 20 wards that met inclusion criteria: close acute inpatient ward, using restraint and seclusion, not involved same kind of research or developing project. Twelve wards applied to participate and were enrolled. Eligible participants were registered nurses working on the study wards for over three months, aged over 18 years, having a sufficient command of Finnish language, and being willing to participate. Participants' attitudes to mental illness were assessed two weeks before the intervention (baseline), as well as 3-month and 9-month follow-ups. **Figure 1** describes the flow of participants.

2.3. Interventions

The intervention was a three-month eLearning course ("ePsychNurse.Net") developed by collaborative work

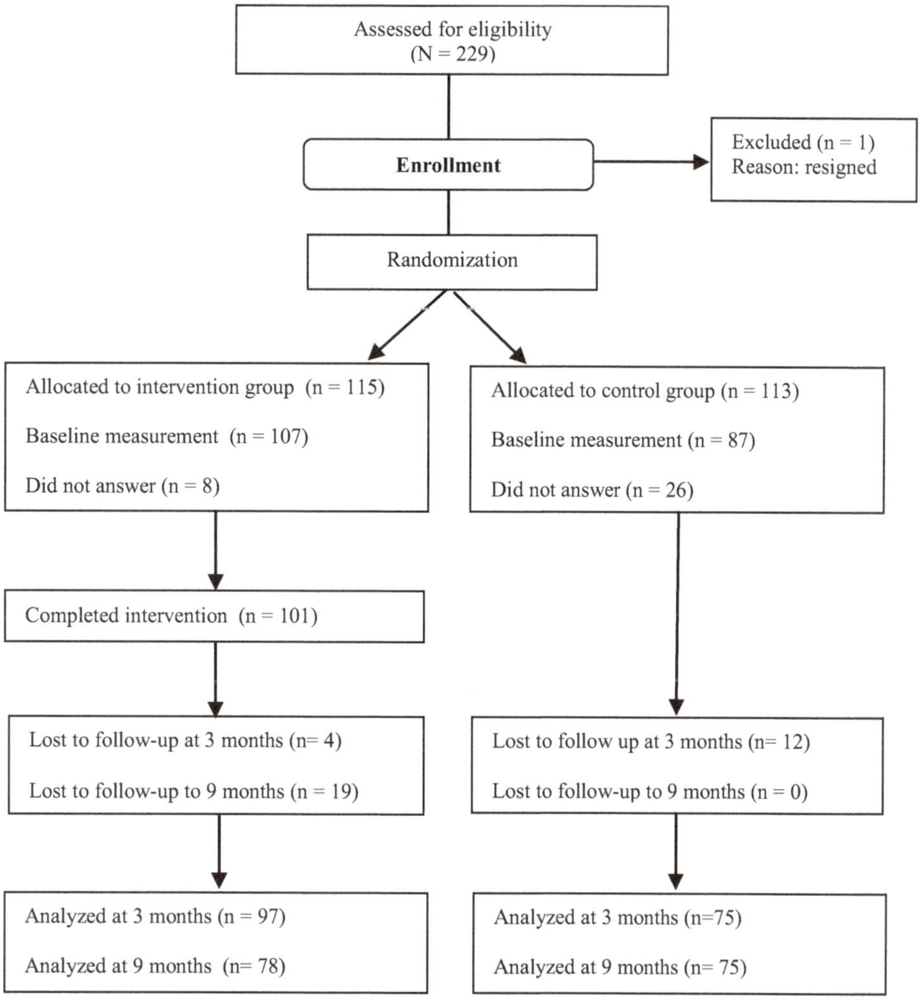

Figure 1. The participant flow diagram.

among experts in Finland, the UK, Ireland, Italy, Lithuania and Portugal in the ePsychNurse.Net project (2006-2008). Although the main aim of the course is to teach nurses to manage distressed and disturbed patients in psychiatric wards, the content of the course includes many elements related psychiatric nurses' attitudes towards mental illness since nurses' positive attitudes are important for treating these patients. The ePsychNurse.Net course cover specific learning methods and includes six modules: 1) legal and ethical issues; 2) behaviour-related factors; 3) therapeutic relationship; 4) self-awareness; 5) teamwork and 6) integrating knowledge with practice. The whole course took 120 h (40 h in working hours and the rest in own time) over three months. It was taken on module-by-module bases in pre-defined order. The main pedagogical approach involved reflective learning [21] because reflection can lead to positive outcomes in students' clinical practice and change their perceptions [22]; for example the self-awareness techniques to gain a more profound understanding of their personal habits and ways of behaving. Several learning methods were used: reading material, Power Point lectures, virtual patients' cases, discussion, online chat option with tutors, reflective writing and assignments. During the course the nurses were supervised by twelve trained tutors. The control group had continuing vocational education as usual. It included different topics of psychiatric care and was irregular and fragmental.

2.4. Outcome Measures

The Community Attitude towards the Mentally Ill (CAMI; [23] [24]) scale was used in this study. The instrument includes 40 items with four subscales: 1) Authoritarianism; 2) Benevolence; 3) Social restrictiveness and 4) Community mental health ideology. Authoritarianism refers to a view of mentally ill persons as someone inferior requiring coercive handling. Benevolence reflects a sympathetic view of those suffering from a mental illness. Social restrictiveness refers to the belief that the mentally ill patients are a threat to society. Community mental health ideology reflects acceptance of mental health services and mental ill patients in the community. Five-point Likert type responses are provided for each item ranging from "strongly agree" (1) to "strongly disagree" (5). Each subscale consists of 10 items, and five of these are reverse-coded. A mean score is calculated for each subscale. Higher scores on the authoritarianism subscale and on the Social Restrictiveness subscale reflect negative attitudes while higher scores on the Benevolence subscale and on the Community Mental Health Ideology subscale suggest a more positive view. The reliability of CAMI ranges from alpha 0.68 to 0.88 for different subscales and the scales correlate highly with each other [24]. Three items were modified to ensure that the language was gender neutral, but still ensuring that the original meaning was retained. CAMI was translated into Finnish according to standard procedures for the purposes of this study [25]. Although CAMI was developed to measure the general population's attitude towards community mental health facilities [23], it has been used during the past 30 years among a wide variety of participants and in a number of differing contexts [26]-[28] also among nurses in psychiatric settings [9] [29].

The background information included the nurses' gender, age, length of working experience in psychiatry, work position, continuing education received on mental health and coercion, and experiences of violence at work.

2.5. Randomization

The study wards were randomized by a coin to allocate them either to the ePsychNurse.Net group or to the training-as-usual group. After wards' randomization the participants (N = 228) were allocated to the intervention (n = 115) or control group (n = 113) according to their baseline ward affiliation. This study was conducted in a real-life clinical setting, therefore we could conceal allocation only until the start of the intervention. Participants and researchers could not be blinded.

2.6. Ethical Considerations

The study was evaluated by the local Ethics Committee (HUS 13.3.2007, §50) and authorized by the directors of the study organizations. It was emphasized that although every nurse in the study wards expected to participate the ePsychNurse.Net course, participation in the study was voluntary and refusal would not affect the working conditions. Data were treated in confidence [30].

2.7. Data Analysis

Sum variables according to theoretical categories were formed. These were obtained by adding up the coded answers and dividing the calculated sum by the number of variables so that the sum variables had the same scale as the individual items. Consequently, the range of the sum variables' was the same as in the original question. The four sum scales of CAMI were analysed and compared at different measuring points (baseline, 3-month and 9-month follow-up). Comparisons were conducted between the two groups for each measurement using two-sample t-test. Repeated measures analysis of variance and Bonferroni corrected contrasts were used to calculate significant changes between groups within time. A P-value of <0.05 was considered statistically significant. Analyses were performed with SPSS 16.0 software.

3. Results

3.1. Baseline Data

The CAMI was completed at baseline by 194 nurses (intervention group n = 107, control group n = 87). One hundred and six (55%) were female, average age was 43 years (range: 24 - 64, SD: 9.2) and working experience in psychiatry varied from one month to 37 years (mean: 15.6 years, SD: 9.3). Most of the participants were registered nurses (n = 116; 60%) or mental health nurses (n = 62; 32%). Sixty-seven percent (n = 122) had received continuing education in psychiatric nursing and 58% (n = 107) in coercion. Only one participant had no experiences of violence at work. There were no statistically significant differences in any characteristics, supporting the effectiveness of the random allocation.

3.2. Outcomes and Estimation

No statistically significant findings were found between the study groups. Only in social restrictiveness at baseline there was a statistically significant difference (p = 0.040) between the study groups (**Table 1**). Both groups were found to have positive attitudes towards mental illness. The control group had slightly more positive attitudes on all four sub-scales at all time-points.

Change in attitudes related to authoritarianism decreased slightly (−0.01) in the intervention group and increased (+0.03) in the control group during the nine months of follow-up. In benevolence both groups showed some decrease at nine months (intervention group −0.04, control group −0.02). Social restrictiveness increased in both groups (intervention group +0.03, control group +0.04). In community mental health ideology there was a slight decrease (−0.03) in the intervention group, while the control group rates were similar at baseline and at 9-month follow-up. In within-group analysis no statistically significant changes were found at three-month (p range from 0.577 to 1) or nine-month (p range from 0.361 to 0.952) follow-ups (**Table 1**).

4. Discussion

Our aim was to explore the impact of the ePsychNurse.Net course on nurses' attitudes related to mental illness. We found the nurses' attitudes in both study groups quite positive, but our hypothesis that nurses completing the ePsychNurse.Net course would have more positive attitudes towards mental illness than the control group was not upheld. In general, education has been shown to have some impact on nurses' attitudes [31] [32]. Our nurses' attitudes were already positive at baseline and this may be one reason why no statistically significant change occurred. Perhaps only a very potent training course would have the capacity to achieve a statistically significant change. On the other hand, reviews of the impacts of e-learning indicate that e-learning is not superior to traditional learning method when educating health care professionals [15] [33].

Change in attitudes is slow [34]. Thus, our study's nine-month time span may have been too short to internalize the new attitude. Moreover, the nurses in our study did not choose to attend the course because all nurses on the intervention wards were expected to take part in it which may have affected some nurses' motivation to study in the course and further to their learning outcomes. However, although the course was obligatory based on directors' decisions, the participation into the study was voluntary.

The lack of attitude change may also have been an expression of the inadequacy of the e-learning course. The e-learning course may be itself a rather new method. The use of eLearning may provoke ambivalence, negative perceptions [35] and some resistance [36]. This may be especially true in psychiatry, where information technologies are not yet as common as in other sectors [37]. Moreover, it has been argued that education alone is insufficient to change nurses' attitudes, especially in acute inpatient facilities [38] [39]. Thus it seems that ePsychNurse.Net alone is not enough to endure changes in staff attitudes but simultaneous use of other interventions is required.

Other research on this ePsychNurse.Net course found that the participating nurses would recommend it to other nurses. Moreover, they reported that knowledge gained during the course was transferrable to daily practice

Table 1. Impact of ePsychNurse.Net on nurses' attitudes towards mental illness.

	Baseline			3 months				9 months			
	Intervention group (n = 107) mean (SD)	Control group (n = 87) mean (SD)	p	Intervention group (n = 97) mean (SD)	Control group (n = 75) mean (SD)	p	Change baseline to 3-months p	Intervention group (n = 78) mean (SD)	Control group (n = 75) mean (SD)	p	Change baseline to 9-months p
Authoritarianism	2.19 (0.42)	2.08 (0.39)	0.055	2.20 (0.42)	2.08 (0.39)	0.113	0.717	2.18 (0.46)	2.11 (0.43)	0.348	0.850
Benevolence	3.94 (0.36)	3.96 (0.36)	0.595	3.89 (0.36)	3.94 (0.36)	0.370	0.577	3.92 (0.38)	3.94 (0.39)	0.716	0.361
Social restrictiveness	2.05 (0.47)	1.91 (0.45)	**0.040**	2.08 (0.46)	1.97 (0.51)	0.131	0.887	2.08 (0.52)	1.95 (0.50)	0.113	0.753
Community mental health ideology	3.69 (0.59)	3.77 (0.53)	0.318	3.66 (0.61)	3.78 (0.60)	0.194	1.000	3.66 (0.66)	3.77 (0.61)	0.277	0.952

and that the course gave them useful ideas for developing their daily work [18]. In future, in light of our results if the object is to improve the nurses attitudes towards mental illness, these different aspects should be focused on more comprehensively in the course. This is important since stigmatization of mental illness is a global problem [5], including psychiatric health care settings [10]. It is also important to note that professionals may be the perpetuators of stigma towards mental illness [10]. Educational interventions are important since although direct impacts on attitudes are not achieved an indirect impact might occur through increased skills to treat psychiatric patients [40]. The ePsychNurse.Net course offers a new educational intervention to be implemented internationally since the course was developed by collaborative work among experts from six European countries.

In interpreting the current results, there are some additional areas of consideration, including how attitudes were assessed, possible contamination bias and capacity of the intervention to change attitudes. First, it may be that the CAMI scale was not sensitive enough to show the attitudinal change. The fact is that the CAMI scale was originally developed to assess the general population's attitudes towards community mental health facilities [24], although it has been used with a wide variety of participants, including nurses in psychiatric settings [9] [30]. Moreover, Morris *et al.* [35] concluded that the validity of the CAMI scale for assessing psychiatric nurses' attitudes is not good. Second, in this study participants and researchers could not be blinded due to the nature of the intervention. Therefore we cannot ensure that no contamination occurred between the study groups. Third, the main aim of the ePsychNurse.Net course was not to change nurses' attitudes to be more positive towards mental illness but to teach nurses to manage distressed and disturbed patients in psychiatric hospitals. Although the ePsychNurse.Net course's modules includes elements related psychiatric nurses' attitudes towards mental illness the strength of the intervention to change nurses' attitudes seems to be too weak. On the other hand, nurses' positive attitudes towards mental illness are in a crucial role when managing distressed and disturbed patients. Thus it is important to explore the ePsychNurse.Net course's impact on nurses' attitudes. It may be that by developing the ePsychNurse.Net course to include more material related to nurses' attitudes towards mental illness the course may be more effective also to change nurses' attitudes.

5. Conclusion

Patients with mental illness are stigmatized and nurses may be the perpetuators of stigma. Thus there is a need to ensure that nurses' attitudes related mental illness are positive. One way to influence nurses' attitudes is education. The ePsychNurse.Net course, which was especially developed for nurses' vocational education on managing disturbed and aggressive psychiatric patients, was not found to be effective. However, it may be that by developing the ePsychNurse.Net course to include more material related to nurses' attitudes and as nurses become more familiar with eLearning, the course may be effective in shaping nurses' attitudes towards mental illness.

Acknowledgements

This study was financially supported by the European Commission (Leonardo da Vinci, FI-06B-F-PP-160701), Hospital District of Helsinki and Uusimaa, and Hyvinkää Hospital Region which are gratefully acknowledged. The authors also wish to acknowledge the contributions of nurses who have taken part in the study.

References

[1] WHO (2008) Policies and Practices for Mental Health in Europe—Meeting the challenges. World Health Organization, Regional Office for Europe, Copenhagen, Denmark. http://apps.who.int/iris/handle/10665/107366

[2] Department of Health (2009) New Horizons: A Shared Vision for Mental Health. Cross-Governments Strategy: Mental Health Division. London, UK. www.apho.org.uk/resource/item.aspx?RID=83954

[3] WHO (2005) Preparing Health Care Workforce for the 21st Century. The Challenge for Chronic Conditions. World Health Organization, Geneva, Switzerland. http://www.who.int/chp/knowledge/publications/workforce_report.pdf

[4] Schulze, B. (2007) Stigma and Mental Health Professionals: A Review of the Evidence on an Intricate Relationship. *International Review of Psychiatry*, **19**, 137-155. http://dx.doi.org/10.1080/09540260701278929

[5] Thornicroft, G., Brohan, E., Rose, D., Sartorius, N. and Leese, M. (2009) Global Pattern of Experienced and Anticipated Discrimination against People with Schizophrenia: A Cross-Sectional Survey. *The Lancet*, **373**, 408-415. http://dx.doi.org/10.1016/S0140-6736(08)61817-6

[6] Corrigan, P.W. and Larson, J.E. (2008) Stigma. In: Mueser, K.T. and Jeste, D.V., Eds., *Clinical Handbook of Schizophrenia*, The Guilford Press, New York, 533-540.

[7] Sartorius, N. (2007) Stigma and Mental Health. *The Lancet*, **370**, 810-811. http://dx.doi.org/10.1016/S0140-6736(07)61245-8

[8] Horsfall, J., Cleary, M. and Hunt, G.E. (2010) Stigma in Mental Health: Clients and Professional. *Issues in Mental Health Nursing*, **31**, 450-455. http://dx.doi.org/10.3109/01612840903537167

[9] Chambers, M., Guise, V., Välimäki, M., Botelho, M.A., Scott, A., Staniuliene, V. and Zanotti, R. (2010) Nurses' Attitudes to Mental Illness: A Comparison of a Sample of Nurses from Five European Countries. *International Journal of Nursing Studies*, **47**, 350-362. http://dx.doi.org/10.1016/j.ijnurstu.2009.08.008

[10] Ross, C.A. and Goldner, E.M. (2009) Stigma, Negative Attitudes and Discrimination towards Mental Illness within the Nursing Profession: A Review of the Literature. *Journal of Psychiatric and Mental Health Nursing*, **16**, 558-567. http://dx.doi.org/10.1111/j.1365-2850.2009.01399.x

[11] Bak, J., Brandt-Christensen, M., Sestoft, D.M. and Zoffmann, V. (2012) Mechanical Restraint—Which Interventions Prevent Episodes of Mechanical Restraint?—A Systematic Review. *Perspectives in Psychiatric Care*, **48**, 83-94. http://dx.doi.org/10.1111/j.1744-6163.2011.00307.x

[12] Epstein, R. and Hundert, E. (2002) Defining and Assessing Professional Competence. *JAMA*, **287**, 226-235. http://dx.doi.org/10.1001/jama.287.2.226

[13] Reed, F. and Fitzgerald, L. (2005) The Mixed Attitudes of Nurse's to Caring for People with Mental Illness in a Rural General Hospital. *International Journal of Mental Health Nursing*, **14**, 249-257. http://dx.doi.org/10.1111/j.1440-0979.2005.00389.x

[14] Välimäki, M., Scott, A., Lahti, M. and Chambers, M. (Eds.) (2008) The Changing Face of Psychiatric Nursing—Care or Control? ePsychNurse.Net. towards Improved Quality—Improving Nurses' Continuing Vocational Training in Psychiatric Hospitals and Inpatient Units. University of Turku, Turku.

[15] Cook, D., Levinson, A. and Garside, S. (2008) Internet-Based Learning in the Health Professions: A Meta-Analysis. *JAMA*, **30**, 1181-1196. http://dx.doi.org/10.1001/jama.300.10.1181

[16] Kontio, R., Lahti, M., Pitkänen, A., Joffe, G., Putkonen, H., Hätönen, H., Katajisto, J. and Välimäki, M. (2011) Impact of eLearning Course on Nurses' Professional Competence in Seclusion and Restraint Practices: A Randomized Controlled Study (ISRCTN32869544). *Journal of Psychiatric and Mental Health Nursing*, **18**, 813-821. http://dx.doi.org/10.1111/j.1365-2850.2011.01729.x

[17] Kontio, R., Hätönen, H., Joffe, G., Pitkänen, A., Lahti, M. and Välimäki, M. (2013) Impact of eLearning Course on Nurses' Professional Competence in Seclusion and Restraint Practices: A 9-Month Follow-Up Results of a Randomized Controlled Study (ISRCTN32869544). *Journal of Psychiatric and Mental Health Nursing*, **20**, 411-418. http://dx.doi.org/10.1111/j.1365-2850.2012.01933.x

[18] Lahti, M., Kontio, R., Pitkänen, A. and Välimäki, M. (2014) Knowledge Transfer from an E-Learning Course to Clinical Practice. *Nurse Education Today*, **34**, 842-847. http://dx.doi.org/10.1016/j.nedt.2013.09.003

[19] Kontio, R., Pitkänen, A., Joffe, G., Katajisto, J. and Välimäki, M. (2014) eLearning Course May Shorten the Duration of Mechanical Restraint among Psychiatric Inpatients: A Cluster-Randomized Trial. *Nordic Journal of Psychiatry*, **68**, 443-449. http://dx.doi.org/10.3109/08039488.2013.855254

[20] Schulz, K., Altman, O. and Moher, D. (2010) CONSORT 2010 Statement: Updated Guidelines for Reporting Parallel Group Randomised Trials. *BMJ*, **340**, c322. http://dx.doi.org/10.1016/j.jclinepi.2010.02.005

[21] Gustafsson, C., Asp, N. and Fagerberg, I. (2007) Reflective Practice in Nursing Care: Embedded Assumptions in Qualitative Studies. *International Journal of Nursing Practice*, **13**, 151-160. http://dx.doi.org/10.1111/j.1440-172X.2007.00620.x

[22] Mann, K., Gordon, J. and MacLeod, A. (2009) Reflection and Reflective Practice in Health Professions Education: A Systematic Review. *Advances in Health Sciences Education*, **14**, 595-621. http://dx.doi.org/10.1007/s10459-007-9090-2

[23] Taylor, S.M., Dear, M.J. and Hall, G.B. (1979) Attitudes toward the Mentally Ill and Reactions to Mental Health Facilities. *Social Science and Medicine*, **13D**, 281-290. http://dx.doi.org/10.1016/0160-8002(79)90051-0

[24] Taylor, S.M. and Dear, M.J. (1981) Scaling Community Attitudes toward the Mentally Ill. *Schizophrenia Bulletin*, **7**, 225-240. http://dx.doi.org/10.1093/schbul/7.2.225

[25] Jones, P.S., Lee, J.W., Phillips, L.R., Zhang, X.E. and Jaceldo, K.B. (2001) An Adaptation of Brislin's Translation Model for Cross-Cultural Research. *Nursing Research*, **50**, 300-304. http://dx.doi.org/10.1097/00006199-200109000-00008

[26] Finkelstein, J., Lapshin, O. and Wasserman, E. (2008) Randomized Study of Different Anti-Stigma Media. *Patient Education and Counseling*, **71**, 204-214. http://dx.doi.org/10.1016/j.pec.2008.01.002

[27] Schafer, T., Wood, S. and Williams, R. (2011) A Survey into Student Nurses' Attitudes towards Mental Illness: Impli-

cations for Nurse Training. *Nurse Education Today*, **31**, 328-332. http://dx.doi.org/10.1016/j.nedt.2010.06.010

[28] Wolff, G., Pathare, S., Craig, T. and Leff, J. (1996) Community Attitudes to Mental Illness. *British Journal of Psychiatry*, **168**, 183-190. http://dx.doi.org/10.1192/bjp.168.2.183

[29] Sévigny, R., Wenying, Y., Peiyan, Z., Marleau, J.D., Zhouyun, Y., Lin, S., Guowang, L., Dong, X., Yanling, W. and Haijun, W. (1999) Attitudes towards the Mentally Ill in a Sample of Professionals Working in a Psychiatric Hospital in Beijing (China). *International Journal of Social Psychiatry*, **45**, 41-55. http://dx.doi.org/10.1177/002076409904500106

[30] World Medical Association (2008) World Medical Association Declaration of Helsinki Ethical Principles for Medical Research Involving Human Subjects. http://www.wma.net/en/30publications/10policies/b3/17c.pdf

[31] McCaffrey, R., Hayes, R.M., Cassell, A., Miller-Reyes, S., Donaldson, A. and Ferrell, C. (2012) The Effect of an Educational Programme on Attitudes of Nurses and Medical Residents towards the Benefits of Positive Communication and Collaboration. *Journal of Advanced Nursing*, **68**, 293-301. http://dx.doi.org/10.1111/j.1365-2648.2011.05736.x

[32] Patterson, P., Whittington, R. and Bogg, J. (2007) Testing the Effectiveness of an Educational Intervention Aimed at Changing Attitudes to Self-Harm. *Journal of Psychiatric and Mental Health Nursing*, **14**, 100-105. http://dx.doi.org/10.1111/j.1365-2850.2007.01052.x

[33] Lahti, M., Hätönen, H. and Välimäki, M. (2014) Impact of E-Learning on Nurses' and Student Knowledge, Skills, and Satisfaction: A Systematic Review and Meta-Analysis. *International Journal of Nursing Studies*, **51**, 136-149. http://dx.doi.org/10.1016/j.ijnurstu.2012.12.017

[34] Kirkpatrick, D.L. (1998) Evaluating Training Programs. The Four Levels. Berrett-Koehler, San Francisco.

[35] Morris, R., Scott, P.A., Cocoman, A., Chambers, M., Guise, V., Välimäki, M. and Clinton, G. (2012) Is the Community Attitudes towards the Mentally Ill Scale Valid for Use in the Investigation of European Nurses' Attitudes towards the Mentally Ill? A Confirmatory Factor Analytic Approach. *Journal of Advanced Nursing*, **68**, 460-470. http://dx.doi.org/10.1111/j.1365-2648.2011.05739.x

[36] Cobb, S. (2004) Internet Continuing Education for Health Care Professionals: An Integrative Review. *The Journal of Continuing Education in the Health Professionals*, **24**, 171-180. http://dx.doi.org/10.1002/chp.1340240308

[37] Ruiz, J.G., Mintzer, M.J. and Leipzig, R.M. (2006) The Impact of E-Learning in Medical Duration. *Academic Medicine*, **81**, 207-212. http://dx.doi.org/10.1097/00001888-200603000-00002

[38] Bowers, L., Brennan, G., Flood, C., Lipang, M. and Oladapo, P. (2006) Preliminary Outcomes of a Trial to Reduce Conflict and Containment on Acute Psychiatric Wards: City Nurses. *Journal of Psychiatric and Mental Health Nursing*, **13**, 165-172. http://dx.doi.org/10.1111/j.1365-2850.2006.00931.x

[39] Duxbury, J., Hahn, S., Needham, I. and Pulsford, D. (2008) The Management of Aggression and Violence Attitude Scale (MAVAS): A Cross-National Comparative Study. *Journal of Advanced Nursing*, **62**, 596-606. http://dx.doi.org/10.1111/j.1365-2648.2008.04629.x

[40] Henderson, C., Noblett, J., Parke, H., Clement, S., Caffrey, A., Gale-Grant, O., Schulze, B., Druss, B. and Thornicroft, G. (2014) Mental Health-Related Stigma in Health Care and Mental Health-Care Settings. *Lancet Psychiatry*, **1**, 467-482. http://dx.doi.org/10.1016/S2215-0366(14)00023-6

16

The Rhythm of the Unit Is the Pace of Life: A Study of Everyday Activities and Sleep in Swedish Residential Care

Amanda Hellström[1*], Anna Condelius[2], Ania Willman[3,4], Cecilia Fagerström[3,5]

[1]Department of Health and Caring Sciences, Linnæus University, Kalmar, Sweden
[2]Department of Health Sciences, Lund University, Lund, Sweden
[3]Department of Health, Blekinge Institute of Technology, Karlskrona, Sweden
[4]Department of Care Science, Malmö University, Malmö, Sweden
[5]Blekinge Centre of Competence, Karlskrona, Sweden
Email: [*]amanda.hellstrom@lnu.se, anna.condelius@med.lu.se, ania.willman@mah.se, cecilia.fagerstrom@bth.se

Abstract

Social and physical activities can improve sleep in older people. However, living in a residential care facility has been associated with a limited potential for activities and increased inactivity, reflected in poor sleep among residents. In turn, poor sleep can impair physical and mental functions. This paper explores sleep habits and everyday activities at three residential care facilities and investigates the link between sleep habits and everyday activities from the perspective of the residents. Data were collected through observations of daily life and interviews with residents. The results showed that fixed times during the day reduced daytime sleep and motivated them to go to the day room, thus enabling social interaction. More impaired residents spent more time in the day room napping or being less active. The residents stated that going outdoors was a desired activity, thought to improve sleep. However, the activity did not occur to the extent the residents wished for. Maintaining mobility and influence over daily activities together with regularity seemed to improve sleep. Awareness among staff of the need for stimulating and enriching activities, as well as access to bright light is requisite. Specific consideration should be given to residents who have difficulties communicating their wishes and/or impaired mobility.

Keywords

Everyday Activities, Older People, Residential Care Facility, Sleep

[*]Corresponding author.

1. Introduction

People at residential care facilities (RCFs) frequently experience sleep disturbances, such as difficulty falling asleep and waking up during the night [1]. This is thought to be affected by levels of physical activity, environmental factors, and health status [2] [3]. Epidemiological studies at RCFs have revealed associations between everyday physical and social activities and improved sleep [4] [5], and insufficient sleep has been associated with adverse health outcomes, such as symptoms of depression and cognitive dysfunction [6]. Activities, rather than extensive use of hypnotics and sedatives, could be used as means to improve sleep in people at RCFs.

Everyday activities could be classified as routines, that is, rigid patterns of behaviour or normal functioning. "Routine" is sometimes used interchangeably with habits, rituals, or rhythms, emphasizing the regularity of the occurrences [7]. Simultaneously, having regular, daily routines may facilitate regulation of the sleep/wake cycle [8]. However, if the routines imply less daytime activity, less exposure to bright light, more time spent in bed, a change in bedtimes, or light and noise disruptions at night, the routines could have a negative effect on sleep [9]. It has been implied that when a person moves to an RCF, he or she is forced to adjust to an environment where the staff mandates daily life [7]. People living in RCFs have expressed dissatisfaction with social relationships and activities [10], which could lead to inactivity and social isolation that negatively affect sleep. Exploring activities in RCFs and how these are perceived to affect sleep are therefore important.

Sleep in Late Life and Its Association with Everyday Activities

In people aged 60 and over, sleep patterns change, with increased night-time waking, less deep sleep, decreased sleep efficiency, and longer sleep onset latency [11]-[13]. These sleep changes are frequently associated with nocturia, pain, and chronic conditions [1] [14] [15]. Other factors that contribute to sleep disturbances are increased time spent in bed, lack of social interaction, disruption of the circadian rhythm, and noise [16]. Sleep is regulated by two processes: one sleep-dependent and a second sleep-independent process. The sleep-dependent process can be influenced by sleep restriction and exhausting activities, increasing sleep propensity. The latter process, however, is an endogenous drive in humans to fall asleep and wake at a certain time, regardless of the time previously spent sleeping or awake [17]. Daytime activities reinforce a diurnal rhythm. Several quantitative studies [5] [18]-[20] have shown positive associations between activity and sleep at advanced age (57 years or older). Because activities play such an important role in sleep and health, it is essential that scheduled activities at the RCF are of interest. Investigation of activity and sleep habits in RCFs, activities requested by the residents, and activities perceived to affect sleep contribute to valuable knowledge when implementing activities at RCFs. Implementation of activities founded in the residents' interests could increase the activity levels, thus improving health factors such as sleep. The aim of the study was to explore sleep habits and everyday activities at residential care facilities and investigate the linkage between sleep habits and everyday activities from the perspective of the residents.

2. Methods

2.1. Design

An explorative, observational design was chosen to identify patterns or themes in everyday activities, behavioural regularities, and daily life [21] among residents in RCFs. Observations of real-world contexts of everyday life facilitate the understanding of complex situations. To increase the completeness of data, semi-structured interviews were undertaken following the observation periods [22].

2.2. Sampling

Convenience sampling of RCFs was carried out; the only inclusion criterion was that the units should be general geriatric units. Six units in three RCFs (X, Y, Z) were included. The RCFs were located in smaller communities in Sweden. The number of residents varied from seven to 16 per unit, and each resident had his or her own apartment. Purposeful sampling was carried out for the interviews. Participants were selected based on physical and mental stability and cognitive ability to answer questions. Staff members recommended that the researcher contact residents whom they found met the inclusion criteria. This approach was chosen in order to include those residents who would be able to share the most information. The researcher sought variations in age, gender, and place of residence. In all, 12 residents were asked to participate in the interviews. Two declined due to pain, advanced age, or lack of interest. The ten residents interviewed were between 72 and 100 years old; seven were women. The spread of interviewees between the RCFs was five, two and three respectively (**Table 1**).

2.3. The Context of Residential Care Facilities in Sweden

RCF are available for those with extensive health and care needs and governed by the municipalities. In the RCF the residents have a rental apartment (a room, toilet and kitchenette) furnished with their own furniture except for the bed which should be vertically adjustable. Food and care is paid separately. The facility also holds joint spaces such as dining room and TV room. Care is mainly performed by nurse aids, but a nurse is employed at the facility and physiotherapist and occupational therapist are available. The facility is staffed 24-7 and care and supervision is provided at all times. The residents interviewed and observed in the present study all had their own apartments with 24-7 care and supervision. All had their meals and coffee in the joint spaces.

2.4. Data Collection

Thirty-nine observations, each lasting 1(1/2) - 2 hours, were performed at different points during the day (8 am - 8 pm) in order to capture the activities that occurred in the day rooms. During observations, field notes were made following a protocol. Observations were made of what activities took place, who participated, when the activities took place, and how and where they were conducted. Participation during observations extended to informal conversations with staff members and residents. The number of observations at each facility was 10, 12, and 17 respectively. Interviews served the purpose of clarifying activities and behaviours that were observed and providing a deeper understanding of the subject matter of the study. The interviews were carried out in the residents' apartments. A semi-structured interview guide was used for the interviews, covering questions about activities and sleep. Interviews were recorded and transcribed verbatim for analysis. All data were collected over a six-month period from September 2011 to January 2012. The first author carried out all observations and interviews. At three occasions, the first author was accompanied by a nurse co-observer to assure the reliability of the observations.

2.5. Data Analysis

Field notes were read through several times and text themes were identified. Open coding of the transcripts, describing the content, was then carried out [23]. Similar codes were gathered into broader categories. The coding system captured the features of the specific categories and revealed differences and similarities [24] (**Table 2**).

Table 1. Description of residents interviewed, n = 10.

Gender (n)	
Male	3
Female	7
Age (median, range)	90, 72 - 100 years
Marital status (n)	
Single	1
Married	1
Widowed	8
Length of interview (range)	19 - 55 minutes
Distribution of respondents between the Residential Care Facilities (n)	
Residential Care Facility X	5
Residential Care Facility Y	2
Residential Care facility Z	3

Table 2. Examples of the steps taken when analysing the data.

Coded section	Code	Sub-category	Category
I don't want to be outdoors freezing. I'd rather stay inside. The last couple of times I chose not to come along outdoors. (Female, 96 years)	I don't want to freeze. So I have stayed inside instead.	Going out depends on the weather.	Time to go outdoors
Sometimes my sons come here....they take me outdoors now and then. I have asked if I may go for a walk on my own, but I am not allowed to. (Male, 91 years)	My children help me go outdoors. I have asked, but am not allowed to leave on my own.	Need and receive help to go outdoors. Feel restricted from going outdoors.	Time to go outdoors
9:06. *The tired woman with the walker is sitting and dozing off. "Would you like to go to bed for a while?" asks a staff member.* (Residential Care Facility Z)	Falling asleep.	Resting, dwelling, sleeping.	Sleep—in or out of pace
In this place? I sit and stare, I suppose. I can't remember anything else. (Female, 89 years)	Sitting and staring.	Lack of things to do.	Letting time go slowly

The researchers independently created lists of categories that were compared and discussed. The first author then created a list of categories in order to reduce the initial number. All the researchers subsequently discussed the labelling of the categories. The transcripts were sorted into codes and sub-categories and were grouped under broader categories [25]. Finally, the transcripts of the interviews were read, coded, and sorted under the sub-categories and categories decided upon, following the same method. The four authors who performed the analysis had experience as registered nurses in hospital care and/or care of older people.

2.6. Ethical Considerations

Verbal and written information about the study was given to the staff and residents at the units. Written consent was obtained from the manager of each facility, the head of the department of geriatric care in the municipality, and the residents who were interviewed. The study was approved by the regional Ethical Review Board in Lund (Ref. No. 308/2011).

3. Results

Six categories emerged from the data. An overarching theme—*The rhythm of the unit is the pace of life*—unfolded during the analysis as being the latent content of data connecting the categories with each other (**Figure 1**). Residents expressed minor sleep complaints in the interviews. However, descriptions of the scheduled activities together with the residents' experiences of the activities enabled the researchers to interpret the link between sleep and everyday activity. It was clear that meals and coffee times created the main structure of the day. This structure, established by the staff, provided the main rhythm of the day for the residents.

3.1. Sleep—In or out of Pace

Most of the residents expressed satisfaction with their sleep and only minor disturbances. Several residents felt that their sleep had become better since they moved to the RCF. Their sleep had become more regular, having a distinct pace. If disturbances did occur, they were mostly problems falling asleep due to thoughts about deceased loved ones or past events in life. Such events were exemplified as loss of a working role or a house or the appearance of illness. At other times it could simply be that the resident went to bed too early and was not sleepy. It was experienced that the difficulties of falling asleep decreased when the bedtime was postponed, indicating that the resident had been put to bed too early in order to be able to fall asleep. One resident stated that it took longer to fall asleep now compared to before he moved in. The man missed his daily walks in the woods and claimed that outdoor walking made him tired and facilitated falling asleep. Lacking the possibility of doing so now put the man off his normal pace and impaired his sleep. Nightly awakenings were considered a minor problem by the residents.

Some residents were quite strict about avoiding sleep during the day and about sleeping only at night. This was founded in a belief that napping would impair their nocturnal sleep and the need for a distinct sleep/wake pattern. Residents who napped commonly retired to their apartment after lunch to rest, nap, or take it easy. The

Theme	**The rhythm of the unit is the pace of life**					
Categories	Sleep—in or out of pace	Able and willing to socialize	Rhythm of movement—mobility or immobility	Time to go outdoors	Mentally escaping the present	Letting time go slowly
	Resting, dwelling, sleeping during the day	*Social interaction or lack thereof in the unit*	*Indoor exercise/ physiotherapy*	*Needs/receives help to go outdoors*	*Watching television, pictures or a film*	*Gazing at activities that are taking place*
	The rhythm of the unit at night	*Social contacts outside the unit*	*Physical activity with a purpose*	*Obstacles to going outdoors*	*Listening to the radio/music*	*Lack of things to do*
Subcategories	*Personal sleep habits*	*Physical contact*	*Twitching, shaking, banging, clapping*	*Moving/walking outdoors*	*Reading*	*Waiting*
	Sleep quality	*Meals and coffee*	*Physical limits*	*Spending time in another place*		*Sitting down*
			Environmental limits	*Likes spending time outdoors*		

Figure 1. The overarching theme, categories and the sub-categories of each category.

residents usually restricted their napping to between lunch and afternoon coffee, which signified an approximate two-hour span. Everyday activities residents emphasized as facilitating sleep were spending time outdoors and the scheduled activities during the day. Thus the time points of the routines at the unit enhanced a stable rhythm.

...if I go to bed during the day, it may well happen that I fall asleep and I don't want to, "cause I want to sleep at night. I believe that if I sleep during the day, I will not be able to sleep at night...Instead I sit here peacefully in my armchair and read, watch something, or solve crosswords, but I won't go to bed." (*Female* 83 *years*)

3.2. Able and Willing to Socialize

Meals and coffee times were fixed points during the day. These motivated the residents to leave their apartments or to finish something they were doing. Meals and coffee times were emphasized continuously in the interviews as creating a time frame for everything else. Coffee was usually intertwined with some social or cultural activity, such as conversations, discussions, or reading circles, whereas the dinner at 5 pm was more quiet and tranquil. Meals and coffee could be interpreted as having two functions: creating a daily rhythm and inviting residents to social interactions. As an example of the social aspect; afternoon coffee was served at one of the facilities. This day, the staff had baked a cake to have with the coffee. The staff sat together with the residents, small-talking about dogs, sleep, coffee and the cake (it was seldom that the staff had the time and opportunity to bake). The residents commented on how good the cake and coffee was.

The ability to talk "resident to resident" was difficult due to residents' impaired hearing or illnesses that affected speech. It was further emphasized in the interviews that the residents did not know anyone at the facility and that the best people to talk to were the staff, because they spoke clearly and loudly.

No, I can't talk so much to the old people here. If I say something they will not answer. They don't hear that well and I am not very chatty myself. So I can't really complain about the others. (*Female* 86 *years*)

3.3. Rhythm of Movement—Mobility or Immobility

Most physical activities took place indoors. The main activity was to walk between the apartment and the day room for meals and coffee. Another common physical activity was cycling on an exercise bike that could also be used by people in wheelchairs. Other activities were individual physiotherapy programs, usually induced by a specific physical injury, which thus were available only for a few.

Mobile residents would also take the daily paper from the day room and read it in the privacy of their own apartment rather than remain in the day room. The behaviour clearly marked the difference between immobile and mobile residents, because the latter had the possibility of choosing where they wanted to spend their time. At one facility it was observed that several of the residents asked for the morning paper right after breakfast. Then they would leave for their apartments and read the paper in privacy. The day room was a place where those residents had their meals or coffee, but other activities were kept private.

3.4. Time to Go Outdoors

All facilities had a patio or balcony for the residents to use. However in the winter especially the balconies were used by residents and staff that smoked, since this is prohibited indoors. Thus smokers could easily come out several times a day together with smoking staff, while non-smokers where left indoors at these times. It was further observed that residents seldom left the facility for a walk or to simply to spend time outdoors. The residents responded that they spent more time outside during the summer but in winter it would be rare due to the weather and icy paths. Going outside for a walk or sitting in the patio usually took place in the mornings between breakfast and coffee or just before lunch, if there was time. One resident explained that he sometimes wheeled to the day room to watch TV, but in the summer when it was hot and sunny, he would rather spend his time outdoors. He enjoyed sitting in the sun and getting tanned. Also taking walks was put forth in the interviews.

I've asked if I can go outdoors by myself, but they won't let me. I do miss... When I had my own apartment [i.e. ordinary housing] I used to go down to the market and do my shopping and...or I would take a stroll. It is nice around here, very beautiful. (Male 91 *years)*

3.5. Mentally Escaping the Present

Several residents enjoyed reading, including books they had read before as well as new detective stories. One resident said that now there was more time to read, more than ever before, and books provided an escape from this world into another. Sitting watching television was quite common but the residents did not always find the programs interesting. They frequently fell asleep in front of the television. Both watching television and reading were mentioned as bedtime routines by several residents. The radio and music were mentioned as ways of keeping the silence away and were sometimes played in the day rooms.

I don't know the people here. They could talk at the dinner table, but it's always quiet. I guess, since it's always quiet, it should be that way. That's why (...) gave me a radio that I can sit and listen to. (Female 96 *years)*

3.6. Letting Time Go Slow

It was common for the day to pass slowly and for some residents to simply sit in silence in the day rooms or in front of the television without watching. However, it was stated during the interviews that remaining in the day room was due to a lack of activities or the perception that the unit was the final station in this life, which could be interpreted as there was no point in engaging in activities.

Some of the passivity arose from waiting for something to happen, such as the start of an activity or for a meal to be served or from an unwillingness to participate in some of the scheduled activities. Immobile residents could remain in the day room from breakfast until bedtime. One of the residents, who was mobile, spent most of the day in the day room just for company and to feel less lonely. However, most of the residents who could walk or operate their wheelchairs on their own left the day room for some privacy.

4. Discussion

Several residents felt that their sleep had become better since they had moved to the RCF. Factors causing the improvement seemed to be an increased feeling of security and more regular bed hours. It was also emphasized that the timing of meals and coffee regulated daytime activities and provided a fixed rhythm for the day. Similarly, a pilot study [8] showed that scheduled activities and fixed times for meals led to more stable sleep/ wake rhythms in institutionalized older people with dementia. When life is no longer about work, mealtimes acquire greater significance in structuring the day, according to [26]. Another reason for sleep satisfaction in the current study could be that most residents were mobile and cognitively preserved. They had greater opportunity to retain their own routines and pace and they were less influenced by the rhythm of the unit.

However, situations were also found that reflected a lack of control and decision-making of the residents. The staff emphasized the importance of scheduled activities for the residents, but the activities did not spring from the wishes of residents or a person centred approach. The residents, on the other hand, had clear opinions about what activities they preferred to do, and the lack of activities of interest was thought to cause a great deal of sleeping and sedentary behaviour during the day, according to the interviewees. Due to discontent with the scheduled activities or as to accentuate the lack of shared decision-making, some residents retired to their apartments instead of participating. Similar attitudes were found towards scheduled activities in British care homes [27]; with limited interest among the residents or that the activities were perceived as trivial or childish. Residents in Swedish RCFs have expressed dissatisfaction with activities as well as their own self-determination, emphasizing the importance of being able to make their own decisions and having the opportunities to engage in freely chosen activities [10] [28].

The overarching theme *the rhythm of the unit is the pace of life* could be interpreted both as a positive structure for the day, but also as a restricting order preventing personalized care. Song *et al.* [8] described positive effects on sleep-wake pattern in dementia. In the present study residents emphasized the structure of the day, but did not express discontent with timing of things, rather the content. Eyers *et al.* [27] also describe a rhythm of the care home, which uniformed sleep-wake patterns in the residents. However, it is further put forth that the rhythm is based on staffing and routines and instead of stressing individuality a hospitalized life-style is introduced [27].

The residents felt that sleep was affected by the possibility of going outdoors and pursuing activities during the day. Environmental cues have proved vital for stabilizing the circadian rhythm [11]. The suprachiasmatic nucleus in the hypothalamus serves as the central pacemaker of the circadian rhythm. Synchronization of the rhythm takes place mainly through environmental light [29]. Many residents were sleepy during the day, even around breakfast time, when they should have been rested. The ageing of the brain results in weaker and more disrupted sleep/wake rhythms as well as decreased secretion of endogenous melatonin [6]. External cues, such as physical inactivity, nocturnal noise/light levels, and low light levels during the day could further impair sleep [30]. Older people in care homes in particular spend little time exposed to bright light, which is one of the most powerful *zeitgebers* of the sleep/wake rhythm, and this may contribute to increased sleepiness during the day [6]. A difficulty for the residents was that they found it inconvenient or unpleasant to go out when the weather was cold, windy, or rainy. Several residents also needed assistance to leave the facility, which was not always provided. The indoor environment was dusky due to dim or sparse lighting, which further could impair the sleep-wake rhythm. Sloane *et al.* [31] introduced high-intensity ambient bright light in public areas of RCFs, and found that those receiving bright-light in the morning or all day increased their night-time sleep. Thus, high-intensity bright light indoors could compensate for not being outdoors, especially in the winter when the opportunities to go outdoors are few.

In the present study, residents who needed to be wheeled by staff usually remained in the day rooms after having breakfast, although they were moved by the staff from the dining table to the television room. No particular activities were introduced to those residents, although sometimes the staff would turn on the television or put on some music to chase the silence away. The residents would sit motionless, shifting between wakefulness and slumber. It has been found that remaining in the day room has an obvious negative effect on sleep [32]. In an observational study [33] conducted at Norwegian RCFs, it was found that residents with a high degree of dependence were left in the day room all day, which is similar to the present study. The threats to sleep as pointed out previously [11]; are not getting enough social interaction with the world outside the facility, little time exposed to outdoor daylight, and excessive daytime sleep that prevents social interaction. Spending time in bed during daylight hours and a lack of social cues may aggravate the changes in the circadian rhythm.

Strengths and Limitations

Trustworthiness of the present study is reflected by credibility and voice. Credibility was achieved through a detailed description of the methods used, through study time lines, and through methodological choices that were made. Furthermore, triangulation of data was used in order to increase the understanding of the phenomenon under study. The advantages of triangulation are confirmation and completeness of data [34]. To accomplish rigour, there was systematic collection of field notes using a protocol. The compliance of the protocol was checked at three occasions through a co-observer simultaneously making notes. Through the analysis, meaning units were selected by the first author (AH) and categories and subcategories were verified by the other authors (AC, AW, CF), which increases the credibility of the results [25] [35].

The sample size of this study could be considered as small. However, qualitative studies emphasize context and the lived experience of the participants; which is why the sample size of a qualitative study could be significantly smaller compared to a quantitative study. No specific guidelines of sample sizes exist. However, Moon *et al.* [36] recommend at least 6 - 7 participants for ethnographic studies and 12 to 15 participants for other qualitative designs, depending on the aim of the study. This study used data triangulation of observations and interviews, which is similar to ethnography, although the data collection was done during a shorter time period and in two-hour intervals. This could motivate a sample larger than that for an ethnographic study. Twelve residents were asked to participate, and ten gave their consent. Data would probably have been richer if all twelve would have agreed to an interview. On the other hand did the categories repeat in the performed interviews, which indicate saturation of data [36].

The inclusion of respondents who were physically and mentally stable for the interviews could imply that the voices of the more dependent and fragile residents were missed. The descriptions of participation in activities and how sleep was perceived might therefore show a more optimistic view than is the case among the general group of residents. Possibly the variety among residents has been achieved only to a limited degree in the present study; however, the observations captured activities of all residents, including those with cognitive impairments. The use of objective measurements such as actigraphs could have enriched the current data with objective measures of sleep and activity levels and provided information about more impaired residents. On the other side, the majority of those living in RCFs in Sweden are women aged 80 or older [10], which was mirrored by the study sample. Another aspect of trustworthiness is voice. It is important to make the voices and experiences of the participants accessible. This has been done through the quotes and field notes, illustrating a link between the data and the interpretation as well as giving insight to the lives and worlds of the participants. This also enhances evaluation of the content in each category [37].

Data were collected in the autumn/winter, which could have had an impact on the results. In the general population, less light physical activity and more sedentary behaviour is reported during autumn/winter [38], possibly due to unpleasant weather and decreasing light levels.

5. Conclusion

The rhythm of the unit sets the pace of life in the RCF—that is, there is a general approach to the scheduled activities, commonly at the expense of the individual wishes of the residents. It is difficult to balance the general routines of a care setting with those of the individual. Residents who have the capacity to make decisions and transport themselves feel that their nocturnal sleep has improved since moving to the RCF. Staff need to be aware of the need for stimulating and enriching activities among residents and to empower self-determination concerning activities. Specific consideration should be given to residents with great impairments that could create difficulties communicating their wishes and moving on their own. It is not solely about being active; it is about being a part of the decision-making, being stimulated, and to have a regular rhythm of the day that promotes sleep.

Disclosure

The authors declare no conflicting interests.

Acknowledgements

We would like to extend our sincere thanks to those who participated in the interviews and to the RCFs and the staff who made this study possible. Many thanks to Doris Bohman for insightful and constructive comments concerning the method. The authors would also like to thank Linnæus University, Lund University and Blekinge Institute of Technology for financial support.

Author Contributions

Amanda Hellström responsible for data collection, leading in the analysis of data and did the drafting. The first author also participated in the conception and design of the study.

Anna Condelius contributed in the interpretation and analysis of data and revised critically on the drafting and provided intellectual content.

Ania Willman contributed in the analysis process and provided with intellectual content in the drafting process. The third author also participated in the conception and design of the study.

Cecilia Fagerström contributed in the analysis process, gave critical comments on drafting and provided with intellectual content. Cecilia Fagerström also participated in the conception and design of the study.

References

[1] Martin, J.L., *et al.* (2010) Sleep Quality in Residents of Assisted Living Facilities: Effect on Quality of Life, Functional

Status, and Depression. *Journal of American Geriatrics Society*, **58**, 829-836. http://dx.doi.org/10.1111/j.1532-5415.2010.02815.x

[2] Ancoli-Israel, S. and Shochat, T. (2010) Insomnia in Older Adults. In: Kryger, M.H., Roth, T. and Dement, W.C., Eds., *Priciples and Practice of Sleep Medicine*, Saunders Elsevier, Philadelphia, 1544-1550.

[3] Herrmann, W.J. and Flick, U. (2011) Nursing Home Residents' Self-Perceived Resources for Good Sleep. *Scandinavian Journal of Primary Health Care*, **29**, 247-251. http://dx.doi.org/10.3109/02813432.2011.628243

[4] Lee, Y. And Kim, S. (2008) Effects of Indoor Gardening on Sleep, Agitation, and Cognition in Dementia Patients—A Pilot Study. *International Journal of Geriatric Psychiatry*, **23**, 485-489. http://dx.doi.org/10.1002/gps.1920

[5] Richards, K.C., *et al.* (2011) Strength Training, Walking, and Social Activity Improve Sleep in Nursing Home and Assisted Living Residents: Randomized Controlled Trial. *Journal of American Geriatrics Society*, **59**, 214-223. http://dx.doi.org/10.1111/j.1532-5415.2010.03246.x

[6] Cooke, J.R. and Ancoli-Israel, S. (2006) Sleep and Its Disorders in Older Adults. *Psychiatric Clinics of North America*, **29**, 1077-1093; Abstract x-xi. http://dx.doi.org/10.1016/j.psc.2006.08.003

[7] Zisberg, A., *et al.* (2007) A Concept Analysis of Routine: Relevance to Nursing. *Journal of Advanced Nursing*, **57**, 442-453. http://dx.doi.org/10.1111/j.1365-2648.2007.04103.x

[8] Song, Y., *et al.* (2009) Rest-Activity Patterns in Institutionalized Korean Older Adults with Dementia: A Pilot Study. *Journal of Gerontological Nursing*, **35**, 20-28; Quiz 30-31. http://dx.doi.org/10.3928/00989134-20091109-99

[9] Bliwise, D.L. (2010) Sleep in Independently Living and Institutionalized Elderly. In: Kryger, M.H., Roth, T. and Dement, W.C., Eds., *Principles and Practice of Sleep Medicine*, Saunders Elsevier, Philadelphia, 1551-1561.

[10] The National Board of Health and Welfare (2010) Vad tycker de äldre om äldreomsorgen?—En rikstäckande undersökning av äldres uppfattning om kvaliteten i hemtjänst och äldreboenden 2010 [What Is the Elderlys' Opinion on Elderly Care?—A National Survey of Elderly Persons' Perceptions of Quality in Home-Help Service and Residential Care Facilities 2010].

[11] Alessi, C.A. and Schnelle, J.F. (2000) Approach to Sleep Disorders in the Nursing Home Setting. *Sleep Medicine Reviews*, **4**, 45-56. http://dx.doi.org/10.1053/smrv.1999.0066

[12] Ancoli-Israel, S., Ayalon, L. and Salzman, C. (2008) Sleep in the Elderly: Normal Variations and Common Sleep Disorders. *Harvard Review of Psychiatry*, **16**, 279-286. http://dx.doi.org/10.1080/10673220802432210

[13] Neikrug, A.B. and Ancoli-Israel, S. (2010) Sleep Disturbances in Nursing Homes. *Journal of Nutrition, Health & Aging*, **14**, 207-211. http://dx.doi.org/10.1007/s12603-010-0051-8

[14] Bliwise, D.L. (1993) Sleep in Normal Ageing and Dementia. *Sleep*, **16**, 40-81.

[15] Fagerström, C. and Hellström, A. (2011) Sleep Complaints and Their Association with Comorbidity and Health-Related Quality of Life in an Older Population in Sweden. *Aging and Mental Health*, **15**, 204-213. http://dx.doi.org/10.1080/13607863.2010.513039

[16] Monjan, A.A. (2010) Perspective on Sleep and Aging. *Frontiers in Neurology*, **1**, 1-9. http://dx.doi.org/10.3389/fneur.2010.00124

[17] Rama, A.N., Cho, S.C. and Kushida, C.A. (2006) Normal Human Sleep. In: Lee-Chiong, T., Ed., *Sleep: A Comprehensive Handbook*, John Wiley & Sons, Hoboken, 3-11.

[18] Chen, K.M., *et al.* (2009) Sleep Quality, Depression State, and Health Status of Older Adults after Silver Yoga Exercises: Cluster Randomized Trial. *International Journal of Nursing Studies*, **46**, 154-163. http://dx.doi.org/10.1016/j.ijnurstu.2008.09.005

[19] Irwin, M.R., Olmstead, R. and Motivala, S.J. (2008) Improving Sleep Quality in Older Adults with Moderate Sleep Complaints: A Randomized Controlled Trial of Tai Chi Chih. *Sleep*, **31**, 1001-1008.

[20] Li, F., *et al.* (2004) Tai Chi and Self-Rated Quality of Sleep and Daytime Sleepiness in Older Adults: A Randomized Controlled Trial. *Journal of American Geriatrics Society*, **52**, 892-900. http://dx.doi.org/10.1111/j.1532-5415.2004.52255.x

[21] Berg, B. (2009) Qualitative Research Methods. 7th Edition, Allyn & Bacon, Boston.

[22] Bolster, D. and Manias, E. (2010) Person-Centred Interactions between Nurses and Patients during Medication Activities in an Acute Hospital Setting: Qualitative Observation and Interview Study. *International Journal of Nursing Studies*, **47**, 154-165. http://dx.doi.org/10.1016/j.ijnurstu.2009.05.021

[23] Burnard, P., *et al.* (2008) Analysing and Representing Qualitative Data. *British Dental Journal*, **204**, 429-432. http://dx.doi.org/10.1038/sj.bdj.2008.292

[24] Downe-Wamboldt, B. (1992) Content Analysis: Method, Applications, and Issues. *Health Care for Women International*, **13**, 313-321. http://dx.doi.org/10.1080/07399339209516006

[25] Burnard, P. (1991) A Method of Analysing Interview Transcripts in Qualitative Research. *Nurse Education Today*, **11**, 461-466. http://dx.doi.org/10.1016/0260-6917(91)90009-Y

[26] Alftberg, Å. (2012) Vad är det att åldras? [What Is It to Grow Old?]. In: Alftberg, Å., Ed., *Humanistiska Fakulteten*, Faculty of Humanities, Lund University, Lund, 176.

[27] Eyers, I., *et al.* (2012) Rhetoric and Reality of Daily Life in English Care Homes: The Role of Organized Activities. *International Journal of Ageing and Later Life*, **7**, 53-78. http://dx.doi.org/10.3384/ijal.1652-8670.11132

[28] Andersson, I., Pettersson, E. and Sidenvall, B. (2007) Daily Life after Moving into a Care Home—Experiences from Older People, Relatives and Contact Persons. *Journal of Clinical Nursing*, **16**, 1712-1718. http://dx.doi.org/10.1111/j.1365-2702.2007.01703.x

[29] Rosenthal, L. (2006) Physiologic Processes during Sleep. In: Lee-Chiong, T., Ed., *Sleep: A comprehensive handbook*, John Wiley & Sons, Hoboken, 19-25.

[30] Martin, J.L. and Alessi, C.A. (2006) Sleep in Institutionalized Older Adults. In: Lee-Chiong, T., Ed., *Sleep: A Comprehensive Handbook*, John Wiley and Sons Inc., Hoboken, 615-621.

[31] Sloane, P.D., *et al.* (2007) High-Intensity Environmental Light in Dementia: Effect on Sleep and Activity. *Journal of American Geriatrics Society*, **55**, 1524-1533. http://dx.doi.org/10.1111/j.1532-5415.2007.01358.x

[32] Chaperon, C.M., Farr, L.A. and LoChiano, E. (2007) Sleep Disturbance of Residents in a Continuing Care Retirement Community. *Journal of Gerontological Nursing*, **33**, 21-28.

[33] Hauge, S. and Heggen, K. (2008) The Nursing Home as a Home: A Field Study of Residents' Daily Life in the Comon Living Rooms. *Journal of Clinical Nursing*, **17**, 460-467.

[34] Casey, D. and Murphy, K. (2009) Issues in Using Methodological Triangulation in Research. *Nurse Researcher*, **16**, 40-55. http://dx.doi.org/10.7748/nr2009.07.16.4.40.c7160

[35] Tobin, G.A. and Begley, C.M. (2004) Methodological Rigour within a Qualitative Framework. *Journal of Advanced Nursing*, **48**, 388-396. http://dx.doi.org/10.1111/j.1365-2648.2004.03207.x

[36] Moon, M.D., *et al.* (2013) Evaluating Qualitative Research Studies for Use in the Clinical Setting. *Journal of Emergency Nursing*, **39**, 508-510. http://dx.doi.org/10.1016/j.jen.2013.06.009

[37] Graneheim, U.H. and Lundman, B. (2004) Qualitative Content Analysis in Nursing Research: Concepts, Procedures and Measures to Achieve Trustworthiness. *Nurse Education Today*, **24**, 105-112. http://dx.doi.org/10.1016/j.nedt.2003.10.001

[38] O'Connell, S.E., Griffiths, P.L. and Clemes, S.A. (2014) Seasonal Variation in Physical Activity, Sedentary Behaviour and Sleep in a Sample of UK Adults. *Annals of Human Biology*, **41**, 1-8. http://dx.doi.org/10.3109/03014460.2013.827737

17

A Comparison between Dietary Habits for Pregnant Women with Preterm and Term Delivery in Khorasan, Iran

Zohreh Teimouri[1], Mahrokh Dolatian[2*], Sara Shishehgar[3], Marjan Ajami[4], Hamid Alavi Majd[5]

[1]Department of Midwifery, International branch of ShahidBeheshti University of Medical Sciences, Tehran, Iran
[2]Department of Midwifery, School of nursing and midwifery, Shahid Beheshti University of Medical Sciences, Tehran, Iran
[3]Faculty of Health, University of Technology, Sydney, Australia
[4]Department of Nutrition Iran University of Medical Sciences, Tehran, Iran
[5]Department of Biostatistics, School of Paramedical Sciences, Shahid Beheshti University of Medical Sciences, Tehran, Iran
Email: zohre_m_teymuri@yahoo.com, *mhdolatian@gmail.com, sara.shishehgar@uts.edu.au, nutritionist80@gmail.com, alavimajd@gmail.com

Abstract

Background: Despite the advances in prenatal care and improving health indicators, preterm delivery and resultant infant mortality rate are still considerable. Emerged financial, social, mental and emotional damages could result in mental and behavioral disabilities for mothers as well as children. Although spontaneous preterm labor is well known as a multifactorial issue, yet poor nutrition is assumed as a strong related factor. Objective: To identify the role of dietary habits on preterm delivery prevalence in Iran, this study was conducted on pregnant women with preterm and term delivery. Methods: In this retrospective case-control study, 70 women with preterm labor and 70 women with term labor were compared in terms of their dietary habits. Women who met the inclusion criteria and referred to two hospitals in North-East of Iran were selected using purposive convenience sampling method and completed 163-item food frequency and dietary habits questionnaire. Results: This study showed that dietary habits of women with preterm labor are more unfavorable compared to women with term labor (P = 0.023). Generally, dietary habit of more than half of the women with preterm labor, in this study, was assessed unfavorable. In terms of different food groups, daily intake of vegetables was significantly lower in women with preterm labor (P = 0.02). Consumption of dairy products was also lower in women with preterm labor than

*Corresponding author.

women with term labor which was significant (P = 0.05). Conclusion: To prevent adverse outcomes of preterm delivery more attention regarding nutritional planning for pregnant women seems to be essential.

Keywords

Dietary Habit, Preterm Delivery, Pregnancy

1. Introduction

Despite the advances in prenatal care and improving health indicators, yet 5% - 10% of all pregnancies are terminated as preterm, and prematurity is still the leading cause of neonatal mortality in developed and developing countries [1] [2]. Preterm infant is defined as the infant who is born before 37 completed weeks of pregnancy [3].

Prevalence of preterm delivery was estimated about 14.9 million globally. About 60% of this occurs in South Asia and sub-Saharan Africa, 18% in African countries, 5% in Europe and 11.1% in the rest of the world [4]. Obviously, higher prevalence of spontaneous preterm labor occurs in poorest countries where people are assumed to be under-nourished [5]. Approximately, 57% of neonatal death occurs at the first month of birth and 36% of them is attributable to preterm delivery [6]. Adverse outcomes of preterm delivery are considered as the greatest social and economic problems causing mental and behavioral disabilities [7].

Multiple pathologic processes such as length of cervix, preeclampsia and maternal stress may be associated with preterm delivery [8] [9] however poor nutrition is still assumed as a substantial related factor [10]-[12]. Based on literature, insufficient intake of food during pregnancy not only leads to increased risk of preterm delivery, fetal growth restriction and low birth weight [13]-[15], but also declined mother's health [15]. Nutritional needs increase during pregnancy due to the fetus growth, placenta, breast and uterus enlargement, increased body fat and blood volume [16]. Therefore, the quantity and quality of nutrition during pregnancy are of particular importance [15].

On the other hand, this is evident in a systematic review that food intake has no effect on preterm birth rate [17].

Since the impact of nutrition during pregnancy on preterm delivery is still controversial, we decided to investigate and compare the pregnant women's nutritional condition in two groups of preterm and term delivery.

2. Methods and Materials

Using a purposive convenience sampling method, 140 women who attended Social Security and Nohome Dey Hospitals and met inclusion criteria were recruited from October 2013 to October 2014. 70 participants were being hospitalized with a diagnosis of preterm delivery and 70 participants had term delivery. The proper sample size was estimated in consultation with a biological statistician (Equation (1): Correlation formula).

$$n \geq 2\frac{\left(z_\alpha + z_\beta\right)^2 \sigma^2}{\left(\mu_1 - \mu_2\right)^2} \tag{1}$$

The study settings were public and referral hospitals located in a city in North-East of Iran.

Women who were between 18 and 35 years of age, Iranian, without any severe trauma or stress leading to preterm delivery were included in this study. They also should have no history of preterm labor and chronic diseases. The selected participants should not be smokers and medication recipients.

Data were collected through face to face interviews by the first author and each interview last about half an hour. Prior to each interview commencement, written consents collected followed by completion of the demographic and obstetric questionnaires. These data were collected after delivery and determining gestational age of the neonate (based on early pregnancy sonography and the neonate's appearance). Nutritional status of the women during recent 12 months was assessed by 168-item food-frequency questionnaire (168-FFQ). Ethics approval was obtained of Shahid Beheshti University and the study settings Ethics Committees.

168-FFQ contains 168 food items with a standard serving size for each food product. The participants were asked to report their consumption frequency of each food product according to standard serving size. Depending on the type of food, the consumption frequency was asked and reported on daily, weekly, monthly and yearly basis. According to the Food Pyramid Guide, then, food items were placed in five major food groups (bread and cereal, vegetables, fruits, dairy, meat and beans).

Standard unit that was considered for daily use for each of the five major food groups was in accordance with the pregnancy nutrition guideline of the Health Ministry of Iran. Dietary habit was considered favorable if daily intake of food products in 4 - 5 main food groups was in accordance with the guideline. Otherwise, it was considered unfavorable. It means that women who intake daily 3 - 4 unit fruits, 7 - 10 units bread and cereals, 4 - 5 units vegetables, 3 - 4 units meat and beans and 3 - 4 units dairy were placed in favorable dietary group.

Validity of 168-FFQ has been determined in previous studies with Spearman coefficient mean of 0.80 [18] [19]. Moreover, reliability of that has been determined examined in previous studies (r = 0.59) [18].

Data analysis:

The collected data from each participant was statistically analyzed using Statistical Package for the Social Science version 22 (SPSS22). The descriptive statistics (frequency-percent, mean ± SD) of Mann-Whitney, chi-square and t-test were used to analyze the collected data. Normal distribution was checked in consultation with a biological statistician. $P < 0.05$ was considered significant.

3. Results

In this study, participants had a mean age of 29 ± 5.7. Most participants, 90 (64.3%), had education level less than diploma, 35 (25%) diploma, and only 15 (10.7%) had an academic education. 12 (8.6%) of the participants' husbands were illiterate, 79 (56.4%) less than diploma, 35 (25%) diploma, and only 14 (10%) had an academic education. Most women 130 (92.9%) were house wives and 10 (7.1%) were employed. Most of the participants in both groups, 86 (more than 60%) were living in urban areas (**Table 1**). In addition, demographic characteristics of women in preterm and term delivery groups were compared using Chi-square test. Accordingly, there was no significant difference between two groups in terms of each character ($P > 0.05$).

In terms of family income, 60% of women with preterm delivery and about half of women with term delivery (48.6%) were categorized in low-income families. Mann-Whitney test showed that the difference between two groups in terms of family income was significant ($P = 0.05$).

Regarding their obstetric characteristics 21.4% experienced their first pregnancy; nearly half (47.9%) were in their second pregnancy; and 25% were in third pregnancy. 36.5% of participants had a history of abortion, 55.1% had intervals less than 4 years with their last pregnancy or abortion.

Respect to participants' BMI prior to pregnancy, there was a significant difference between two case and control groups ($P = 0.01$). Women with lower BMI at the beginning of pregnancy had the higher possibility of preterm delivery (**Table 2**). Notably, about half of women in case group reported an unfavorable dietary habit during pregnancy.

Nutritional status in two case and control groups has been shown in **Table 3**. Evaluation of dietary habits in two groups showed that women with preterm delivery had more unfavorable dietary habits during pregnancy than women with term delivery ($P = 0.023$).

Based on the Health Ministry guideline, daily intake of vegetables was less in women with preterm delivery than women in control group (**Table 4**). The results of chi-square test showed a significant difference between two groups in terms of daily intake of vegetables ($P = 0.01$). A significant difference also was recognized in terms of dairy intake in two groups ($P = 0.05$) while bread, fruit, meat and beans consumption seems to not be different significantly in two groups ($P > 0.05$).

Moreover, 60% and 50% of women with preterm and term delivery, respectively, intake 3 or less food groups on a daily basis. This was emerged from this study that about one third (32.9%) of women in both groups intake only one food group. Notably, 4.3% of women in case group didn't consume food products according the guideline (**Table 5**).

4. Discussion

Unfavorable dietary habits were relatively sensible in women with preterm delivery. There are some studies that affirm this study's findings. In a study by Kamalifard *et al.* (2010), food consumption in term delivery group is

Table 1. Demographic characters of participants.

Age (year)	N (%)	Mean ± SD
<20	12 (8.5)	29 ± 5.7
20 - 24	46 (32.8)	
25 - 29	31 (22.3)	
≤30	51 (36.9)	
Education		
Lower than Diploma	90(64.3)	
Diploma	35 (25)	
Higher than Diploma	15 (10.7)	
Education (Husband)		
No Education	12 (8.6)	
Lower than Diploma	79 (56.4)	
Diploma	35 (25)	
Higher than Diploma	14 (10)	
Occupation		
Housewives	130 (92.9)	
Employed	10 (7.1)	
Monthly Income		
<6,000,000 R	21 (15)	
6,000,000 - 9,000,000 R	55 (39.3)	
>9,000,000 R	64 (45.7)	
Residential Area		
City	86 (61.4)	
Rural	54 (38.6)	

Table 2. Distribution of body mass index of participants.

Body Mass Index before pregnancy		P-value
Preterm	Term	
22/33 ± 2/78	23/34 ± 2/09	P = 0/01

Table 3. Comparison of dietary habits between two groups of preterm and term delivery.

	Delivery		P-value[1]
	Preterm	Term	
Unfavorable	45 (64.3%)	32(45.7%)	0.023
Favorable	25 (35.7%)	38(54.3%)	

[1]The chi-square test was used.

Table 4. Comparison and frequency distribution of food groups' intake between two groups of preterm and term delivery.

food groups	Delivery		P-value
	Preterm	Term	
Bread	57 (81.4)	57 (81.4)	1.00
Fruit	33 (47.1)	39 (55.7)	0.31
Vegetable	26 (37.1)	40 (57.1)	0.01
Dairy	40 (57.1)	50 (71.4)	0.05
Meat and beans	47 (67.1)	42 (60.0)	0.38

The chi-square test was used

Table 5. Comparison and frequency distribution of food intake between two groups of preterm and term delivery.

Number of consumed food groups	Delivery		P-value
	Preterm	Term	
None	3 (4.3)	0	0.391
One case	13 (18.6)	10 (14.3)	
Two cases	12 (17.1)	9 (12.9)	
Three cases	14 (20.0)	16 (22.9)	
Four cases	16 (22.9)	23 (32.9)	
Five cases	12 (17.1)	12 (17.1)	

The chi-square test was used

more favorable than preterm delivery group [20]. Another study on women with twin pregnancies showed a significant relationship between appropriate nutrition along with regular prenatal care and decrease of preterm delivery prevalence [21].

About the importance of nutrition, it should be noted that the woman's body during pregnancy needs very various food products with adequate calories. Growth of the fetus, placenta, uterus and breasts and increasing the blood volume demand different food products especially protein. Lack of adequate and qualified nutrition causes health problems for the mother and fetus and considerably increases the risk of preterm delivery and resultant adverse outcomes for mothers and children [22] [23].

Comparison of daily intake of five major food groups indicated that vegetable intake was significantly lower in women with preterm delivery than other counterparts in term delivery group. This is well documented by previous studies that Mediterranean diet which is rich in fruits, vegetables, fish and olive oil could reduce the incidence of preterm delivery [24]-[26] due to antioxidants [27] by preventing the damaging effects of oxidative stress along with protection of the connective tissues and increase the strength of membranes [28]. So, concerning this fact that about half of preterm deliveries are resulted from premature rupture of membranes, consumption of vegetables should be of importance [29].

Awareness of the benefits of taking these food groups may increase the tendency to use them. Along with vegetables, milk and dairy consumption also seems to be of importance due to the influence of calcium deficiency on membrane permeability and uterus contractions that may contribute to preterm delivery [30].

Contrary to this study, Bakhtiari *et al.* (2007) concluded that the majority of pregnant women have relatively favorable dietary pattern during pregnancy [31]. However, others assessed pregnant women's dietary habits moderate and less than standard [32] [33]. This inconsistency may relate to the different regions of studies. The Bakhtiari's study was conducted in north of Iran where is green and rainy and food products are varied and affordable while this study was undertaken in an arid area where vegetables are expensive to afford.

According to the present study, the majority of women in case group had unfavorable dietary habits that can be attributable to their low socio-economic status and resultant low awareness of nutrition requirements during pregnancy [33]. This is documented that higher socio-economic status may improve pregnant women's health and decrease adverse effects of poor diet through increase the knowledge and life skills [34] although this study has found only a nearly significant relationship ($P = 0.08$). However better dietary habits and term delivery could be attributable to higher socio-economic status [35]-[38], relationship is still controversial [20].

Having a higher BMI prior to pregnancy has a determining role in gestational age at the delivery time [39]. Inability to afford adequate food resources as a result of low socio-economic status may continue during pregnancy and contribute to restricted fetal growth and preterm delivery [40].

Generally, we expected to find some relationship between observing the daily intake of food groups and reduction of prevalence of preterm delivery. However we found this relationship, studies that confirm the current findings are still rare. Inconsistencies between the current study and Bakhtiari study in a same country [31] overshadow the results of both studies. So, further studies are worthwhile to cover limitations with this study. A limitation of this study is related to the memory of the participants. Since dietary habits were assessed by food frequency questionnaire for one year, the participants might not remember all the used food products. Another limitation is due to convenience sampling method. Further randomized control studies should be conducted to affirm the results of this study and make them generalizable to all Iranian pregnant women.

This study, however, was the first study conducted to explore relationship between dietary habits of pregnant women and prevalence of preterm delivery in Iran.

Acknowledgements

This article is the result of a Master's Degree Dissertation in Midwifery from the International branch of Shahid Beheshti University of Medical Sciences We thank the staff of Tamin Ejtemaei and NohomDey Hospitals in Torbat Heidarieh and the women who participated in the study and answered the questionnaires.

References

[1] Karimi, R., Shabani, F., Dehghan Nayeri, N., Zareii, K., Khalili, G. and Chehrazi, M. (2012) Effect of Music Therapy on Physiological Pain Responses of Blood Sampling in Premature Infants. *Hayat*, **18**, 76-86.

[2] Sangkomkamhang, U.S., Lumbiganon, P., Prasertcharoensook, W. and Laopaiboon, M. (2015) Antenatal Lower Genital Tract Infection Screening and Treatment Programs for Preventing Preterm Delivery. Cochrane Database of Systematic Reviews Issue, 2. http://dx.doi.org/10.1002/14651858.CD006178.pub3

[3] Bastek, J.A., Sammel, M.D., Srinivas, S.K., McShea, M.A., Foreman, M.N., Elovitz, M.A., *et al.* (2012) Clinical Prediction Rules for Preterm Birth in Patients Presenting with Preterm Labor. *Obstetrics & Gynecology*, **119**, 1119-1128. http://dx.doi.org/10.1097/AOG.0b013e31825503e5

[4] Blencowe, H., Cousens, S., Oestergaard, M.Z., Chou, D., Moller, A.-B., Narwal, R., *et al.* (2012) National, Regional, and Worldwide Estimates of Preterm Birth Rates in the Year 2010 with Time Trends since 1990 for Selected Countries: A Systematic Analysis and Implications. *The Lancet*, **379**, 2162-2172. http://dx.doi.org/10.1016/S0140-6736(12)60820-4

[5] Beck, S., Wojdyla, D., Say, L., Betran, A.P., Merialdi, M., Requejo, J.H., *et al.* (2010) The Worldwide Incidence of Preterm Birth: A Systematic Review of Maternal Mortality and Morbidity. *Bulletin of the World Health Organization*, **88**, 31-38. http://dx.doi.org/10.2471/BLT.08.062554

[6] Dorling, J.S. and Field, D.J. (2008) Value and Validity of Neonatal Disease Severity Scoring Systems. *Archives of Disease in Childhood-Fetal and Neonatal Edition*, **93**, F80-F82.

[7] Newnham, C.A., Milgrom, J. and Skouteris, H. (2009) Effectiveness of a Modified Mother-Infant Transaction Program on Outcomes for Preterm Infants from 3 to 24 Months of Age. *Infant Behavior and Development*, **32**, 17-26. http://dx.doi.org/10.1016/j.infbeh.2008.09.004

[8] Hestiantoro, A. (2013) Preterm Labor and Preeclampsia: Time to Make Good News. *Indonesian Journal of Obstetrics and Gynecology*, **36**, 54.

[9] Shishehgar, S., Mahmoodi, A., Dolatian, M., Mahmoodi, Z., Bakhtiary, M. and Majd, H.A. (2013) The Relationship of Social Support and Quality of Life with the Level of Stress in Pregnant Women Using the PATH Model. *Iranian Red Crescent Medical Journal*, **15**, 560-565. http://dx.doi.org/10.5812/ircmj.12174

[10] Muglia, L.J. and Katz, M. (2010) The Enigma of Spontaneous Preterm Birth. *New England Journal of Medicine*, **362**, 529-535. http://dx.doi.org/10.1056/NEJMra0904308

[11] Plunkett, J. and Muglia, L.J. (2008) Genetic Contributions to Preterm Birth: Implications from Epidemiological and Genetic Association Studies. *Annals of Medicine*, **40**, 167-179. http://dx.doi.org/10.1080/07853890701806181

[12] Goldenberg, R.L., Culhane, J.F., Iams, J.D. and Romero, R. (2008) Epidemiology and Causes of Preterm Birth. *The Lancet*, **371**, 75-84. http://dx.doi.org/10.1016/S0140-6736(08)60074-4

[13] Rodríguez-Bernal, C.L., Rebagliato, M., Iñiguez, C., Vioque, J., Navarrete-Muñoz, E.M., Murcia, M., *et al.* (2010) Diet Quality in Early Pregnancy and Its Effects on Fetal Growth Outcomes: The Infancia y Medio Ambiente (Childhood and Environment) Mother and Child Cohort Study in Spain. *The American Journal of Clinical Nutrition*, **91**, 1659-1666. http://dx.doi.org/10.3945/ajcn.2009.28866

[14] Rocco, P.L., Orbitello, B., Perini, L., Pera, V., Ciano, R.P. and Balestrieri, M. (2005) Effects of Pregnancy on Eating Attitudes and Disorders: A Prospective Study. *Journal of Psychosomatic Research*, **59**, 175-179. http://dx.doi.org/10.1016/j.jpsychores.2005.03.002

[15] Delvarian-Zadeh, M., Bolbol Haghighi, N. and Ebrahimi, H. (2007) The Relationship between Nutritional Status of Mothers in Their Third Trimester and Delivery of Low Birth Weight Infants. *Arak Medical University Journal*, **10**, 54-63.

[16] Fowles, E.R. (2004) Prenatal Nutrition and Birth Outcomes. *Journal of Obstetric, Gynecologic, & Neonatal Nursing*, **33**, 809-822. http://dx.doi.org/10.1177/0884217504270599

[17] Imdad, A. and Bhutta, Z.A. (2012) Maternal Nutrition and Birth Outcomes: Effect of Balanced Protein-Energy Supplementation. *Paediatric and Perinatal Epidemiology*, **26**, 178-190. http://dx.doi.org/10.1111/j.1365-3016.2012.01308.x

[18] Haftenberger, M., Heuer, T., Heidemann, C., Kube, F., Krems, C. and Mensink, G. (2010) Relative Validation of a Food Frequency Questionnaire for National Health and Nutrition Monitoring. *Nutrition Journal*, **9**, 36. http://dx.doi.org/10.1186/1475-2891-9-36

[19] Mirmiran, P., Hosseini Esfahani, F., Mehrabi, Y., Hedayati, M. and Azizi, F. (2010) Reliability and Relative Validity of an FFQ for Nutrients in the Tehran Lipid and Glucose Study. *Public Health Nutrition*, **13**, 654-662. http://dx.doi.org/10.1017/S1368980009991698

[20] Kamali Fard, M., Alizadeh, R., Sehati Shafaei, F. and Gojazadeh, M. (2010) The Effect of Lifestyle on the Rate of Preterm Birth. *Journal of Ardabil University of Medical Sciences*, **10**, 55-63.

[21] Luke, B., Brown, M.B., Misiunas, R., Anderson, E., Nugent, C., van de Ven, C., *et al*. (2003) Specialized Prenatal Care and Maternal and Infant Outcomes in Twin Pregnancy. *American Journal of Obstetrics and Gynecology*, **189**, 934-938.

[22] Khatun, S. and Rahman, M. (2008) Socio-Economic Determinants of Low Birth Weight in Bangladesh: A Multivariate Approach. *Bangladesh Medical Research Council Bulletin*, **34**, 81-86.

[23] Burris, H.H., Mitchell, A.A. and Werler, M.M. (2010) Periconceptional Multivitamin Use and Infant Birth Weight Disparities. *Annals of Epidemiology*, **20**, 233-240. http://dx.doi.org/10.1016/j.annepidem.2009.12.003

[24] Haugen, M., Margrete Meltzer, H., Lise Brantsæter, A., Mikkelsen, T., Louise Østerdal, M., Alexander, J., *et al*. (2008) Mediterranean-Type Diet and Risk of Preterm Birth among Women in the Norwegian Mother and Child Cohort Study (MoBa): A Prospective Cohort Study. *Acta Obstetricia et Gynecologica Scandinavica*, **87**, 319-324. http://dx.doi.org/10.1080/00016340801899123

[25] Khoury, J., Henriksen, T., Christophersen, B. and Tonstad, S. (2005) Effect of a Cholesterol-Lowering Diet on Maternal, Cord, and Neonatal Lipids, and Pregnancy Outcome: A Randomized Clinical Trial. *American Journal of Obstetrics and Gynecology*, **193**, 1292-1301. http://dx.doi.org/10.1016/j.ajog.2005.05.016

[26] Haggarty, P., Campbell, D.M., Duthie, S., Andrews, K., Hoad, G., Piyathilake, C., *et al*. (2009) Diet and Deprivation in Pregnancy. *British Journal of Nutrition*, **102**, 1487-1497. http://dx.doi.org/10.1017/S0007114509990444

[27] Loy, S.-L., Marhazlina, M., Nor Azwany, Y. and Hamid Jan, J. (2011) Higher Intake of Fruits and Vegetables in Pregnancy Is Associated with Birth Size. *Southeast Asian Journal of Tropical Medicine and Public Health*, **42**, 1214-1223.

[28] Siega-Riz, A.M., Promislow, J.H., Savitz, D.A., Thorp, J.M. and McDonald, T. (2003) Vitamin C Intake and the Risk of Preterm Delivery. *American Journal of Obstetrics and Gynecology*, **189**, 519-525. http://dx.doi.org/10.1067/S0002-9378(03)00363-6

[29] Abedini, Z. and Gaini, M. (2011) Dietary Food Intake of Pregnant Women Based on Food Guide Pyramid and Its Related Factors. *Iran Journal of Nursing*, **24**, 36-46.

[30] Mahmoodi, Z., Karimlou, M., Sajjadi, H., Dejman, M. and Vameghi, M. (2013) Development of Mother's Lifestyle Scale during Pregnancy with an Approach to Social Determinants of Health. *Global Journal of Health Science*, **5**, 208-219. http://dx.doi.org/10.5539/gjhs.v5n3p208

[31] Bakhtiari, A., Sajadi, P. and Hajian, K. (2007) Nutrient Consumption Pattern in Pregnant Women Referred to Health Care Centers in Babol.

[32] Fadakar Soogheh, K., Ghav, A., Niknami, M. and Kazemnejad Leili, E. (2012) Relationship between Mothers' Nutritional Status and Weight Gain during Pregnancy with Low Birth Weight. *Journal of Guilan University of Medical Sciences*, **21**, 27-35.

[33] Shaikh, F., Zeeshan, F., Hakeem, R., Basit, A., Fawwad, A. and Hussain, A. (2014) Maternal Dietary Intake and Anthropometric Measurements of Newborn at Birth. *The Open Diabetes Journal*, **7**, 14-19. http://dx.doi.org/10.2174/1876524601407010014

[34] Adler, N.E. and Newman, K. (2002) Socioeconomic Disparities in Health: Pathways and Policies. *Health Affairs*, **21**, 60-76. http://dx.doi.org/10.1377/hlthaff.21.2.60

[35] Dolatian, M., Mirabzadeh, A., Forouzan, A.S., Sajjadi, H., Majd, H.A. and Moafi, F. (2012) Preterm Delivery and Psycho-Social Determinants of Health Based on World Health Organization Model in Iran: A Narrative Review. *Global Journal of Health Science*, **5**, 52-64. http://dx.doi.org/10.5539/gjhs.v5n1p52

[36] Park, M.-J., Son, M., Kim, Y.-J. and Paek, D. (2013) Social Inequality in Birth Outcomes in Korea, 1995-2008. *Journal of Korean Medical Science*, **28**, 25-35. http://dx.doi.org/10.3346/jkms.2013.28.1.25

[37] Moster, D., Lie, R.T. and Markestad, T. (2008) Long-Term Medical and Social Consequences of Preterm Birth. *New England Journal of Medicine*, **359**, 262-273. http://dx.doi.org/10.1056/NEJMoa0706475

[38] Zarbakhsh Bhari, M.R., Hoseinian, S., Afrooz, G. and Hooman, H. (2012) The Comparison of Many Biological Characteristics, Economical Conditions, General Health (Mental), of Mothers with Low and Normal Birth Weight at Guilan Province. *Payavard Salamat*, **5**, 67-78.

[39] Sukalich, S., Mingione, M.J. and Glantz, J.C. (2006) Obstetric Outcomes in Overweight and Obese Adolescents. *American Journal of Obstetrics and Gynecology*, **195**, 851-855. http://dx.doi.org/10.1016/j.ajog.2006.06.070

[40] Viengsakhone, L., Yoshida, Y. and Sakamoto, J. (2010) Factors Affecting Low Birth Weight at Four Central Hospitals in Vientiane, Lao PDR. *Nagoya Journal of Medical Science*, **72**, 51-58.

18

Consequences of Working in Eldercare during Organizational Changes and Cut Backs While Education and Clinical Supervision Was Provided: A Mixed Methods Study

Birgitta Fläckman[1], Kirsti Skovdahl[2], Ingegerd Fagerberg[1,3], Mona Kihlgren[4], Annica Kihlgren[5*]

[1]Department of Health Care Sciences, Ersta Sköndal University College, Stockholm, Sweden
[2]Faculty for Health Sciences, Buskerud and Vestfold University College, Drammen, Norway
[3]Department of Neurobiology, Care Sciences and Society, Karolinska Institute, Stockholm, Sweden
[4]Centre for Caring Sciences, Örebro University Hospital, Örebro, Sweden
[5]School of Health and Medical Sciences, Örebro University, Örebro, Sweden
Email: Birgitta.Flackman@esh.se, Kirsti.Skovdahl@hbv.no, Ingegerd.Fagerberg@esh.se, Mona.Kihlgren@telia.com, *Annica.Kihlgren@oru.se

Abstract

Background: Reorganization and downsizing can disrupt a competent staff and conflicts can arise between what the employee is being asked to do and their knowledge and competences. Reduced job satisfaction among nursing home staff with increased workload and strain can occur. Aim and Objectives: The aim was to investigate the organizational climate and prevalence of burnout symptoms among caregivers over time in three Swedish nursing homes (NH I-III) undergoing organizational changes, while education and clinical supervision were provided. Design: The study design combines qualitative and quantitative methods in a longitudinal two-year follow-up project in NH I-III. Methods: Support through education and clinical supervision was provided for caregivers only at NH I and NH II. At NH I-III caregiver self-assessments and interviews were completed and analysed three different times. Results: NH I revealed improvement and increased innovation over time, while NH II showed a decline with no ability to implement new knowledge. NH III retained a more status quo. Conclusions: Organizational changes and cutbacks, occurring at different times, appeared to cause major stress and frustration among the three personnel groups. They felt

*Corresponding author.

guilty about not meeting their perceived obligations, seemed to have lost pride in their work but kept struggling. The changes seemed to over-shadow attempts to improve working conditions through education and clinical supervision initially. Implications for practice: It will be important to learn from reorganizations and the consequences they will have for the staff and quality of care. Important topics for future research are to study financial cutbacks and changes in organizational processes in care of older people to be able to develop a more person centered care for older people.

Keywords

Nursing Home, Organizational Climate and Burnout, Education and Clinical Supervision, Cutbacks and Organizational Changes

1. Introduction

The focus in this study is to investigate through caregivers' self- assessments and experiences, the organizational climate and burnout relative to changes and cut backs in elder care; while education and clinical supervision was provided. In the last decades, the care of older people has increasingly come to be viewed as a primarily public matter in Sweden. Divergent and opposite views to mobilise a reorganization of public services and identities of workers have been discussed in the Nordic countries [1] [2]. When interviewing employees at different nursing homes, they regarded their job as meaningful and were proud of their work but revealed that a moral uneasiness existed between the care they were able to provide and what they would like to provide [3]. Häggström *et al.* [4] have also found mixed feelings toward work. The caregivers experienced a committed relationship to older people but felt guilty when organizational structures forced them to rush their daily care and did not allow enough time for each person. It is difficult for caregivers to balance all demands successfully and Suhonen *et al.* [5] as well as Fagerberg and Engström [6] suggest that key aspects are ethical discussions within their work.

Organizational changes have been addressed as a factor that prevents learning interventions in the care of older people [7] and this is unfortunate, considering the importance of development in the care of older people. Within the context of nursing health care, supervision has been viewed as a valuable means of supporting and developing professional practice [8] and one way of recruiting and keeping personnel aimed at developing professional competence and personal identity [9]. Another way to develop staff members' lack of formal competence can be with e-learning and e-assessment [10]. Furthermore, ethical dilemmas are present in almost every nursing care situation and clinical supervision makes it possible for reflection on these ethical dilemmas [11] resulting in a process leading to increased quality of care [12].

As people live longer nowadays, they consume an increasing amount of various forms of health care. At the same time, the financial resources in society are decreasing, necessitating efficient usage of health care resources [13] [14]. Among those working in elder care, licensed practical nurses (LPNs) and nurse's aides (NAs) make up the largest group, with registered nurses (RNs) numbering only a few [14] [15]. Weak leadership is thought to be a prominent problem in municipal care of the old [6] [16]. There is also a problem with illness absenteeism and staff turnover, which have increased markedly during recent years. In municipal health care, a lack of well-educated personnel and difficulties in retaining personnel are well-known facts that have an immense impact [17].

Burnout is most commonly defined as a syndrome that includes feelings of emotional exhaustion, depersonalization and reduced personal accomplishment [18]. In Sweden, burnout has been cited as one of the major causes of the sharp increase in long-term disability [19]. When meaningfulness and manageability are not balanced, feelings of fatigue and symptoms of burnout appear. Likewise, high job involvement plays paradoxically a part in burnout [20].

According to Ekvall [21], the work climate is regarded as an attribute of the organization, such that attitudes, feelings and behaviours characterize life in the organization. These exist, independent of the perceptions and understandings held by organization members. The work climate influences organizational processes such as problem-solving, decision-making, communication, co-ordination and control [21] [22]. In times of downsizing and reorganization, challenges emerge regarding ways of keeping and motivating those affected [23].

The literature review shows that changes in the health care system exist today and has done so previously as well. Changes will always likely be present in elder care and necessary if they contribute to the development of health care in a positive manner. However, little is known about how caregivers are influenced by these changes and cutbacks in the elder care context during clinical supervision. Presumably these changes can undermine caregivers' ability to do good work and to feel good about their work. It therefore seems important to focus on caregivers' experiences when threats of organizational change and closing of facilities occur during clinical supervision.

The aim of the present study was to investigate the organizational climate and prevalence of burnout symptoms among caregivers over time in three Swedish nursing homes undergoing organizational changes, while education and clinical supervision was provided. This study addressed a research question: What are the consequences for the caregivers when organizational changes are a fact?

2. Methods and Material

The present study is part of a two-year, annual follow-up, longitudinal project in three Swedish municipal nursing homes of older people (NH I, NH II and NH III). At the outset of the project, promises were made that no organizational changes were planned. Despite this, as a result of political decisions, administrative reorganization and personnel reductions on all shifts were instituted at all three of the NHs, though at different times during the two-year period. At the onset of the present study a quantitative approach was chosen in order to explore organizational climate and prevalence of burnout among caregivers in three nursing homes. Due to the organizational changes that led to subjects dropping out, we decided to include interview data with the same focus from the caregivers working at the involved NHs.

2.1. Design and Settings

The present study has combined quantitative and qualitative methods to facilitate acquisition of knowledge and improved understanding. Certain questions required a mixed methods approach; mixed-method research can expand and improve analytical power in studies [24]. Organizational climate and prevalence of burnout symptoms were studied at the group level at three different nursing homes. After collection of the initial baseline data at NH I, NH II and NH III a two-year support through education and clinical supervision started at NH I and NH II. Caregivers were able to request the educational topics and could give their input regarding the approach taken to the education and clinical supervision. A voluntary training program was offered about once a month and delivered by physicians and nurse specialists during the two years. Caregivers sought more knowledge about different diseases, as well as additional training in communication, seeking literature, team cooperation, and conflict management. This staff support is further described by Fläckman *et al.* [25].

In an effort to be more comprehensive, the NHs were followed over a two years period. NH I, with 40 residents, was situated in a municipality with a population of over 100,000. NH II and NH III, with 40 and 52 residents respectively, were located in a municipality with 20,000 inhabitants. Several residents had dementia diagnoses and multiple diseases, some in advanced stages including behavioural and psychiatric symptoms of dementia (BPSD). Each of the NHs had one RN and the total ratio, including LPNs and NAs, was 1.0 staff member per bed (including night staff). The staff members were distributed so as to cover all the shifts.

The time frame for the announcement of the politicians' decisions for reorganization and financial cutbacks at the respective NHs is presented in **Figure 1**. For example, nine RNs from NH I who resigned were replaced by LPNs. Additionally, a simultaneous reduction in the number of employees and an increase in the number of residents took place at NH II, and when personnel were absent, they were not replaced. NH III was still in its original form at the end of the study, but the number of residents and personnel had decreased markedly.

2.2. Sample

The personnel at the three NHs gave their informed consent to participate in the study. The Regional Research Ethics Committees (§ 803/99, § 00-070) approved this project. Information was given verbally that participation was voluntary, confidentiality was guaranteed and that participants had the right to leave the study at any time without giving a reason. The caregivers who volunteered to participate, performed the self-assessments and were interviewed are further presented in **Table 1**, **Table 2**. The participating caregivers varied at the three data collection points, but no new caregivers were included during the study time. Caregivers dropped out due to illness, personnel turnover, inability to respond for personal reasons and undefined reasons.

Table 1. Caregivers at NH I-III and their response rate on CCQ with mean values and standard deviations (SD) versus normative data on innovative and stagnated organizations according to Ekvall [22].

		I			II			III		
		Baseline	12 month	24 month	Baseline	12 month	24 month	Baseline	12 month	24 month
Caregiver		n = 19	n = 13	n = 12	n = 16	n = 13	n = 13	n = 11	n = 14	n = 11
RNs and LPNs		1/15	1/11	0/11	0/7	0/6	0/7	0/2	0/1	0/2
NAs and SS		2/0	1/0	1/0	8/1	6/1	6/0	9/0	13/0	9
Female/male		17/1	12/1	10/2	15/1	12/1	11/2	11/0	14/0	11/0
Age (years)	18 - 34	5	2	2	4		2	2	2	1
	35 - 44	8	7	7	8	7	6		1	1
	45 - 54	2	2	2	2	3	3	4	5	4
	55 - 64	3	2	1	2	3	2	5	6	5
Day/night shift		16/2	12/1	9/3	13/3	13/0	12/1	11/0	12/2	10/1
Years of	<1	1								
health care	1 - 10	2	2	2	5	3	4	2	1	2
experience	>10	15	11	10	11	10	9	9	13	9
Missing data		1								
Challenge		2.13	2.65	2.42	2.03	1.86	1.65	2.02	1.89	1.82
Innov.org.	Stagna.org	(0.69)	(0.55)	(0.56)	(0.50)	(0.46)	(0.45)	(0.29	(0.30)	(0.47)
2.38	1.63									
Freedom		1.72	1.94	2.00	1.79	1.74	1.69	1.76	1.98	1.96
Innov.org.	Stagna.org	(0.36)	(0.59)	(0.40)	(0.32)	(0.45)	(0.41)	(0.40)	(0.49)	(0.65)
2.10	1.53									
Idea support		1.74	2.25	2.37*	1.95	1.72	1.37	1.87	1.78	1.80
Innov.org.	Stagna.org	(0.75)	(0.79)	(0.59)	(0.69)	(0.61)	(0.63)	(0.34)	(0.70)	(0.66)
1.83	1.08									
Trust		1.69	2.05	2.16	1.56	1.45	1.03	1.87	1.76	1.96
Innov.org.	Stagna.or	(0.84)	(0.84)	(0.51)	(0.67)	(0.54)	(0.68)	(0.30)	(0.69)	(0.59)
1.78	1.28									
Dynamism		2.00	2.50	2.45	1.76	1.68	1.48	1.95	1.85	1.69
Innov.org.	Stagna.org	(0.71)	(0.61)	(0.63)	(0.63)	(0.45)	(0.44)	(0.34)	(0.46)	(0.55)
2.20	1.40									
Playfulness		2.55	2.55	2.58	1.95	1.95	1.83	1.98	1.98	2.05
Innov.org.	Stagna.org	(0.73)	(0.73)	(0.55)	(0.56)	(0.56)	(0.57)	(0.59)	(0.59)	(0.69)
2.30	1.40									
Debates		1.66	2.10	2.08	1.74	1.66	1.58	1.67	1.65	1.64
Innov.org.	Stagna.org	(0.53)	(0.64)	(0.57)	(0.43)	(0.42)	(0.34)	(0.22)	(0.44)	(0.62)
1.58	1.05									
Conflicts		0.98	0.58	0.38	0.86	1.11	1.49	0.73	0.77	0.82
Innov.org.	Stagna.org	(0.94)	(0.88)	(0.45)	(0.61)	(0.67)	(0.97)	(0.40)	(0.45)	(0.53)
0.78	1.40									
Risk taking		1.52	1.98	1.90	1.39	1.48	1.15	1.33	1.29	1.29
Innov.org.	Stagna.org.	(0.56)	(0.57)	(0.56)	(0.44)	(0.38)	(0.45)	(0.38)	(0.48)	(0.65)
1.95	0.53									
Idea time		1.24	2.08**	2.15*	1.51	1.46	1.25	1.56	1.52	1.33
Innov.org.	Stagna.org	(0.68)	(0.69)	(0.53)	(0.49)	(0.55)	(0.42)	(0.45)	(0.52)	(0.56)
1.48	0.97									

*Significant at ≤0.05; **Significant at ≤0.01 within nursing home. Registered nurse (RNs), Licensed Practical Nurses (LPNs), Nurse Aides (NAs), Social service (SS).

Table 2. Caregivers at NH I-III and their response rate on MBI with mean values and standard deviations (SD) versus normative data on low, average and high burnout according to Maslach *et al.* [18].

			I			II			III		
				12	24		12	24		12	24
			Baseline	month	month	Baseline	month	month	Baseline	month	month
			n = 13	n = 13	n = 10	n = 16	n = 13	n = 13	n = 10	n = 14	n = 11
Caregivers											
RNs and LPNs			0/10	1/11	1/9	0/7	0/6	0/6	0/2	0/2	0/2
NAs and SS			2/0	1/0	0/0	8/1	6/1	6/1	8/0	12/0	9/0
Female/male			12/0	12/0	8/2	15/1	12/1	11/2	10/0	14/0	11/0
Age (years)		18 - 34	4	3	2	4	3	2	1	2	1
		35 - 44	4	6	6	8	5	6		1	1
		45 - 54	1	2	2	2	3	3	4	6	4
		55 - 64	3	2		2	2	2	5	5	5
Day/night shift			10/2	12/1	8/2	13/3	12/1	12/1	10/0	12/2	10/1
Years of		<1	1								
health care		1 - 10	2	2	2	5	2	4	1	2	2
experience		>10	9	11	8	11	11	9	9	12	9
Missing data			1								
Emotional exhaustion			23.08	17.46	15.78	12.12	14.38	12.31	12.40	12.86	8.55
Low	Average	High	(7.18)	(10.52)	(10.61)	(7.97)	(7.73)	(9.46)	(7.53)	(9.16)	(6.95)
0 - 16	17 - 27	28+									
Depersonalization			3.85	3.46	2.30	1.31	2.77	2.23	3.40	2.71	2.82
Low	Average	High	(3.65)	(2.57)	(4.74)	(1.85)	(1.96)	(2.01)	(3.17)	(3.00)	(3.63)
0 - 5	6 - 10	11+									
Personal accomplishment			40.46	40.62	42.33	37.31	35.08	31.62	37.50	32.50	38.09
Low	Average	High	(5.94)	(7.45)	(8.79)	(7.80)	(7.79)	(8.06)	(5.13)	(13.40)	(13.46)
37+	30 - 36	0 - 29									

Registered Nurse (RNs), Licensed Practical Nurses (LPNs), Nurse Aides (NAs), Social service (SS).

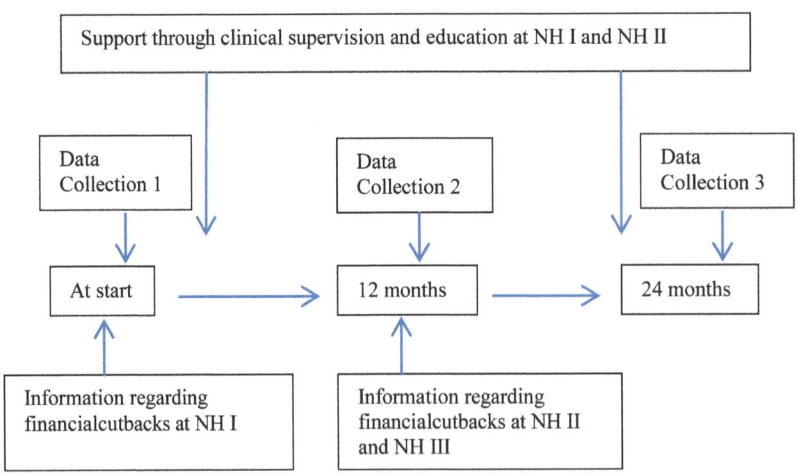

Figure 1. Design of the study and time frame for information regarding financial cutbacks at the respective nursing homes, NH I, NH II and NH III.

2.3. Self-Assessment Questionnaires

The self-assessment questionnaires were distributed three times: before the intervention (baseline) and after 12 and 24 months, respectively. The completed questionnaires were returned individually in postage-paid envelopes addressed to the research team. Two different instruments of Lickert type were used: the Creativity and Innovative Climate Questionnaire (CCQ) [21] and the Maslach Burnout Inventory (MBI) [18].

2.3.1. Creativity and Innovative Climate Questionnaire

The CCQ is a self-assessment instrument, earlier used in Sweden [26]-[28] for measuring the degree of creativity and innovativeness in an organization. The CCQ contains 50 items covering 10 dimensions: challenge; freedom; idea support; trust/openness; safety dynamics/liveliness; playfulness/humour; debates; conflicts; risk-taking; idea-time [22]. Each dimension includes five statements assessed on a four-point Likert scale from absolutely not applicable (0) to applicable to some extent (1), fairly applicable (2) and highly applicable (3). The points for these five statements are added up and then divided by the number of statements. The dimensions were developed in connection with several large-factor analytic studies. The stability and internal consistency reliability have been tested and are considered high [22]. Mean reference values for innovative and stagnated organizations are presented in **Table 1**. The instrument is described as being an organizational rather than individual measure, as changes are measured at the organizational level [22]. The mean value in each dimension can vary from a strong and dynamic (3.0) to an extremely weak and stagnating organization (0.0). The scales are not reciprocally calibrated, for example the value 2.0 in one dimension is not necessarily higher than 1.5 in another. Comparisons can only be made dimension by dimension. Cronbach's alpha reliability coefficient for the CCQ subscales in the present study is 0.85.

2.3.2. Maslach Burnout Inventory

MBI has become one of the most widely used and validated instruments for assessing burnout and was translated into Swedish by Hallsten [29]. The scale consists of 22 items divided into three subscales. The first subscale, Emotional Exhaustion (EE), uses nine items to assess "feelings of being emotionally overextended and exhausted by one's work". Depersonalization (DP), another subscale, consists of five items and assesses "unfeeling and impersonal response towards recipients of one's care". The Personal Accomplishment (PA) subscale, with eight items, assesses "feeling of competence and successful achievement in one's work with people" [18] [30]. The MBI is scored on a 7-point scale from never (0) to every day (6). Responses are summed to give separate scores for each of the three subscales and are categorized into low, average or high degrees of burnout according to normative data presented in **Table 2** [18]. High levels of EE and DP and low levels of PA are associated with burnout. The reliability coefficient for the MBI subscale in the present study was 0.75.

2.4. Interviews

The caregivers at the three NHs were interviewed at the start, after 12 months and after 24 months, giving in total 30 + 21 + 13 interviews at NH I, 16 + 11 + 17 interviews at NH II and 18 + 19 + 13 interviews at NH III. The individual interviews lasted 30 - 60 minutes and took place in a setting chosen by the interviewees, where there would be no interruptions. They were asked about their expectations and experiences of work at the NH and were encouraged to speak freely about the joys and difficulties of their working situation as well as how they envisioned the future. To investigate changes over time the same questions were asked at all three occasions. To clarify and develop the content of what the interviewees said, questions such as "please tell me more about this situation" or "can you tell me more about how you felt about that situation" were asked cf. [31]. The interviews were tape-recorded with the participants' permission and transcribed verbatim by an experienced secretary. For the present study, five interviews were chosen at random from each interview occasion within the three groups of caregivers (5 × 3 from NH I- III), which resulted in a total of 45 interviews.

2.5. Data Analysis

2.5.1. Quantitative Data

Because the sample was small and those taking part were not always the same at the three data-collection points, group mean scores rather than individual scores have been used in the quantitative data analysis. Further, the

Kruskal-Wallis non-parametric method was used to analyse the differences within the three independent NHs at baseline and both follow-up measurements. Descriptive analysis using means and standard deviations was used for all responses. When significant differences emerged, the Mann-Whitney U-test was used [32]. The analyses were carried out using the SPSS computer program (SPSS, version 17). Because a P value of ≤0.05 was considered statistically significant, the majority of the results were not significant. When the quantitative analyses were finalized it appeared that the results were statistically weak due to the number of drop outs. Thus, qualitative analyses were deemed important to explore how the caregivers expressed the domains in the scales.

2.5.2. Qualitative Data

The interviews were analyzed by two of the authors who had not performed the interviews and the procedure was a directed content analysis [33], using the 10 dimensions in CCQ and the three subscales in MBI as a raster. All text from the three interview periods were read several times and coded immediately using the predetermined codes [33]. Notes were made indicating whether and how the interviews changed over time dependent on occurrences and intensity. To validate the outcome, all authors discussed the findings until a consensus was reached.

3. Results

Results from interviews and caregivers' self-assessments will be presented and described separately for the respective NHs. The numbers of included caregivers from the three NHs with their response rate of CCQ are presented in **Table 1** and **Figure 2(a)**, **Figure 3(a)** and **Figure 4(a)**. MBI scores are presented in **Table 2** and **Figure 2(b)**, **Figure 3(b)**, and **Figure 4(b)**.

3.1. NH I

3.1.1. Creative Climate Questionnaire

The majority of the baseline scores from the CCQ demonstrated that NH I functioned at the innovative organizational level and an improvement from baseline was seen, which suggests a more innovative organization. The scores for "conflict" and "trust" improved at NH I (**Table 1**, **Figure 2(a)**).

3.1.2. Maslach Burnout Inventory

The scores from the MBI measurement in NH I did not suggest burnout, but the degree of burnout changed for the better. The caregivers estimated their symptom as average in the EE subscale at baseline, but demonstrated more favourable scores after 24 months. In the PA subscale, the caregivers at NHI estimated favourable scores throughout the study (**Table 2**, **Figure 2(b)**).

3.1.3. Interviews

The *first* interviews showed that conflicts were prevalent in the personnel group due to different opinions about prioritizing work and indecisive leadership. Challenges were seen with their expectations of something new, and there was a foreboding that the implementation of new ideas would be limited due to lack of time and support from management. The interviews showed a high degree of emotional frustration among the caregivers. "*It was going to be so new and great here. But we don't get on and there's always some argument among the staff. You don't work in the same way. What's worse is that nobody deals with it. The manager says we have to accept that it takes time to start something new, but I mean really we can't continue like this*".

The *second* interviews showed that conflicts still existed among the caregivers as well as frustrations over the weak leadership. Several of the personnel had quit and a lack of dynamics existed due to untrained and insecure replacements. They reported that several in the personnel group had been on sick leave for a shorter or longer period due to emotional distress or exhaustion. The caregivers expressed exhaustion, fatigue and resignation. They tried to do their job, but had no creative ideas or solutions for developing the care they were giving at work. The caregivers felt unable to fully utilize their competence in their work and felt that they worked without planning. The conflicts and lack of time created a lack of freedom. "*I've never been at a workplace as bad as this one and we don't have any leadership. One after the other quits or gets burned out. I have no use for my education here. You can't plan and do activities and you don't have time for anything because you never know what your day will be like*".

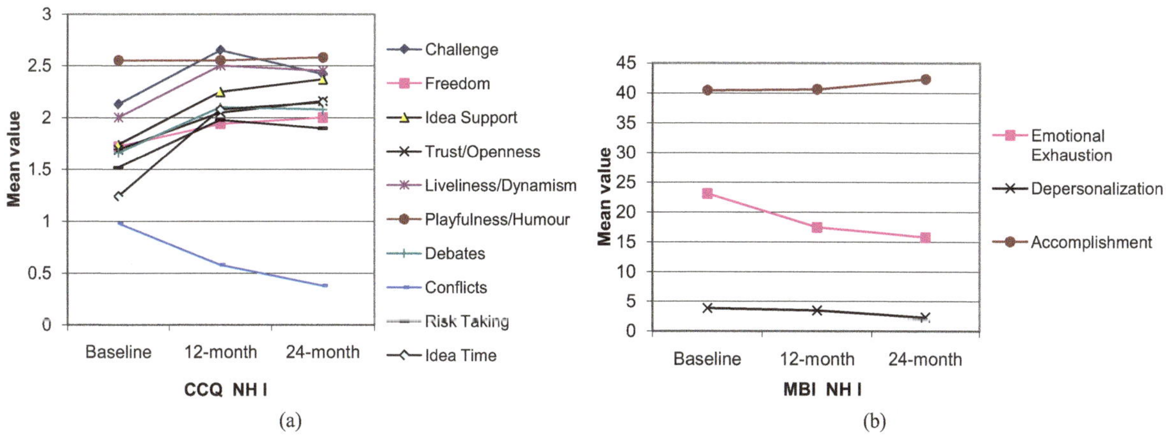

Figure 2. (a) Caregivers' (NH I) response rate from CCQ with mean values. High values (except conflicts) are representative of a more positive climate; (b) Caregivers' (NH I) response rate from MBI with mean values. Low values (except accomplishment) are representative of a more favourable score.

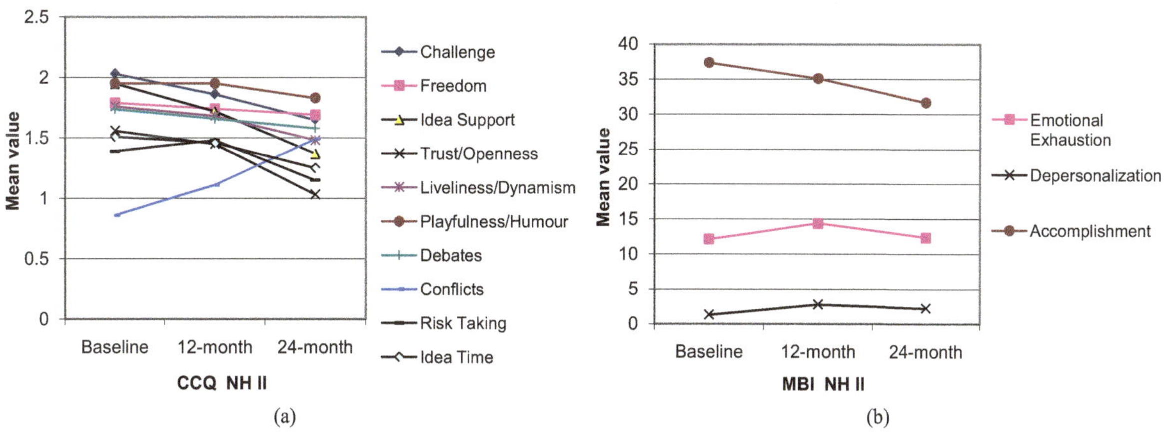

Figure 3. (a) Caregivers' (NH II) response rate from CCQ with mean values. High values (except conflicts) are representative of a more positive climate; (b) Caregivers' (NH II) response rate from MBI with mean values. Low values (except accomplishment) are representative of a more favourable score.

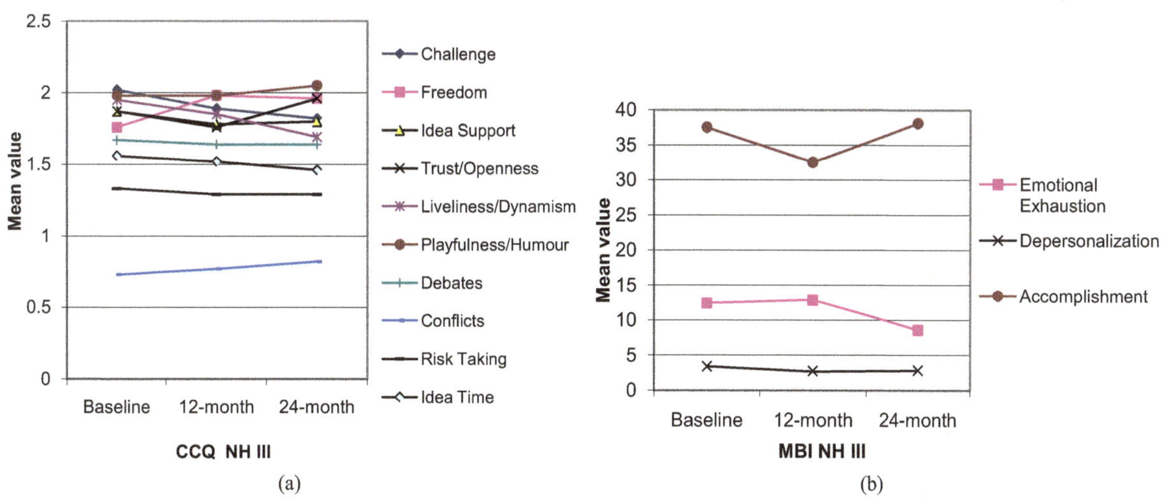

Figure 4. (a) Caregivers' (NH III) response rate from CCQ with mean values. High values (except conflicts) are representative of a more positive climate; (b) Caregivers' (NH III) response rate from MBI with mean values. Low values (except accomplishment) are representative of a more favourable score.

The *third* interviews showed that many in the primary work group had left their employment. The remaining caregivers attempted to find new challenges and possibilities in their work. The interviews indicated an ability among the caregivers to tolerate uncertainty and disparity, despite the conflicts that still existed due to poor leadership. The personnel had divided themselves into informal groups attempting to support each other. They used playfulness and humour and avoided discussions in an effort to cope with their work. Some said they could cope with the work situation because they "did not care" or "just didn't think about it". "*Our expectations were much higher than how things turned out. Dementia care here was going to be really super, but that hasn't happened. There's been quite a bit of friction, but things have got better. We try to stick together and laugh about the craziness, otherwise you can't cope. Of course it's always so that you don't like everybody, but what does that matter? I don't care about things like that, as long as you can work together*".

3.2. NH II

3.2.1. Creative Climate Questionnaire

The caregivers from NH II had scores that progressed negatively from baseline to the 24-month follow up. Some of the scores suggested stagnation in the organization. The scores for "conflict" and "trust" worsened over the period (**Table 1**, **Figure 3(a)**).

3.2.2. Maslach Burnout Inventory

The caregivers from NH II had a low mean score on DP and EE, which changed after 12 months, but still indicated a low degree of burnout. NH II had a mean score at 24 months on the PA subscale that was considered "average" (**Table 2**, **Figure 3(b)**).

3.2.3. Interviews

The *first* interviews showed that challenge, freedom and playfulness were prevalent, with positive feelings and expectations regarding their new work. The caregivers felt they had idea-support from management when they were given the opportunity to implement a positive milieu for themselves and the older people and they showed independence in their decisions. Time was available to work on new ideas and the climate suggested easiness in the workplace atmosphere. The relationship with colleagues and the residents showed emotional involvement with security. Nevertheless some anxiety existed about the unfamiliar milieu due to the vast physical layout of the NH. "*I try to do my best for the residents so they will thrive. Meet their needs to the extent I can*".

After one year, the interviews showed uncertainty, and the caregivers' trust and openness with regard to the management had decreased. There were increasing conflicts in work groups, and the freedom and independence in decision-making that was seen in the first interviews was no longer prominent. From having been focused on their work, the personnel were now more focused on their individual situations. Nevertheless, they still had hope that they could continue to influence their work and some emotional involvement still existed. "*We've heard rumors that another facility will be closed and that more residents will come here without any increase in staff. What happened to everything they promised us, for example, that we'd be part of a project, get supervision and support? Do we dare believe that we can continue as we planned and as we were promised*"?

Emotional involvement and trust in management were not prominent in the *third interviews*, and the caregivers were more watched over in their work. They were frustrated about conflicts that existed in the groups and the lack of idea-support. Signs of fatigue and exhaustion now appeared in the interviews when the caregivers described their work as more hectic. They realized that their expectations of giving good care would not been fulfilled, but they were not willing to give up. "*What's missing is a discussion about what duties we should have in relation to the staff we are. Now we're supposed to clean, do laundry, take care of purchasing, call in staff and give residents personal care, food and such, but does the individual older person have a right to individual time*"?

3.3. NH III

3.3.1. Creative Climate Questionnaire

The scores from NH III were stable throughout the study, however half of the CCQ dimensions demonstrated less favourable conditions at the 24-month follow-up. The scores for "conflict" and "trust" remained stable (**Table 1**, **Figure 4(a)**).

3.3.2. Maslach Burnout Inventory

In the EE and PA subscales from NH III, the mean scores worsened at 12 months, but eventually improved from baseline after 24 months (**Table 2**, **Figure 4(b)**).

3.3.3. Interviews

The *first* interviews showed that trust, safety dynamics and playfulness predominated. The caregivers were preoccupied with their work and showed self-confidence when describing a workplace that was familiar to them. They knew their colleagues and management well and did not feel tension in their work groups. They showed pride when describing that the residents and management appreciated them. The atmosphere was relaxed, even though there was a great deal of work to do and sometimes no time for doing that "little extra". "*I think it works fine, we can bring up problems, new suggestions and we often get responses to what we bring up. We're going to change the schedule and food provision, and I think that's good. Our supervisor lets us decide more and more for ourselves how we want to work*".

After one year, the interviewees expressed feelings of insecurity and increasing conflict. Their degree of freedom was reduced by the changes that had occurred. Not knowing where to go in the morning, which residents they would be responsible for or with whom they would work created the feeling they were losing control. The tension in the work groups was increasing and they felt forced to cooperate. The playfulness and humour present in the first interview was not prominent, and they missed colleagues who had left. The discussions about reduction and termination notices filled their days, and according to the caregivers, these had given rise to an unpleasant atmosphere. "*Now we think there's no reason for us after knowing we're going to be closed down—well we do what has to be done, nothing more, and I feel dissatisfied with not being able to plan my work*".

Resignation was shown in *the third* interviews, and the caregivers talked about making the best of the situation. They were safeguarding themselves and the residents. Conflicts and irritations existed in the work groups. Lack of commitment was seen when they described the discussions about planning their work. Nevertheless, their feelings of responsibility for the residents, a belief in the future or in new work made them continue to struggle. The appreciation they received from the residents, relatives and management helped them carry out their work. "*I wouldn't have anything against leaving this place, the work situation is insecure. In elder care there must be people who are interested and there must be commitment to working with the old people. As it is now it's difficult to feel motivated. You can't lose your patience when you work with old people*".

4. Discussion

The present mixed methods study investigates consequences experienced over time by the caregivers at three NHs when organizational changes are an actuality; and when caregivers at two of these NHs received support. Interesting findings include the negative outcome from both assessment instruments and the interviews at all three NHs when they were anticipating and undergoing organizational changes and cutbacks (**Figure 1**). Cutbacks appeared to cause much stress and frustration among the personnel groups, and they felt guilty about not fulfilling their perceived obligations. The caregivers from all three NHs gave the impression of continuing to struggle, but seemed to have lost something important: their pride in giving good care. Juthberg *et al.* [34] have described similar results in a study; not being able to provide the care residents need, experiencing shortcomings and caregivers having to silence one's conscience in order to continue working. Likewise stress from a troubled conscience can lead to emotional exhaustion and a risk for burnout [35]. Jones [36] concluded that clinical supervision challenges nurses to think differently about their professional work. This has also been highlighted as a possible strategy for recruitment and retention within all levels of nursing personnel [37]. Therefore, supervision can help nurses to achieve a number of valuable objectives. In a literature review, Butterworth *et al.* [38] found that most clinical supervision was seen as an educative and supportive process, in addition they also found in some studies that clinical supervision can be cost-effective and improve care.

NHs I and II received support through education and clinical supervision for two years, but the outcome with regard to their scores was different. The scores at NH III were more constant compared with the others. The announcement of planned cutbacks and their realization may have been mirrored in the scores. The support provided in the present study seemed to have helped the caregivers at NH I, but was not able to alter the situation for caregivers at NH II, who were informed of the changes later in the study. A second analysis of all NH II interviews was reported by Fläckman *et al.* [25], with the conclusion that after two years the caregivers' willingness to care continued, despite their disappointment in the worsened working conditions. The main theme that resulted was that despite shattered expectations, a willingness to care for older people remained. The continued education and clinical supervision seem to be one factor behind this continued commitment. These findings demonstrate that support and caregiver involvement in educational programs are important during times of change and when disappointments arise in the workplace. Other aspects such as the work climate and support and inclusion of all those that work in the nursing homes are also important when education and clinical supervision are offered to produce good outcomes [39].

At NHs II and III, the MBI scores worsened at the 12-month assessment, which corresponded to the time when they began discussing financial cutbacks (**Figure 1**). The 24-month scores improved for "feelings of competence and successful achievement in one's work" at NH III. By that time, the personnel at NH III were familiar with the plan for staff reduction. Research regarding the correlations and a manifestation of burnout is quite difficult to interpret because the theories vary a great deal and the research findings often contradict each other [40] [41]. Different patterns of possible causes and consequences imply that different intervention strategies need to be used [42].

The interviews from NH I-II revealed a disappointment with the leadership and the staffs there were not as stable as those at NH III who were more pleased with their leaders. Hannigan *et al.* [43] revealed that poor support from management was associated with higher emotional exhaustion and that longer work experience in a field was associated with lower depersonalization scores. This is consistent with the BMI result of NH I in this study. Hyrkäs *et al.* [44] claimed that even first-line leaders need support in their work. Several organizational changes and scarce economic resources in the health care system have also challenged nursing leaders.

Using a quantitative design, Edwards *et al.* [45] found a lower level of burnout among community mental health nurses when clinical supervision was effective. Similarly, Begat and Severinsson [46] reported that clinical supervision had an influence on nurses' experiences of well-being. Based on a quantitative design, Choi and Johantgen [47] showed that supportive supervision was important for job satisfaction among certified nursing assistants in nursing homes. This confirmed findings reported by Hyrkäs [44] and Hyrkäs *et al.* [48] who also found that levels of stress decreased when supervision was available.

In a creative climate, organization members are emotionally involved in their work [22]. Furthermore, a question can be raised about the nursing care quality during the two-year period. According to Ekvall [21], the work climate influences organizational processes such as problem-solving, decision-making, communication, co-ordination and control. Providing care in the context of organizational change can lead to conflicts between what the employee is being asked to do and the employee's knowledge and competences. Creative work climate has a strong relationship to job satisfaction [49]. The present study followed the personnel group over time from an organizational rather than an individual perspective, which is in accordance with Ekvall [22]. The results presented in the present study have similarities with Trydegård [2] indicating that changes have not been appreciated.

5. Study Limitations

In this study due to reorganizations and cut backs the quantitative research originally intended was not possible; so a mixed method design was chosen. Changes are common in elder care [1]-[5] and there is much that can interfere and influence ongoing research projects. This can be seen as a challenge for future research in elder care especially for longitudinal studies. A mixed method that included a combination of methods was chosen to meet this challenge, add strength to the study and facilitate a deeper understanding into the experiences of caregivers of older people. Data from the qualitative analysis provided insights and facilitated interpretation of statistical findings based on the self-assessment instruments [50]. The approach also provided an opportunity to maximize the richness of the narratives [51]. The divergent results in the quantitative and qualitative data among caregivers in NH I are interesting. One question is whether questionnaires are sensitive enough to capture the necessary dimensions in an organizational climate. The present findings demonstrate, however, how the use of mixed methods [24] can lead to accounts that strengthen and/or complement each other. One contributory factor may also be lack of time needed to respond to and reflect on the questions in the questionnaires. Another issue is what kind of situations the caregivers assessed and what kind of situations they reported. The questionnaires were directed towards the work climate, and the interviews were more focused on the work situation as a whole. In the interviews, most of the frustrations expressed were over the leadership, which the assessment scales did not capture. This can be understood in that the leader and their leadership are more important than the staff as individuals when change is to be executed [12].

The interviews were analyzed by two of the authors who had not performed the interviews. In the present study, this can be viewed as a strength, as the authors were able to consider the interviews as a whole and without any pre-understandings based on the interview situations or earlier analyses of quantitative data. The personnel groups were largely comparable. NHs II and III were, however, located in a smaller municipalities than NH I, which may have limited staff members' opportunities for job change. This may have affected the results as well as the structural changes and reductions in staff due to political decisions. During an intervention period of two years, many unexpected events can occur, as was the case in the present study. The unplanned changes in the NHs, due to the organizational changes and uncontrolled factors influencing the study, created another threat to internal validity [52].

6. Conclusions and Practical Implications

The results of the present study showed negative outcomes at all three NHs when the organizational changes and cutbacks were announced. The new situation caused major stress and frustrations among the personnel groups, and they felt guilty about not meeting their perceived obligations. Providing education and clinical supervision during such a time constituted a challenge, but it is interesting to speculate on what would have happened without such an intervention. The present study emphasizes the need for more research in this area to further investigate factors for preventing burnout, improving creativity and innovation in an effort to help people stay in their occupations as caregivers of older people. More research is also needed on how these factors such as reorganization and cutbacks influence person-centered care and the support the staff requires to provide good quality care to older people. Further research is also necessary in the area of the working environment and its effects on recruiting and retaining health care staff in elder care.

Acknowledgements

The authors wish to express their gratitude to the Swedish Association of Local Authorities in Gävleborg, the Centre for Caring Sciences, Örebro University Hospital and to the University of Gävle for their financial support during the study. Our thanks also go the personnel from the nursing homes for their cooperation and extra efforts.

Contributions

Study design: AK, BF, KS, MK; data collection: BF; data analysis: AK, BF, KS and manuscript preparation: BF, AK, KS, IF, MK

Conflict of Interest

No conflict of interest has been declared by the authors.

References

[1] Dahl, H.M. (2009) New Public Management, Care and Struggles about Recognition. *Critical Social Policy*, **29**, 634-654. http://dx.doi.org/10.1177/0261018309341903

[2] Trydegård, G.-B. (2012) Care Work in Changing Welfare States: Nordic Care Workers' Experiences. *European Journal of Ageing*, **9**, 119-129. http://dx.doi.org/10.1007/s10433-012-0219-7

[3] Dwyer, L.-L., Andershed, B., Nordenfeldt, L. and Ternestedt, B.-M. (2009) Dignity as Experienced by Nursing Home Staff. *International Journal of Older People Nursing*, **4**, 185-193. http://dx.doi.org/10.1111/j.1748-3743.2008.00153.x

[4] Häggström, E., Mamhidir, A.-G. and Kihlgren, A. (2010) Caregiver's Strong Commitment to Their Relationship with Older People. *International Journal of Nursing Practice*, **16**, 99-105. http://dx.doi.org/10.1111/j.1440-172X.2010.01818.x

[5] Suhonen, R., Stolt, M., Virtanen, H. and Leino-Kilpi, H. (2011) Organizational Ethics: A Literature Review. *Nursing Ethics*, **18**, 285-303. http://dx.doi.org/10.1177/0969733011401123

[6] Fagerberg, I. and Engström, G. (2012) Care of the Old—A Matter of Ethics, Organization and Relationship. *International Journal of Qualitative Studies on Health and Well-Being*, **7**, 9684. http://dx.doi.org/10.3402/qhw.v7i0.9684

[7] Petterson, I.-L., Donnersvärd, H.Å., Lagerström, M. and Toomingas, A. (2006) Evaluation of an Intervention Programme Based on Empowerment for Eldercare Nursing Staff. *Work and Stress*, **20**, 353-369. http://dx.doi.org/10.1080/02678370601070489

[8] Kihlgren, M. and Hansebo, G. (2014) Organizational Change and Supervision. In: Watkins Jr., C. and Milne, D.L., Eds., *The Wiley International Handbook of Clinical Supervision*, John Wiley & Sons, Ltd., West Sussex, 155-176. http://dx.doi.org/10.1002/9781118846360.ch7

[9] Berggren, I. and Severinsson, E. (2003) Nurse Supervisors' Actions in Relation to Their Decision-Making Style and Ethical Approach to Clinical Supervision. *Journal of Advanced Nursing*, **41**, 615-622. http://dx.doi.org/10.1046/j.1365-2648.2003.02573.x

[10] Nilsson, A. and Engström, M. (2015) E-Assessment and an e-Training Program among Elderly Care Staff Lacking Formal Competence: Results of a Mixed-Methods Intervention Study. *BMC Health Services Research*, **15**, 189 http://dx.doi.org/10.1186/s12913-015-0843-y

[11] Berggren, I., Barbosa da Silva, A. and Severinsson, E. (2005) Core Ethical Issues of Clinical Nursing Supervision. *Nursing and Health Services*, **7**, 21-28. http://dx.doi.org/10.1111/j.1442-2018.2005.00224.x

[12] Johansson, G., Andersson, L., Gustafsson, B. and Sandahl, C. (2010) Between Being and Doing—The Nature of Leadership of First-Line Nurse Managers and Registered Nurses. *Journal of Clinical Nursing*, **19**, 2619-2628. http://dx.doi.org/10.1111/j.1365-2702.2010.03211.x

[13] The Swedish National Board of Health and Welfare (2004) Vård och omsorg om äldre—En läges rapport 2004 [Caring for Older People—A Situation Report 2004]. Socialstyrelsen, Stockholm. (In Swedish) http://www.socialstyrelsen.se/publikationer2004/2004-131-5

[14] The Swedish National Board of Health and Welfare (2012) Vård och omsorg om äldre—En läges rapport 2012 [Caring for Older People—A Situation Report 2012]. Socialstyrelsen, Stockholm. (In Swedish) http://www.socialstyrelsen.se/publikationer2012/2012-2-2

[15] The Swedish National Board of Health and Welfare (2009) Vård och omsorg om äldre—En läges rapport 2009 [Caring for Older People—A Situation Report 2009]. Socialstyrelsen, Stockholm. (In Swedish) http://www.socialstyrelsen.se/publikationer2009/2009-126-44

[16] Josefsson, K. and Hansson, M. (2011) To Lead and to Be Led in Municipal Elderly Care in Sweden as Perceived by Registered Nurses. *Journal of Nursing Management*, **19**, 498-506. http://dx.doi.org/10.1111/j.1365-2834.2011.01228.x

[17] Fagerberg, I. and Gilje, F. (2007) A Comparison of Curricular Approaches of Care of the Aged in Swedish and US Nursing Programs. *Nurse Education in Practice*, **7**, 358-364. http://dx.doi.org/10.1016/j.nepr.2006.11.007

[18] Maslach, C., Jackson, S.E. and Leiter, P. (1996) Maslach Burnout Inventory Manual. Consulting Psychologists Press, Palo Alto.

[19] Ekstedt, M. and Fagerberg, I. (2005) Lived Experiences of the Time Preceding Burnout. *Journal of Advanced Nursing*, **49**, 59-67. http://dx.doi.org/10.1111/j.1365-2648.2004.03264.x

[20] Vinje, H.F. and Mittelmark, M.B. (2007) Job Engagement's Paradoxical Role in Nurse Burnout. *Nursing and Health Sciences*, **9**, 107-111. http://dx.doi.org/10.1111/j.1442-2018.2007.00310.x

[21] Ekvall, G. (1987) The Climate Metaphor in Organization Theory. In: Bass, B. and Drenth, P., Eds., *Advances in Organizational Psychology*, Sage, Beverly Hills, 177-190.

[22] Ekvall, G. (1996) Organizational Climate for Creativity and Innovation. *European Journal of Work and Organizational Psychology*, **5**, 105-123. http://dx.doi.org/10.1080/13594329608414845

[23] Hertting, A., Nilsson, K., Theorell, T. and Sätterlund Larsson, U. (2004) Downsizing and Reorganization: Demands, Challenges and Ambiguity for Registered Nurses. *Journal of Advanced Nursing*, **45**, 145-154. http://dx.doi.org/10.1046/j.1365-2648.2003.02876.x

[24] Cresswell, J.W. and Plano Clark, V.L. (2007) Designing and Conducting Mixed Method Research. Sage Publications Inc., Thousand Oaks.

[25] Fläckman, B., Fagerberg, I., Häggström, E., Kihlgren, A. and Kihlgren, M. (2007) Despite Shattered Expectations a Willingness to Care for Elders Remains with Education and Clinical Supervision. *Scandinavian Journal of Caring Science*, **21**, 379-389. http://dx.doi.org/10.1111/j.1471-6712.2007.00478.x

[26] Lövgren, G., Rasmussen, B.H. and Engström, B. (2002) Working Conditions and the Possibility of Providing Good Care. *Journal of Nursing Management*, **10**, 201-209. http://dx.doi.org/10.1046/j.1365-2834.2002.00290.x

[27] Norberg, K.-G., Hellzén, O., Sandman, P.-O. and Asplund, K. (2002) The Relationship between Organizational Climate and the Content of Daily Life People with Dementia Living in a Group-Dwelling. *Journal of Clinical Nursing*, **11**, 237-246. http://dx.doi.org/10.1046/j.1365-2702.2002.00579.x

[28] Söderlund, M., Norberg, A. and Hansebo, G. (2014) Validation Method Training: Nurses' Experiences and Ratings of Work Climate. *International Journal of Older People Nursing*, **9**, 79-89. http://dx.doi.org/10.1111/opn.12027

[29] Hallsten, L. (1985) Burnout. A Study about Adaption and Development Processes in a Bureaucracy [Burnout. En studie kring anpassning och utvecklings processer I en byråkrati]. Rapport 18:2, LAMI Arbetsmarknadsinstitutet,

Länsarbetsnämnden I Stockholms Läns, Stockholm. (in Swedish)

[30] Maslach, C. and Jackson, S.E. (1981) The Measurement of Experienced Burnout. *Journal of Occupational Behaviour*, **2**, 99-113. http://www.aagbi.org/sites/default/files/Maslach.pdf http://dx.doi.org/10.1002/job.4030020205

[31] Kvale, S. (1997) The Qualitative Research Interview [Den kvalitativa forsknings intervjun]. Studentlitteratur, Lund. (in Swedish)

[32] Polit, D.F. and Beck, C.T. (2008) Nursing Research. Principles and Methods. 7th Edition, Lippincott Williams & Wilkins, Philadelphia.

[33] Hsieh, H.-F. and Shannon, S.E. (2005) Three Approaches to Qualitative Content Analysis. *Qualitative Health Research*, **15**, 1277-1288. http://dx.doi.org/10.1177/1049732305276687

[34] Juthberg, C., Eriksson, S., Norberg, A. and Sundin, K. (2008) Stress of Conscience and Perceptions of Conscience in Relation to Burnout among Care-Providers in Older People. *Journal of Research in Nursing*, **17**, 1897-1906. http://dx.doi.org/10.1111/j.1365-2702.2007.02184.x

[35] Glasberg, A.L., Eriksson, S. and Norberg, A. (2007) Burnout and "Stress of Conscience" among Healthcare Personnel. *Journal of Advanced Nursing*, **57**, 392-403. http://dx.doi.org/10.1111/j.1365-2648.2007.04111.x

[36] Jones, A. (2006) Clinical Supervision: What Do We Know and What Do We Need to Know? A Review and Commentary. *Journal of Nursing Management*, **14**, 577-585. http://dx.doi.org/10.1111/j.1365-2934.2006.00716.x

[37] Cummins, A. (2009) Clinical Supervision: The Way Forward? A Review of the Literature. *Nurse Education in Practice*, **9**, 215-220. http://dx.doi.org/10.1016/j.nepr.2008.10.009

[38] Butterworth, T., Bell, L., Jackson, C. and Pajnkihar, M. (2008) Wicked Spell or Magic Bullet? A Review of the Clinical Supervision Literature 2001-2007. *Nurse Education Today*, **28**, 264-272. http://dx.doi.org/10.1016/j.nedt.2007.05.004

[39] Nolan, M., Davies, S., Brown, J., Wilkinson, A., Warnes, T., McKee, K., Flannery, J. and Stasi, K. (2008) The Role of Education and Training in Achieving Change in Care Homes: A Literature Review. *Journal of Research in Nursing*, **13**, 411-433. http://dx.doi.org/10.1177/1744987108095162

[40] Schaufeli, W.B. and Buunk, B.P. (1996) Burnout: An Overview of 25 Years of Research and Theorizing. In: Schabracq, M.J., Winnubst, J.A.M. and Cooper, C.L., Eds., *Handbook of Work and Health Psychology*, John Wiley & Son Ltd., Chichester, 383-425.

[41] Schaufeli, W.B., Bakker, A.B. and Van Rhenen, W. (2009) How Changes in Job Demands and Resources Predict Burnout, Work Engagement, and Sickness Absenteeism. *Journal of Organizational Behavior*, **30**, 893-917. http://dx.doi.org/10.1002/job.595

[42] Schaufeli, W.B. and Bakker, A.B. (2004) Job Demands, Job Resources, and Their Relationship with Burnout and Engagement: A Multi-Sample Study. *Journal of Organizational Behavior*, **25**, 293-515. http://dx.doi.org/10.1002/job.248

[43] Hannigan, B., Edwards, D., Coyle, D., Fothergill, A. and Burnard, P. (2000) Burnout in Community Mental Health Nurses: Findings from the All-Wales Stress Study. *Journal of Psychiatric and Mental Health Nursing*, **7**, 127-134. http://dx.doi.org/10.1046/j.1365-2850.2000.00279.x

[44] Hyrkäs, K. (2005) Clinical Supervision, Burnout, and Job Satisfaction among Mental Health and Psychiatric Nurses in Finland. *Issues in Mental Health Nursing*, **26**, 531-556. http://dx.doi.org/10.1080/01612840590931975

[45] Edwards, D., Burnard, P., Urnard, P., Hannigan, B., Cooper, L., Adams, J., Juggessur, T., Fothergil, A. and Coyle, D. (2006) Clinical Supervision and Burnout: The Influence of Clinical Supervision for Community Mental Health Nurses. *Journal of Clinical Nursing*, **15**, 1007-1015. http://dx.doi.org/10.1111/j.1365-2702.2006.01370.x

[46] Begat, I. and Severinsson, E. (2006) Reflection on How Clinical Nursing Supervision Enhances Nurses' Experiences of Well-Being Related to Their Psychosocial Work Environment. *Journal of Nursing Management*, **14**, 610-616. http://dx.doi.org/10.1111/j.1365-2934.2006.00718.x

[47] Choi, J.S. and Johantgen, M. (2012) The Importance of Supervision in Retention of CNAs. *Research in Nursing & Health*, **35**, 187-199. http://dx.doi.org/10.1002/nur.21461

[48] Hyrkäs, K., Appelqvist-Schmidlechner, K. and Haataja, R. (2006) Efficacy of Clinical Supervision: Influence on Job Satisfaction, Burnout and Quality of Care. *Journal of Advanced Nursing*, **55**, 521-535. http://dx.doi.org/10.1111/j.1365-2648.2006.03936.x

[49] Sellgren, S.F., Ekvall, G. and Tomson, G. (2008) Leadership Behaviour of Nurse Managers in Relation to Job Satisfaction and Work Climate. *Journal of Nursing Management*, **16**, 578-587. http://dx.doi.org/10.1111/j.1365-2934.2007.00837.x

[50] Morgan, D.G. and Stewart, N.J. (2002) Focus on Research Methods, Theory Building through Mixed-Method Evaluation of a Dementia Special Care Unit. *Research in Nursing & Health*, **25**, 479-488. http://dx.doi.org/10.1002/nur.10059

[51] Szabo, V. and Strang, V.R. (1997) Secondary Analysis of Qualitative Data. *Advances in Nursing Science*, **20**, 66-74. http://dx.doi.org/10.1097/00012272-199712000-00008

[52] Burns, N. and Grove, S.K. (2001) The Practice of Nursing Research, Conduct, Critique, and Utilization. 4th Edition, W.B. Saunders Company, Philadelphia.

19

Pilot Study on an Integrated Pilates and Yoga Program for Decreasing Postpartum Depression in Women

Yi-Li Ko[1*], Pi-Chu Lin[2], Chi-Li Yang[3], Chie-Pein Chen[4], Huai-Jung Shih[5]

[1]Department of Nursing, College of Medicine, Fu-Jen Catholic University, Taiwan
[2]School of Nursing and Master Program in Long-Term Care, College of Nursing, Taipei Medical University, Taiwan
[3]Department of Physical Education, Shih Chien University, Taiwan
[4]Department of Obstetrics and Gynecology, Mackay Memorial Hospital, Taiwan
[5]Department of Dentistry, University of Szeged, Szeged, Hungary
Email: *071462@mail.fju.edu.tw, pclin02@gmail.com, chili@mail.usc.edu.tw, cpchen@mmh.org.tw, sunplay77712@hotmail.com

Abstract

Objective: This study evaluated the effectiveness of a 10-week exercise intervention in reducing depression and fatigue in women with postpartum depression. Design: A one-group pretest/posttest quasi-experiment was conducted. Setting: A postpartum ward in a medical center in Taipei city was used. Participants: Nineteen women at 7 - 12 weeks postpartum with an Edinburgh Postnatal Depression Scale score ≥ 9 were recruited. Methods: The women participated in a postpartum exercise support program 1 hour per week for 10 weeks. The program was led by a professional coach; it integrated yoga, Pilates, elastic band exercise, low-intensity aerobics, and motherhood role experience sharing. Results: After the postpartum exercise support program intervention, depression scores decreased from 10.4 ± 3.29 to 7.80 ± 2.73 (t = 3.632, P = 0.003); fatigue scores decreased from 8.73 ± 5.02 to 5.40 ± 3.89 (t = 2.988, P = 0.010). Conclusion: PESP administered to women with postpartum depression appeared to benefit their psychological wellbeing.

Keywords

Exercise, Women with Postpartum Depression, Fatigue, Depression

*Corresponding author.

1. Introduction

Postpartum depression (PPD) is a prominent health issue. Few multidisciplinary studies, combining physical-exercise and nursing, have been conducted. The prevalence of PPD reports 10% - 15% in Western country [1]. In Taiwan, a 40% prevalence of mild-to-severe PPD has been reported at 6 weeks postpartum [2]. In a meta-analysis of 30 studies based only on structured clinical interview assessments, the point prevalence is estimated to be approximately 6.5% - 12.9%, involving both major and minor depression at various times during the first postpartum year [3]. PPD is characterized by episodes of irritability, insecurity, anxiety, fatigue, guilt, obsessive thoughts, and physical symptoms, which have negative effects on mother-infant interactions [4] [5]. Research has determined that 44% - 95% of postpartum mothers in the United States experience postpartum fatigue [6] [7]. Postpartum fatigue is also a common problem in Taiwan [8] [9]. Postpartum fatigue is a predictor of PPD [9]. Postpartum psychological problems can interfere with a new mother's ability to care for her child and may adversely affect her quality of life [9].

In Taiwan, if postpartum women exhibit depressive symptoms, physicians often consult psychiatrists to prescribe antidepressants; however, mothers are typically worried about exposing infants to the adverse side effects of drugs through breastfeeding; they are generally afraid to take medicine. Epidemiological research has suggested that physical activity may be associated with reduced symptoms of depression. Few studies have investigated the effect of exercise programs on women's psychological health during the postpartum period. However, concerns have been expressed regarding the methodological quality of these studies [10]-[12]. In Taiwan, only one study has been conducted on PPD intervention [12]. Heh evaluated whether an exercise program (consisting of one hour-long session per week at a hospital and two sessions per week at home for 3 months) was more effective than routine care for alleviating depression symptoms in women with an Edinburgh Postnatal Depression Scale (EPDS) score > 10 [12]. The results indicated that women with PPD ($n = 33$) who attended an exercise support program were less likely to exhibit high depression scores at 5 months postpartum than the women in the control group ($n = 30$). Da Costa *et al.* examined 88 Women with PPD who underwent a 12-week home-based exercise program and determined that the program constituted an effective intervention for alleviating postpartum depressive symptoms, particularly in women with greater depression at baseline (EPDS; score > 13). The intervention group exhibited a significantly lower post-treatment EPDS score than the usual—care group did (mean difference 4.06 points, 95% confidence interval 1.51 - 6.61, $p < 0.001$) [11]. Armstrong and Edwards developed a 12-week pram-walking exercise program (for mothers and their babies) and compared the outcomes to those of a social support group (nonstructured session, similar to a playgroup). The results suggested that members of the pram-walking group reduced their level of depressive symptomatology significantly more than the members of the social support group did [10].

Chinese culture considers "postpartum preservation" as critical to the overall wellness of a woman who has given birth. In Chinese culture, postpartum women should eat high-calorie and high-protein food, rest, and avoid the outdoor environment in addition to caring for their infants. In this period, mothers may reduce or stop exercising, which can affect subsequent exercise habits [13]. Ko *et al.* [14] developed a community-based "Yoga and Pilates Exercise Program" for general postpartum women (*i.e.* not targeted at specifically women with PPD) in Taiwan. The exercise program was conducted in group sessions of 60 min, once a week for 3 months (12 times in total) by a professional coach. A total of 23 women at 2 - 6 months postpartum completed the entire program and it was determined that the program was effective in improving the women's PPD. This study used only a small sample size, and the authors found that it was difficult to encourage women to go outdoors for exercise because of the traditional ideas about postnatal care in Taiwan.

Despite limited evidence regarding women with PPD, the National Institute for Health and Clinical Excellence in the United Kingdom recommended in their postnatal mental-health guidelines that health professionals should consider exercise as a management strategy for women experiencing mild-to-moderate PPD.

The purpose of this study was to evaluate the effectiveness of a postpartum exercise support program (PESP) in reducing fatigue and depression in women with PPD.

2. Materials and Methods

2.1. Study Design

This study adopted a quasi-experimental one-group pretest/posttest design and a convenience sampling method.

Study participants, who were at 7 - 12 weeks postpartum, participated in a 10-week exercise program developed in this study, one session perweek.

2.2. Participants and Setting

Participants were recruited between May and July 2013 at a medical center in Taipei. The inclusion criteria were as follows: being postpartum, aged between 20 and 40 years, exhibiting no maternal or neonatal complications, having an EPDS score ≥ 9, and willing to participate in the study.

Research assistants (RAs) used the EPDS to assess women at 1 - 3 days after giving birth in the postpartum ward. When women exhibited an EPDS score ≥ 9, Ras obtained written consent after explaining research the purpose and process, and left a contact telephone number. Researchers arranged women to participate in a PESP until 7 - 12 weeks postpartum.

After the initial recruited, 50 women with an EPDS score ≥ 9 accepted the invitation; however, after 1 - 2 months, having completed 1 month, several women left the program, causing a small sample size in this study. The reasons of withdrawal from the study included the following: women were living in Southern Taiwan (their parents' home, which was far from the study site); women had to work on the day of class; women felt tired, had no motivation, and did not feel comfortable letting others take care of their baby.

Overall, 19 women were enrolled, 15 of whom completed the entire program and answered the questionnaires (a 79% valid response rate). Four women did not complete the 10-week exercise program for work or childcare reasons.

2.3. Experimental Intervention

2.3.1. Postpartum Exercise Support Program

The PESP was designed for women who were considered to have mild PPD. The exercise support program consisted of the following: 1) 10-minute warm-up and 10-minute cool-down; 2) a 40-minute whole body stretching exercise, integrated Pilates, yoga, and elastic band exercise, which achieved a target heart rate (HR) of 60% - 75% of maximal HR; 3) after-exercise program with a 30-minute experience-sharing session, including breastfeeding and talking about adapting to the new role as a mother; 4) RAs created an exercise program video and upload edit to Facebook; the participants were encouraged to practice the exercises based on the video at home at least twice perweek. In addition, the RAs reminded the participants to attend the exercise class every week using Line (a mobile device application).

2.3.2. Professional Coach-Led Program

The postpartum exercise program was led by a professional coach who was one of researchers. The coach has a doctor of philosophy degree and is licensed to teach postpartum yoga and Pilates. The postpartum exercise program was conducted in a group once per week; it lasted from 10:30 to 11:30 a.m. every Saturday for a 3-month period (total 10 sessions) in a gym at a university.

2.3.3. Facilitators

Ras used Line to maintain weekly contact with the postpartum women to monitor home exercise, provide remote care, and remind the women to continue with the program. To encourage participation: a gift was presented after each week (e.g. a pedometeror gift certificate).

The stadium is a professional venue with wooden floor classrooms and spacious, comfortable areas; there is a beautiful surrounding landscape with numerous trees and large areas of grassland that provide bright and sunny spaces. The researcher and Ras joined the weekly program, to help with taking care of the babies when necessary; in addition, female family members of the participants were allowed to attend classes.

2.4. Instruments

The study tools comprised a structured questionnaire designed in this study, including basic information, postpartum exercise status, the Fatigue Symptoms Checklist (FSC), and the EPDS.

Basic Information: The basic information obtained was age, height, prepregnancy weight, weight gain during pregnancy, current weight, education level, occupation, family type, annual household income, pregnancy history, childbirth history, and the current infant feeding method.

Postpartum Exercise Status: The data obtained were used to evaluate whether participants were engaging in regular exercise, their exercise intensity, exercise conditions, and barriers to exercise after giving birth.

FSC: The FSC, developed by Yoshitake, [15] was designed for the National Institute of Occupational Safety and Health in Japan to assess fatigue symptoms. The checklist contains 30 common fatigue symptoms that are categorized into three categories as follows: sleepy and powerless (Items 1 - 10), difficulty concentrating (Items 11 - 20), and partial abnormalities of the body (Items 21 - 30). Each item permits a dichotomous yes/no (0 to 1) response. Possible scores range between 0 and 30, and a high score is indicative of severe fatigue.

The FSC is a multidimensional scale that exhibits strong reliability and validity and is not excessively taxing to complete. Milligan *et al.* [7] used the FSC to measure postpartum fatigue among 285 mothers immediately after birth, during the hospitalization period, and 6 weeks postpartum. Their results indicated that the internal consistency of the scale ranged from 0.82 to 0.95.

EPDS: The EPDS has been determined to exhibit higher validity than the BDI regarding sensitivity and specificity [16] [17]. The EPDS consists of 10 short statements and requires less than 5 minutes to complete. A cutoff score of 9 is recommended for identifying genuine cases of postnatal depression [16].

Study Tools and Tests of Reliability and Validity: The scales adopted in this study were widely used domestic and international scales, all of which exhibit good reliability. In this study, the Cronbach α obtained for both the FSC and the EPDS was 0.86.

2.5. Ethical Considerations

This study was approved by the institutional review board of the hospital where the study was conducted (IRB No. 12MMHIS161). The purpose and process were explained to the participants, and after signing an informed consent form, they were enrolled in the study. In addition, participants were informed that they could withdraw from the study at any time without a loss of benefits. The women were assured that involvement in the study would not affect their medical care and that all information obtained from the questionnaire would be treated confidentially and used only for research purposes.

2.6. Data Collection Procedure

Our RA recruited eligible women with PPD in the postpartum ward in a medical center in Taipei by describing the purpose of the study. Because Taiwanese have a "doing-the-month" culture whereby, after delivery, postpartum women are discharged from the hospital and expected to stay at home for an entire month; therefore, our RA called the women regarding follow-up care during this month.

A pretest was conducted before the first session of the exercise program. The pretest was used to collect basic participant information, postpartum exercise habits, postpartum fatigue, and body composition. After the participants had attended 10 sessions of the program, a posttest was conducted to obtain measurements regarding postpartum fatigue and depression.

2.7. Data Analysis

SPSS version 19.0 was used to analyze data and significant level was set as 0.05 (SPSS, Chicago, IL, USA). Participants' basic information was exhibited according to frequency, percentage, mean, and standard deviation (SD). A paired *t* test was employed to identify differences in fatigue and depression before and after the exercise program.

3. Results

3.1. Basic Participant Information

The average age of the 15 postpartum women was 34.3 ± 3.8 years. The average number of pregnancies among the participants was 1.27 ± 0.46; 12 participants (80%) were primiparas. All participants had a college degree or above (100%). In addition, most participants had a full-time job (60%). Twelve (80%) participants had NSDs, whereas 20% had CS. Six (40%) participants breastfed exclusively, and the others adopted mixed feeding methods. Only four (26.7%) of the participants exercised after childbirth. Six of the participants (40%) lived in a nuclear family (**Table 1**).

3.2. Depression and Fatigue of Participants

The mean score of depression in the pretest was 10.40 ± 3.29 points; the scores ranged between 0 and 30. Three women (20%) scored ≥12 points on the EPDS. The mean depression score was 7.80 ± 2.73 points in the posttest. The decrease of 2.60 points was significant ($t = 3.632$, $P = 0.003$).

The mean score of fatigue in the pretest was 8.73 ± 5.02 points, and 5.40 ± 3.89 points in the posttest. A paired t test was used to compare feelings of fatigue before and after the exercise intervention; the decrease of 3.33 points was significant ($t = 2.988$, $P = 0.010$). Comparing the scores of fatigue subscales revealed significant differences in physical and psychological scores before and after the intervention ($t = 2.525$, $P = 0.024$; $t = 2.824$, $P = 0.014$). No significant difference was observed in the symptom score before and after the test ($t = 1.234$, $P = 0.238$; **Table 2**).

Table 1. Basic information of study participants ($n = 15$).

Characteristic	n (%)	$M \pm SD$
Age (year)		34.33 ± 3.84
Gravida		1.27 ± 0.46
Primipara	12 (80%)	
Education level		
≥University	13 (86.7%)	
≤College	2 (13.3%)	
Work status		
—Full-time job	9 (60%)	
—Housewife	6 (40%)	
Method of delivery		
—NSD	12 (80%)	
—Cesarean section	3 (20%)	
Breastfeeding		
—Exclusive	6 (40%)	
—Formula	1 (6.7%)	
—Mixed feeding	8 (53.3%)	
Exercise habits (pretest)		
—Yes	4 (26.7%)	
—No	11 (73.3%)	
Family structure		
—Nuclear family	6 (40%)	
—Other	9 (60%)	

Note. NSD: normal spontaneous delivery; C: section, cesarean section.

Table 2. Participants depression and fatigue scores ($n = 15$).

Dimensions and subscales	Pretest $M \pm SD$	Post-test $M \pm SD$	t	P
Fatigue				
—Physical (items 1 - 10)	4.13 ± 2.13	2.40 ± 1.77	2.525	0.024*
—Psychological (items 11 - 20)	2.40 ± 2.20	1.47 ± 1.77	2.824	0.014*
—Symptoms (items 21 - 30)	2.20 ± 2.15	1.53 ± 1.51	1.234	0.238
—Total score	8.73 ± 5.02	5.40 ± 3.89	2.988	0.010*
Depression scores ($n = 15$)	10.40 ± 3.29	7.80 ± 2.73	3.632	0.003*

*$P < 0.05$; **$P < 0.001$.

4. Discussion

In this study, 20% of participants who were 7 - 12 weeks postpartum exhibited a depression score of ≥12 points in the pretest, which is the cutoff point indicating depression in Taiwan; this suggests that these women were prone to depression. However, the depression scores obtained in this study were lower than those obtained by Chen's *et al.* study, [2] who found that in Taiwan, 40% of women 6 weeks postpartum received a diagnosis of postnatal depression. Robertson *et al.* reported that the prevalence rate of PPD was 30% - 75% [18], which is higher than that exhibited in this study. The occurrence of depressive illnesses following childbirth can be detrimental to mothers, marital relationships, and children, and can have adverse long-term effects if left untreated. Certain studies have indicated that postpartum moods are associated with changes in hormone levels, including progesterone, estrogen, cortisone, beta-endorphins, oxytocin, and prolactin [17]; therefore, many postpartum women experience depression. In addition, psychosocial factors play key roles; Robertson *et al.* indicated that the most critical period for detecting postnatal depression is within 6 weeks of delivery [18]. Daley, MacArthur, and Winter stated that the peak incidence of depression is within the first 4 - 6 weeks after giving birth [19]. When hormone levels stabilize, depressive moods may improve. The period of data collection in this study was 7 - 12 weeks after delivery; therefore, the prevalence of depression should have been lower than that demonstrated immediately after delivery.

The results of this study demonstrated that our PESP reduced physical and psychological fatigue and depression. This finding is consistent with those reported by previous studies, they suggested that exercise reduces depression severity [12] [20]. Heh *et al.* investigated the effectiveness of exercise in reducing the severity of postnatal depression. In their study, 80 primiparas in Taiwan exhibiting an EPDS score of >10 at 4 weeks postpartum were allocated into either an intervention group (provided with exercise support) or a control group (provided with standard care) at 6 weeks postpartum. The main measured outcome was the EPDS score at 5 months postpartum. The results revealed that women who participated in the exercise support program were less likely to exhibit high depression scores after childbirth than the women in the control group ($P = 0.01$). By contrast, among participants in the low-score group, the exercise program did not result in any significant differences in depression scores [12]. Daley *et al.* reviewed five RCT or quasi-RCT studies that targeted postnatal depression management intervention for treating postpartum women. The results showed that compared with participants who did not exercise, in participants who did exercise, symptoms of postnatal depression were reduced (obtaining a standardized mean difference in effect of −0.8% and a 95% confidence interval from −1.53 to −0.10) [20].

Dritsa, *et al.* indicated that exercise reduced tension and raised exercise-related energy consumption, thereby relieving postpartum fatigue [21]. Researchers have suggested that a proportion of postpartum fatigue depends on the characteristics of the infant and breastfeeding behavior, [22] and exercise may be ineffective regarding those factors. However, this study's finding was consistent with that of Dritsa *et al.*'s study [21]. The participants exhibited a significant relieve off atigue after 3 months of participating in the exercise program.

In addition, in the after-program experience-sharing sessions, postpartum women stated that participating in the exercise program had the following advantages: the location was near an Mass Rapid Transit (MRT) station; the teacher and venue were professional; the program content was interesting; the surroundings were beautiful and helped participants to relax; the elastic band could be taken home and used to exercise there; there was a full-time assistant to help take care of babies during exercises; and after they completed the PESP program, the women received a gift voucher. The intimate design of this program can be adapted for future interventions to enhance the recruitment rate.

5. Conclusions

The results of this study indicate that among women who are 7 - 12 weeks postpartum, the 10-week exercise intervention significantly reduces the fatigue and depression levels in those who are prone to depression.

This is the first trial study of women with PPD at 7 - 12 weeks postpartum who participate in a PESP in a gym. The results of this study are limited by the single-group pretest/posttest design, a study length of only 10 weeks, and a small sample size; therefore, the results should be generalized with caution. Encouraging women with PPD to leave their homes to engage in exercise is difficult. Therefore, recruiting numerous women with PPD who are willing to attend an exercise program is difficult. Further research that adopts a quasi-experimental design and involves a control group to enable comparing the effectiveness is necessary. In addition, the sample size and amount of exercise can be increased to improve the generalizability of the results. Regarding the high loss of participants in this study, future studies should consider how to encourage women with depressive tendencies to leave their homes to participate in an exercise program.

Acknowledgements

I hereby, thank all the pregnant women who participate in this research for their cooperation. The financial support from the National Science Council (NSC 101-2410-H-030-085) is greatly appreciated.

References

[1] Sierra Manzano, J.M. (2002) Variables Associated with the Risk of Postpartum Depression. Edinburgh Postnatal Depression Scale. *Atención Primaria*, **30**, 101-111.

[2] Chen, C.H., Tseng, Y.F., Wang, S.Y. and Lee, J.N. (1994) The Prevalence and Predictors of Postpartum Depression. *The Journal of Nursing Research*, **2**, 263-274.

[3] Gaynes, B.N., Gavin, N., Meltzer-Brody, S., Lohr, K.N., Swinson, T., *et al.* (2005) Perinatal Depression: Prevalence, Screening Accuracy, and Screening Outcomes. Agency for Healthcare Research and Quality, Rockville.

[4] Logsdon, M.C., Wisner, K.L. and Pinto-Foltz, M.D. (2006) The Impact of Postpartum Depression on Mothering. *Journal of Obstetric Gynecology and Neonatal Nursing*, **35**, 652-653. http://dx.doi.org/10.1111/j.1552-6909.2006.00087.x

[5] Manchon, C.A., Barnett, B., Kowalenko, N.M. and Tennant, C.C. (2006) Maternal Attachment State of Mind Moderates the Impact of Postnatal Depression on Infant Attachment. *Journal of Child Psychology and Psychiatry*, **47**, 660-669. http://dx.doi.org/10.1111/j.1469-7610.2005.01547.x

[6] Atkinson, L.S. and Baxley, E.G. (1994) Postpartum Fatigue. *American Academy of Family Physicians*, **50**, 113-118.

[7] Milligan, R.A., Rarks, P.L., Kitzman, H. and Lenz, E.R. (1997) Measuring Women's Fatigue during the Postpartum Period. *Journal of Nursing Measurement*, **5**, 3-16.

[8] Chen, C.H., Wang, S.Y., Chung, U.L. and Seng, Y.F. (2006) Being Reborn: The Recovery Process of Postpartum Depression in Taiwanese Women. *Journal of Advanced Nursing*, **54**, 450-456. http://dx.doi.org/10.1111/j.1365-2648.2006.03843.x

[9] Ko, Y.L. (2004) Postpartum Fatigue. *The Journal of Nursing*, **51**, 75-79. (In Chinese)

[10] Armstrong, K. and Edwards, H. (2004) The Effectiveness of a Pram-Walking Exercise Programme in Reducing Depressive Symptomatology for Postnatal Women. *International Journal of Nursing Practice*, **10**, 177-194. http://dx.doi.org/10.1111/j.1440-172X.2004.00478.x

[11] Da Costa, D., Lowensteyn, I., Abrahamowicz, M., Ionescu-Ittu, R., Dritsa, M., *et al.* (2009) A Randomized Clinical Trial of Exercise to Alleviate Postpartum Depressed Mood. *Journal of Psychosomatic Obstetrics & Gynecology*, **30**, 191-200. http://dx.doi.org/10.1080/01674820903212136

[12] Heh, S.S., Huang, L.H., Ho, S.M., Fu, Y.Y. and Wang, L.L. (2008) Effectiveness of Exercise Support Program in Reducing the Severity of Postnatal Depression in Taiwan Women. *Birth*, **35**, 60-65. http://dx.doi.org/10.1111/j.1523-536X.2007.00192.x

[13] Ko, Y.L., Yang, C.L. and Chiang, L.C. (2008) Effects of Postpartum Exercise Program on Fatigue and Depression during Doing the Month Period. *Journal of Nursing Research*, **16**, 177-186. http://dx.doi.org/10.1097/01.JNR.0000387304.88998.0b

[14] Ko, Y.L., Yang, C.L., Fang, C.L., Lee, M.Y. and Lin, P.C. (2013) Community-Based Postpartum Exercise Program. *Journal of Clinical Nursing*, **22**, 2122-2131. http://dx.doi.org/10.1111/jocn.12117

[15] Yoshitake, H. (1971) Relations between the Symptoms and the Feeling of Fatigue. *Ergonomics*, **14**, 175-186. http://dx.doi.org/10.1080/00140137108931236

[16] Cox, J.L., Holden, J.M. and Sagovsky, R. (1987) Detection of Postnatal Depression Development of the 10-Iten Edinburgh Postnatal Depression Scale. *The British Journal of Psychiatry*, **150**, 782-786. http://dx.doi.org/10.1192/bjp.150.6.782

[17] Harris, B., Huckle, P., Thomas, R., Johns, S. and Fung, H. (1989) The Use of Rating Scales to Identify Post-Natal Depression. *The British Journal of Psychiatry*, **154**, 813-817. http://dx.doi.org/10.1192/bjp.154.6.813

[18] Robertson, E., Grace, S., Wallington, T. and Stewart, D.E. (2004) Antenatal Risk Factors for Postpartum Depression: A Synthesis of Recent Literature. *General Hospital Psychiatry*, **26**, 289-295. http://dx.doi.org/10.1016/j.genhosppsych.2004.02.006

[19] Daley, A.J., MacArthur, C. and Winter, H. (2007) The Role of Exercise in Treating Postpartum Depression: A Review of the Literature. *Journal of Midwifery & Women's Health*, **52**, 56-62. http://dx.doi.org/10.1016/j.jmwh.2006.08.017

[20] Daley, A., Jolly, K. and MacArthur, C. (2009) The Effectiveness of Exercise in the Management of Post-Natal Depression: Systematic Review and Meta-Analysis. *The Journal of Family Practice*, **26**, 154-162. http://dx.doi.org/10.1093/fampra/cmn101

[21] Dritsa, M., Dupuis, G., Lowensteyn, I. and Da Costa, D. (2009) Effects of Home-Based Exercise on Fatigue in Postpartum Depressed Women: Who Is More Likely to Benefit and Why? *Journal of Psychosomatic Research*, **67**, 159-163. http://dx.doi.org/10.1016/j.jpsychores.2009.01.010

[22] Ko, Y.L. and Lu, C.M. (2003) Psychophysiologic and Situational Correlates of Postpartum Fatigue. *Journal of Health Education*, **19**, 137-153.

20

Effects of a Health Promotion Program on Elementary Students' Physical and Mental Health

Insook Lee[1], Kyung-Sook Bang[1*], Sungjae Kim[1], Heeseung Choi[1], Inju Hwang[2]

[1]College of Nursing, The Research Institute of Nursing Science, Seoul National University, Seoul, Korea
[2]College of Nursing, Seoul National University, Seoul, Korea
Email: *ksbang@snu.ac.kr

Abstract

Many health promotion programs have been implemented to prevent obesity and mental health problems among school-aged children. However, only a few programs included both physical and psychological measures to assess the effects of the program. The present study was designed to test the effects of a 6-week health promotion program on physical and mental health among school-aged children using physiological and psychological measures. A total of 74 elementary school students (4th and 5th grade) recruited from urban (n = 51) and rural areas (n = 23) participated in the study. We used the Korean version of the Kovacs' Children's Depression Inventory and the Conners-Wells' Adolescent Self-Report Scale-Short Form (CASS-S) to measure levels of depression and hyperactivity, respectively. To assess children's physical health, we measured body mass index (BMI), body fat percentage, and heart rate variability. In addition, children's health-related behaviors (e.g., eating and exercise habits) were assessed using the health promotion behavior scale. A total of 63 students (13 in the experimental and 50 in the control group) who completed both physiological and psychological measures were included in the final analysis. Compared to children in the control group, children in the experimental group showed a significant decrease in their level of hyperactivity ($t = -2.01$, $p = 0.049$) and increase in heart rate variability ($t = -2.35$, $p = 0.022$). No significant group differences were noted for depression, BMI, body fat percentage, and health promotion behaviors between the two groups. Findings of this study provided preliminary evidence of the effectiveness of a 6-week school-based health promotion program for improving emotional health among school-aged children living in a rural area. Future studies testing the effects of health promotion programs with longer sessions and programs focusing on social-emotional skill development are needed.

*Corresponding author.

Keywords

Health Promotion, Heart Rate Variability, Mental Health, School-Aged Children

1. Introduction

In Korea, the physical and mental health of elementary students is of concern. Approximately 10% - 20% of school-aged children in Korea have been categorized as overweight, and 5% - 20% as obese [1]. In addition, physical activity and fitness have decreased and the mean height and weight for children and adolescents have increased over the past 10 years [2]. Based on a recent report on the mental health of Korean children and adolescents, 20 percent had suicidal ideation and 3 percent had attempted suicide during the past year, and one third of middle and high school students had experienced depressed mood [3]. Recently, the prevalence rate of ADHD symptoms among 4th - 6th grade elementary students was reported to be up to 22.3% [4], and the high level of bullying and violence among elementary school students warned of the risk for mental health problems [5] [6]. Hence, the development of school-based health promotion programs and related policies is needed.

Many intervention programs have been implemented to promote physical and mental health among children and adolescents and have shown promising results in individual studies. The intervention, "Maum Meditation program" had positive effects on the promotion of self-esteem and school adjustment of children in the early grades of primary school in Korea [7]. However, a meta-analysis on the effects of school-based and after-school intervention programs on the BMIs of children and adolescents reported a low magnitude of effect size of 0.068 [8]. Thus, more efficient and sustainable health promotion programs and policies are required. In a meta-analysis on the effect of school-based anti-bullying programs, a small to moderate effect was found for victimization, suggesting that effective school-based anti-bullying programs should include training in emotional control, peer counseling, and the establishment of a school policy on bullying [6].

To date, most intervention programs have relied on self-report data and very few studies have included both psychological and physical measures to assess the effects of intervention programs. Even studies that have used objective measures for identifying the effect of school based health promotion programs in Korea used only weight change or BMI [9]-[11]. Recently, heart rate variability (HRV) has been used as an indicator for emotional stability as well as a valuable tool for assessing heart health. HRV is a non-invasive quantitative marker of cardiac autonomic function derived from continuous electrocardiogram (ECG) recordings [12]. Little change in HRV means a stable autonomic nerve system (*i.e.*, stable emotional state). Even though HRV has been increasingly used as a stress marker, less research is available examining HRV in children, especially in Korea.

To address the gaps in current knowledge, this study aimed to examine the effect of a school-based health promotion program on both physical and mental health among late school-aged children. Changes in health status were assessed using both self-report measures and physiological measures, including HRV. Also, based on previous evidence of a positive effect of nature on physical and mental health [13] [14], we included nature-related activities for the experimental group, and tested the effect of this program.

2. Methods

2.1. Study Design

This study used a quasi-experimental, non-equivalent pretest-post design to test the effect of a 6-week school-based health promotion program on school-aged children's health.

2.2. Description of the Program

Based on the Information-Motivation-Behavior (IMB) model [15], we developed the "Physical & Mental Health" program to improve physical and mental health (*i.e.*, body fat, HRV, depression, and hyperactivity) among school-aged children. The contents of the program were developed based on an extensive review of the literature and other health promotion programs for children. We provided information about various health topics and motivated participants to engage in health promotion activities and self-monitoring. "Physical & Mental Health" consisted of three physical health promotion sessions and three mental health promotion sessions. The physical health sessions focused on the improvement of lifestyle habits including eating habits, exercise habits, and sleeping habits. The mental health promotion sessions addressed self-reflection and understanding others' perspectives, communication skills, and regulation of emotion (**Table 1**).

2.3. Study Procedure and Participants

2.3.1. Procedure

After obtaining approval from the principals and school health teachers of the two elementary schools, we recruited prospective participants. The two elementary schools were selected as a convenience, and assigned to either the experimental or the control group. A total of 74 elementary school students (4th and 5th grade) participated in the study; the total number of 4th and 5th grade in one school who agreed to participate were 23, and assigned to the experimental group, and the number of 1 class for each 4th and 5th grade who agreed to participate

Table 1. Main contents of the "Physical & Mental Health" program for the experimental group.

Theme	Session	Topic	Main content		
			Goal	Activities	Evaluation
Physical health	Session 1	Eating habits	· Practicing healthy eating habits	·Recording present eating habits ·Learning about the harmfulness of an imbalanced diet, overeating, and skipping meals ·Planning healthy eating habits	·Recording everyday eating habits in the workbook ·Making healthy food with parents at home
	Session 2	Exercise habits	· Practicing healthy exercise habits	·Recording my present exercise habits ·Learning about the benefits of exercise and how to exercise in everyday life ·Planning exercise to maintain an appropriate weight	·Recording everyday exercise habits in the workbook ·Exercising with friends and family
	Session 3	Sleep habits	· Practicing healthy sleep habits	·Recording present sleeping habits ·Learning about the function of sleep and the benefits of sound sleep ·Planning feasible sleeping habits	·Recording everyday sleep habits in the workbook ·Waking up early and having time before going to school
Mental health	Session 4	Understanding the mind	·Recognizing thoughts and feelings on diverse situations ·Understanding the other person's situation and perspective and shifting one's own perspective	·Sharing thoughts and feelings about diverse situations ·Shifting one's perspective and learning about different perspectives ·Becoming the tree on gathered together	·Talking about thoughts and feelings while looking at paintings and pictures of diverse situations in the workbook (over 2 minutes) ·Sharing thoughts and feelings with parents
	Session 5	Communication	·Understanding the concept of communication ·Knowing your own communication style ·Learning how to communicate effectively	·Play games to learn about communication ·Communicating while changing headbands	·The most used words ·5 words from friends that made you feel better ·5 words from friends that made you feel worse
	Session 6	Controlling the mind	·Understanding how to control stress effectively ·Understanding how to control conflict and anger	·Making the leaf of feeling ·Tearing the leaf of feeling ·Accepting diverse feelings ·Anger control training	·Practicing relaxation ·Reporting the experience of anger control

were 51 in the other school, and assigned to the control group. The study was conducted from August to December 2013. For the experimental group, we provided intervention sessions every Friday for 6 weeks. Each intervention session took place for 45 minutes after school. No intervention was applied to the control group. The post test was carried out in December 2013. Participants in the experimental group were assessed before and after receiving the 6-week health promotion program. At the same interval, individuals in the control group were also assessed. Data were collected by the author and the research assistants who were well-trained and thoroughly understood the study. It took about 30 minutes for participants to fill out the self-questionnaire and complete the physiology procedure.

2.3.2. Self-Report Measures

1) Depression

Depression was measured using the Kovacs' Children's Depression Inventory (CDI) [16], which was translated into Korean [17]. This self-report inventory is composed of five subcategories: depressed mood (5 questions), behavior disorder (7 questions), loss of interest (7 questions), self-degradation (4 questions), and physiological symptoms (4 questions). It is assessed on a 3-point scale (0, 1, and 2). Total scores range from 0 to 54 points and the higher the CDI total score, the more severe the depression is. The internal consistency reliability in this study, measured with Cronbach's α, was 0.868.

2) Hyperactivity

The Conners-Wells' Adolescent Self-Report Scale: Short Form (CASS: S) translated into Korean [18] was used to measure the level of hyperactivity. The scale is composed of 27 items and is rated on a 4-point scale (0, 1, 2, and 3). A higher score means a higher level of hyperactivity. The data collected using this inventory had a Cronbach's α of 0.880.

3) Health promotion behavior

Health promotion behavior was measured using the questionnaire originally developed by Walker, Sechrist, and Pender [19] and then revised and supplemented in Korea [20] [21]. The questionnaire is composed of 36 questions: 11 items on eating habits, 8 items on exercise habits, 7 items on healthy living conditions, 5 items on personal relations, and 5 items on self-realization. The internal consistency reliability in this study (Cronbach's α) was 0.909.

2.3.3. Physiological Measures

1) Body Mass Index (BMI) and body fat percentage

Body weight, height, and body fat percentage were measured with the J10 (Biospace, Seoul, Korea), a body composition analyzer. Juvenile body mass index was calculated by dividing the child's body weight (kg) by the square of the child's height (m^2). We measured the participant's body fat percentage, which is an indicator of the ratio of body fat to body weight.

2) Heart Rate Variability (HRV)

Autonomic nervous system function was assessed using Heart Rate Variability (HRV) analysis. Participants in the experimental group were assessed before and after receiving the 6-week health promotion program. HRV was measured with PolyG-I (Laxtha, Daejeon, Korea) in a quiet room. During the test, we let participants lie quietly and attached 2 electrodes on their wrists for 3 minutes. Participants were instructed to close their eyes but not to fall asleep. If the participants moved and an abnormal wave was shown, we stopped the test and re-measured.

2.4. Ethical Considerations

This study was approved by the S University Institutional Review Board (Approval No.: 2013-64). Written Informed consent was obtained from all participants and their parents. Parental consent and child assent were obtained before students completed the pretest. Children who participated in this study were assured of anonymity and confidentiality.

2.5. Data Analysis

SPSS 21.0 for Windows was used for analysis. To test homogeneity between the two groups, a t-test and chi-square test were applied. To confirm the effect of the intervention, the pretest-posttest difference was calculated and compared between the two groups using a t-test. The normality of the physiological variables was confirmed using the Kolmogorov-Smirnov test. Two-tailed p-values < 0.05 were considered significant.

3. Results

3.1. Participants' Demographic Characteristics and Homogeneity Test Results

The participants' demographic and biological characteristics assessed at baseline are shown in **Table 2** and **Table 3**. Homogeneity tests were also performed on the dependent variables between the experimental and control groups at the time of the pretest. No significant differences were reported in demographic characteristics and dependent variables between the two groups at baseline.

Among the 84 participants, only 13 of 23 children in the experimental group completed the physiological measures for both the pre- and posttest, whereas all 50 participants in the control group completed the physiological measures both times. Therefore, we included only 63 students (13 in the experimental and 50 in the control group) in further analysis.

3.2. Effects of Health Promotion Program on Dependent Variables

Findings for analyses of the overall program effects on physical and mental health outcomes by self-report questionnaire are shown in **Table 4**. For mental health, no significant difference was shown between two groups. Only changes in the level of hyperactivity were significantly different between the experimental and control groups ($t = -2.01$, $p = 0.049$). Also, health promotion behavior was not different between two groups.

In biological index, children in the experimental group showed significant changes in LF ($t = -2.35$, $p = 0.022$) and HF of HRV ($t = 2.35$, $p = 0.022$) after the intervention compared to the control group. This meant that the experimental group's parasympathetic nerve was more activated than that of the control group after the intervention. No significant group differences were noted in BMI and body fat percentage (**Table 5**).

Table 2. Homogeneity tests of general characteristics and self-report questionnaire between the two groups at the pretest.

Variable	Categories	Experimental (n = 23) n(%) or Mean ± SD	Control (n = 51) n(%) or Mean ± SD	χ^2 or t	p
Gender	Boy	11 (47.8)	25 (49.0)	0.01	0.924
	Girl	12 (52.2)	26 (51.0)		
Grade	4th grade	12 (52.2)	27 (52.9)	0.00	0.951
	5th grade	11 (47.8)	24 (47.1)		
Perceived health status	Healthy	16 (69.6)	45 (88.2)		
	Moderate	7 (30.4)	5 (9.8)	5.28*	0.071
	Unhealthy	0 (0)	1 (2.0)		
Perceived body shape	Thin	9 (39.1)	11 (21.6)		
	Moderate	6 (26.1)	22 (43.1)	3.03	0.220
	Fat	8 (34.8)	18 (35.3)		
Economic status	High	11 (47.8)	30 (58.8)		
	Middle	11 (47.8)	19 (37.3)	0.79*	0.674
	Low	1 (4.4)	2 (3.9)		
Walking time/day (minutes)		55.43 ± 51.05	69.58 ± 49.17	−1.13	0.260
Self-report questionnaire	Depression	7.78 ± 4.66	7.12 ± 6.46	0.44	0.659
	ADHD	13.44 ± 8.31	11.82 ± 8.32	0.77	0.443
	Health promotion behavior	109.70 ± 13.68	112.25 ± 15.88	−0.71	0.480

*Fisher's exact test.

Table 3. Homogeneity tests of biological characteristics between the two groups at the pretest.

Variables		Experimental (n = 13)	Control (n = 50)	t	*p*
		Mean ± SD	Mean ± SD		
BMI		19.45 ± 4.97	19.08 ± 2.85	0.255	0.802
Body fat		26.40 ± 13.49	25.03 ± 7.79	0.353	0.729
Heart rate variability	LF/HF	1.38 ± 0.87	1.24 ± 1.18	0.410	0.683
	LF (sympathetic nerve activation)	0.53 ± 0.15	0.47 ± 0.18	1.132	0.262
	HF (Parasympathetic nerve activation)	0.47 ± 0.15	0.53 ± 0.18	−1.132	0.262

LF = Low Frequency, HF = High Frequency, BMI = Body Mass Index.

Table 4. Comparisons of differences between the pre- and posttest (posttest-pretest) for the two groups on the self-report questionnaire.

Variable	Experimental (n = 23)	Control (n = 51)	t	*p*
	Mean ± SD	Mean ± SD		
Depression	−1.52 ± 2.87	−0.37 ± 3.03	−1.49	0.142
Hyperactivity	−3.96 ± 5.66	−0.86 ± 6.31	−2.01	0.049
Health promotion behaviors	0.59 ± 10.87	0.73 ± 10.95	−0.05	0.961

Table 5. Comparisons of differences between the pre- and posttest (posttest-pretest) for the two groups on the biological index.

Variable		Experimental (n = 13)	Control (n = 50)	t	*p*
		Mean ± SD	Mean ± SD		
	BMI	0.45 ± 0.54	−0.28 ± 3.50	0.74	0.461
	Body fat	1.58 ± 8.53	−0.75 ± 1.55	0.98	0.345
HRV	LF/HF	−0.63 ± 0.96	−0.01 ± 1.03	−1.94	0.057
	LF (sympathetic nerve activation)	−0.12 ± 0.17	0.00 ± 0.18	−2.35	0.022
	HF (Parasympathetic nerve activation)	0.12 ± 0.17	0.00 ± 0.18	2.35	0.022

BMI = Body Mass Index, HRV = Heart rate variability, LF = Low Frequency, HF = High Frequency.

4. Discussion

This study was conducted to assess the effects of a 6-week school-based health promotion program for late school-aged children. The results of this study showed a significant decrease in the level of hyperactivity and increase in relaxation expressed by parasympathetic activation.

In terms of HRV, vital variability reflects the heart's ability to respond to physiological and environmental stimuli. Because of the specific autonomic nervous innervations of the heart, HRV is recognized as a quantitative marker of the autonomic nervous system: it is influenced by sympathetic activity (SA) and vagal parasympathetic activity (PA). For children, studies measuring HRV have not been frequently reported. One study reported short-term HRV in a population-based sample of 10-year-old children [12], and low HRV (*i.e.*, low PA, HF) has previously been linked to poor emotion regulation, high stress, decreased stress reactivity, and increased stress vulnerability, also in children [22] [23].

In this study, the experimental group showed more decrease in LF compared to the control group. This implied that the intervention was effective in decreasing children's stress (e.g., resulting from peer problems) and negative emotions such as anger and anxiety. A previous study also showed a positive correlation between anxiety and higher LF and the stress marker cortisol [24]. This meant that high stress among children was associated with higher LF/HF, which may reflect more sympathetic activation over parasympathetic activation. This might explain why overweight/obese children demonstrated lower HF compared to normal weight children in previous a study [25].

Even though we could not find a relationship between depression and LF/HF scores, this health promotion program might help improve emotional stability among elementary school students. Other evidence in support of this proposition is the greater decrement in hyperactivity scores seen in the experimental group compared to that of the control group.

However, this health promotion program showed no significant effect on BMI or body fat proportion. It may be possible that two to three months was not enough time to elicit a change in weight. One study reported positive effects of a 12-week24-session after-school health promotion program for Hispanic elementary school children on BMI and eating habits [26], and using jazz in school program showed improving physical strength and self- efficacy of the Korean elementary school students [27]. In this study, interventions consisted of health education and indoor activity. We encouraged regular outdoor activities, but did not include outdoor physical activity in the intervention program. In addition, we focused more on emotional health, emphasizing peer relationships and communication. This may explain why we found more obvious changes in emotional outcomes than physical outcomes. In addition, this program was applied mostly to normal weight student, not obese children. Still, we observed greater reductions in BMI in the experimental group than the control group, but the sample size for the experimental group was too small to show a significant effect.

This study has several limitations. First, the regions for the experimental and control group were selected as a convenience, and not comparable: the region for the experimental group was a rural area whereas the region for the control group was a capital city. However, the general characteristics between the two groups at baseline were homogeneous. Secondly, only 13 among 23 children in the experimental group participated in the post test. The high attrition rate in the experimental group could have affected the results. Also, because we did not measure directly the effect of education on diet and sleep, we could not conclude that this program had effects on compliance with good eating and sleeping habits.

Although this study had some limitations, it is meaningful in assessing the possibility of emotional health promotion using school-based health programs. Additional research with a more sufficient sample size is suggested.

5. Conclusion

The findings of this study provided preliminary evidence of the effectiveness of a 6-week school-based health promotion program for improving emotional health among school-aged children living in a rural region. Future research should examine whether the effectiveness of physical and mental health promotion programs can be enhanced through refinements such as more focused attention to social-emotional skill development.

Acknowledgements

This work was supported by a Research Grant of the Korea Forest Service.

Conflict of Interest

No potential conflict of interest relevant to this article was reported.

References

[1] Ahn, Y., Choi, S. and Sohn, M. (2013) Adiposity of Korean School-Age Children Measured by National and International Growth Charts. *Research in Nursing and Health*, **36**, 16-25. http://dx.doi.org/10.1002/nur.21510

[2] Heo, J. (2009) An Examination of the Relationships among Body Shape, Physical Fitness and Body Composition in Elementary School Students. *The Korean Journal of Growth and Development*, **17**, 201-209.

[3] Mo, S.H., Kim, H.J., Lee, S.Y., Kim, J.H. and Yoon, K.M. (2013) Study on the Policy for Mental Health Promotion of Children and Adolescents III: Combined Report. National Youth Policy Institute, Seoul, 1-338.

[4] Song, Y.J. (2014) Estimated Prevalence of ADHD Symptoms and Relationships among ADHD Symptoms, Environmental Variables, and Peer Relationships in Elementary School Students. *Asian Journal of Education*, **15**, 189-217.

[5] Kim, D., Park, A. and Lee, K. (2008) Effect of PC Game to Improve Interpersonal Abilities for Prevention of Bullying and Violence in Elementary School Environment. *Asian Journal of Education*, **9**, 49-65. http://dx.doi.org/10.15753/aje.2008.9.2.003

[6] Lee, S., Kim, C.J. and Kim, D.H. (2013) A Meta-Analysis of the Effect of School-Based Anti-Bullying Programs. *Journal of Child Health Care: For Professionals Working with Children in the Hospital and Community*, 3 October.

[7] Yoo, Y.G. and Lee, I.S. (2013) The Effects of School-Based Maum Meditation Program on the Self-Esteem and School Adjustment in Primary School Students. *Global Journal of Health Science*, **5**, 14-27.

[8] Vasques, C., Magalhaes, P., Cortinhas, A., Mota, P., Leitao, J. and Lopes, V.P. (2014) Effects of Intervention Programs on Child and Adolescent BMI: A Meta-Analysis Study. *Journal of Physical Activity and Health*, **11**, 426-444. http://dx.doi.org/10.1123/jpah.2012-0035

[9] Lee, K.Y., Nam, H.M. and Lee, J.R. (2007) Effect of Elementary School Based Intervention to Prevent Obesity in Children. *Journal of Korean Society for the Study of Obesity*, **16**, 125-129.

[10] Hong, Y.H., Park, J.K. and Lee, D.H. (2010) The Evaluation of Obese Control Program in Elementary School. *Journal of the Korean Society for the Study of Obesity*, **19**, 9-15.

[11] Nam, S.M. (2013) Effects of Club Obesity Management Program for Obese Children on Body Composition, Self-Efficacy, and Health Promotion. *Journal of Korean Public Health Nursing*, **27**, 619-632. http://dx.doi.org/10.5932/JKPHN.2013.27.3.619

[12] Jarrin, D.C., McGrath, J.J., Poirier, P., Séguin, L., Tremblay, R.E., Montplaisir, J.Y., *et al.* (2015) Short-Term Heart Rate Variability in a Population-Based Sample of 10-Year-Old Children. *Pediatric Cardiology*, **36**, 41-48.

[13] Kim, D.J. and Lee, S.J. (2014) Effects of Forest Therapy Program in School Forest on Employment Stress and Anxiety of University Students. *Journal of the Korean Society for Plants, People and Environment*, **17**, 107-115. http://dx.doi.org/10.11628/ksppe.2014.17.2.107

[14] Park, H.J., Jung, Y.O. and Kim, J.P. (2014) The Effect of the Eco-Experience Learning on the Fostering of Elementary School Students' Sociality. *Journal of the Korean Society for Plants, People and Environment*, **13**, 101-108.

[15] Fisher, W.A., Kohut, T., Schachner, H. and Stenger, P. (2011) Understanding Self-Monitoring of Blood Glucose among Individuals with Type 1 and Type 2 Diabetes. An Information-Motivation-Behavioral Skills Analysis. *The Diabetes Educator*, **37**, 85-94. http://dx.doi.org/10.1177/0145721710391479

[16] Kovacs, M. (1985) The Children's Depression Inventory (CDI). *Psychopharmacology Bulletin*, **21**, 995-998.

[17] Cho, S.C. and Lee, Y.S. (1990) Development of the Korean Form of the Kovacs' Children's Depression Inventory. *Journal of Korean Neuropsychiatric Association*, **29**, 943-956.

[18] Bahn, G.H., Shin, M.S., Cho, S.C. and Hong, K.-E. (2001) A Preliminary Study for the Development of the Assessment Scale for ADHD in Adolescents: Reliability and Validity for CASS(S). *Journal of Child & Adolescent Psychiatry*, **12**, 218-224.

[19] Walker, S.N., Sechrist, K.R. and Pender, N.J. (1987) The Health-Promoting Lifestyle Profile: Development and Psychometric Characteristics. *Nursing Research*, **36**, 76-81. http://dx.doi.org/10.1097/00006199-198703000-00002

[20] Kim, M.H. (2000) A Study on the Relations of Health Promoting Daily Life Style and Self-Efficiency about Boys' Obesity. Central University Social Education Development Institute, Seoul.

[21] Jung, S.H. (2006) The Effects of Weight Management Educational Program Based Problem-Based Learning (PBL) on Self-Efficacy, Health Promotion Behavior and Obesity Index in Obese Children. Korea University Graduate School of Education, Seoul.

[22] Porges, S.W. (1995) Cardiac Vagal Tone: A Physiological Index of Stress. *Neuroscience and Biobehavioral Reviews*, **19**, 225-233. http://dx.doi.org/10.1016/0149-7634(94)00066-A

[23] Porges, S.W., Doussard-Roosevelt, J.A. and Maiti, A.K. (1994) Vagal Tone and the Physiological Regulation of Emotion. *Monographs of the Society for Research in Child Development*, **59**, 167-186. http://dx.doi.org/10.2307/1166144

[24] Michels, N., Sioen, I., Clays, E., *et al.* (2013) Children's Heart Rate Variability as Stress Indicator: Association with Reported Stress and Cortisol. *Biological Psychology*, **94**, 433-440. http://dx.doi.org/10.1016/j.biopsycho.2013.08.005

[25] Birch, S.L., Duncan, M.J. and Franklin, C. (2012) Overweight and Reduced Heart Rate Variability in British Children: An Exploratory Study. *Preventive Medicine*, **55**, 430-432. http://dx.doi.org/10.1016/j.ypmed.2012.09.015

[26] de Heer, H.D., Koehly, L., Pederson, R. and Morera, O. (2011) Effectiveness and Spillover of an After-School Health Promotion Program for Hispanic Elementary School Children. *American Journal of Public Health*, **101**, 1907-1913. http://dx.doi.org/10.2105/ajph.2011.300177

[27] Nam, H.Y. and Lee, D.K. (2009) The Effects of Jazz Dance Program on the Physical Strength and Self-Efficacy of the Elementary School Students. *The Korean Journal of the Elementary Physical Education*, **15**, 123-133.

21

Construction and Validation of an Educational Technology for Mammary Health Promotion

Izabel Cristina Falcão Juvenal Barbosa, Ana Fátima Carvalho Fernandes, Camila Brasil Moreira, Míria Conceição Lavinas Santos, Altamira Mendonça Félix Gomes, Ivna Silva Andrade, Anna Paula Sousa da Silva

Department of Nursing, Federal University of Piauí, Floriano, Piauí, Brazil
Email: izabelbarbosa@ufpi.edu.br

Abstract

Mammary health is issue faced by public health nurses and the science follows new ways into this thematic area of learning course wares. The purpose of this study was to construct and to validate a distance course for mammary health promotion for nurses. Methodological proposal has been composed of five stages: 1) analysis and planning, 2) modeling, 3) implementation, 4) evaluation and maintenance and 5) distribution. A total of nine experts as research population were consulted who were expert judges of nursing, pedagogy and web designer, three of each specific area, which were included in the study. The variables that had concordance index of 50% were: graphic designer pages favors learning, the user has easy navigation, the learning of the student experience, the environment provides interdisciplinary, content is built on process rather than there is a unique sequence, allows access to the available environment and holds a discussion on the subject. The distance learning course is intended to broaden and to enrich the living spaces and construct their own knowledge, favors interactivity, communication, autonomy and cooperation between the participants and provides access to educational technologies.

Keywords

Distance Education, Educational Technology, Breast Neoplasms, Health Promotion, Nursing

1. Introduction

The production of care in clinical practice requires combinations of technology of materials and not material dimensions to be resolute. Continuing Education should work to break the hegemonic mode of production of care, reduce the biologicism, promote discussions with professionals and users with regard to extended clinic which includes beyond the disease, the person, the context and to charge for both healing and rehabilitation [1].

Knowing the basic issues of women's health, the ability of breast cancer result in mastectomy, the risk factors and their determinants, the main clinical manifestations due to surgery, the innovations of reconstructive techniques are issues that deserve attention in health for the construction and implementation of a satisfactory physical and organizational infrastructure of health services, of a better quality of care provided by the health staff and nursing professionals, because it is an important public health problem in Brazil [2] [3].

Thus, it is necessary an continuous improvement in breast health, of the professionals of primary care network, as the most effective ways for early detection of breast cancer are clinical breast examination and mammography, which are offered at the entrance door of health services in Family Health Centres.

Some previous studies in the area of women's health and on the problems faced by women who underwent mastectomy and by primary care nurses sought new paths in the theme of distance education. From the foregoing the objective of this study is to design and to validate an updating distance course on breast health for nurses.

2. Method

2.1. Participants

The study sample was composed of nine specialist judges in nursing, pedagogy and web designer, three of each specific area, who evaluated the distance course on breast health, in the educational and pedagogical technique, communication/social and administrative perspectives, as showed in **Table 1**.

2.2. Instruments

To collect data, two instruments were used by questionnaire, one to evaluate content, technique, pedagogical-didactic, communicational and social that included three (3) items, distributed in 24 criteria where each item consisted of five categories of answers, like the Likert scale: (TA) totally agree; (PA) partially agree, (U) undecided, (TD) totally disagree e (PD) partially disagree. The other instrument for the assessment of the technical and administrative perspective contained two (02) items distributed in 50 criteria, where each item presented a value scale with five response categories: (1) poor, (2) regular, (3) good, (4) very good and (5) Excellent.

2.3. Data Analysis

The Statistical Package for the Social Sciences 15.0 software was used for statistical analysis. The significance level for all analyses was set at 5%. For descriptive analysis, data were organized into categorical and numerical variables. For categorical variables, the absolute frequencies were used, the percentages and confidence interval (95%) and for numerical variables the mean, median and standard deviation were used. The Bloom's Taxonomy was used to guide the development of educational materials and assist in the evaluation of the teaching-learning process [4].

3. Results

For the elaboration of educational material developed, Curso de Atualização em Saúde Mamária-CASM (a continuing course on breast health) 100% compliance of the judges was obtained in full agreement as to the question referred to the compatibility of the information with the objectives previously established, 66.7% reported they strongly agreed that the contents of the references add value to information and only (2) 33.3% agreed partially. When analyzing the topic for the organization of information clearly to facilitate learning (5) 83.3% of the judges completely agreed and (1) 16.7% agreed partially.

Regarding the content, (4) 66.7% partially agreed that the content is appropriate to users, (2) 33.3% agreed completely, (5) 83.3% of the judges partially agreed with the consistency of content (4) 66.7% fully agreed with the content stream, (5) 83.3% stated that they totally agree with the objectivity of content.

As for the pages graphic designer promoting the learning of users and the facility for users to navigate on the page, 50% of the judges completely agreed, and 100% totally agreed that the pictures and images add knowledge, (5) 83.3% said the images and prints match those texts. Concerning the arrangement of modular units

Table 1. The demographic and other characteristics of the specialists.

Sociodemographic information	Value		
	Frequency	%	Mean
Age			
28 ⊢⊣ 40	4	44.4	42 SD[a] = ± 11.02
41 ⊢⊣ 51	3	33.3	
52 ⊢⊣ 62	2	22.2	
Marital Status			
Single	1	11.1	
Married	4	44.4	
Separated/Divorced	1	11.1	
Did not answer	3	33.3	
Titles			
Specialty	3	33.3	
Master	2	22.2	
Doctorate	3	33.3	
Pos Doctorate	1	11.1	
Graduation year			
1975 ⊢⊣ 1984	1	11.1	
1985 ⊢⊣ 1994	3	33.3	
1995 ⊢⊣ 2004	3	33.3	
≥2005	2	22.2	
Graduation period (year)			
4 ⊢⊣ 13	5	55.6	
14 ⊢⊣ 23	2	22.2	
24 ⊢⊣ 33	1	11.1	
34 ⊢⊣ 43	1	11.1	
Experience in EAD			
student	2	22.2	
tutor	4	44.4	
know it	2	22.2	
work with it	1	11.1	
Period of experience in EAD			
0 ⊢⊣ 4	6	66.7	4.0 SD[a] = ± 3.2
5 ⊢⊣ 9	2	22.2	
Did not answer	1	11.1	

a. SD (±) = Standard Deviation.

content contributes to the user learning (5) 83.3% of the judges completely agreed.

When analyzing the reliability of provided information and, if they are updated and add knowledge about breast cancer, 66.7% of the judges fully agreed that the sources used in the course construction are credible and are free of typographical and grammatical errors.

What concerns the description of the learning assessment, 50% of nursing and pedagogy judges totally agreed that the course allows learning from the user experience, 66.7% of the judges completely agreed that evaluations at the end of each module are useful for reviewing the course material.

As noted, 66.7% of the judges fully agreed that evaluations at the end of each module are useful for reviewing the course material. In this sense it is noteworthy that at the end of each CASM modular unit there are multiple choice questions with only one correct answer for each question, with mutually option excluded. There are no restrictions and limits on the maximum number of attempts to the student to get the correct answer.

As the paradigm of interactional and constructivist learning (4) 66.7% of the judges completely agreed and (2) 33.3% partially agreed. With regard to the question of focus on learning-based, autonomy and respect for the pace of development system (4) 66.7% of the judges completely agreed and (2) 33.3% partially agreed.

With regard to collaboration (3) 50% of the judges totally agree and (3) 50% partially agree, (6) 100% of the judges fully agreed that the system focus is based on the development of skills and abilities and the construction of knowledge, (5) 83.3% of the judges fully agreed that the focus of the system is in cooperation.

The learning environment was considered by the judges participative and centered on interaction. It promotes the exchange of experiences and the construction of knowledge, is cooperative and provides an interdisciplinary environment.

Regarding the description of the learning environment methodology, 83.3% of judges fully agreed that the methodology is cooperative, 66.7% completely agreed in the question referred to the methodology being interactive and problematizing and based on the identification and resolution of problems.

It was found that 100% of the judges completely agreed that the assessment is formative, continuous and allows troubleshooting situations, study of cases highlighted in the spaces of interaction. The evaluation is focused on the process, observation and development and values the interaction to the understanding and application of concepts.

It was observed that all the judges fully agreed that autonomous learning allows students to access their own sources expanding their learning. As regards the reflection item, 83.3% of the judges fully agreed with this topic stating it allows teachers to assist students on feedback from their actions with the goals.

Regarding the description of the information space and sources of trading of the learning environment, 83.3% of judges completely agreed it allows the access to general information about the course and communities, 100% completely agreed in the question regarding the possibility of holding a participatory and flexible planning and define responsibilities and mutual agreements.

It is observed that 83.3% of the judges strongly agreed that communication tools are integrated, 66.7% state that they fully agreed that the tools (e-mail and conferencing) allow one to attach and extract files.

In items related to the learning objectives being specified and could be recorded on the basis of conversation and the question that allows access within the same environment the available material and conduct a discussion on the subject, 50% of the judges agreed completely. In the question referred to allow the objectives being shown with their learning topic, 83.3% judges completely agreed that both teacher and student conceptions are affordable for everyone, 100% of completely judges agreed it enables cooperative goal setting learning and (4) 66.7% of judges completely agreed it enables action, production and receiving feedback on the defined objectives.

Finally, a modular structure presented in four learning modules which includes fifteen thematic units, containing items and sub-items was obtained (**Table 2**).

4. Discussion

The biggest challenge for a constructivist and social interactionist practice requires a break of the teaching and students posture from the traditional teaching practice. The pedagogical proposal should be challenging and problematizing and should involve the participating subjects in the teaching and learning process [5].

The specialized judges in nursing and pedagogy rated and mostly (65%), completely or partially agreed the educational proposal included the criteria items of the technical, pedagogical educational, communicational and social perspective of the distance education in the breast health.

In the technical perspective the items that obtained more than 65% of satisfactory evaluation were: authority; presentation, organization, evaluation, coherence, sequence, objectivity and reliability of the contents; used tools and evaluation of learning. Except for this last aspect, "assessment of learning" whose topic referring to promote learning from the user experience, evaluation obtained less than 65%.

In the pedagogical didactic perspective the topics also obtained top rating to 65%, ranging from fully and partially agree on the following aspects: paradigm of interactionist and constructivist learning, focus on learning-based system, autonomy and respect for the pace of development, development competences and skills,

Table 2. Educational content of each class in the CASM.

Module	Frequency
I	Class 01—Cancer: Historical background and definitions Class 02—Breast anatomy Class 03—Cancer pathophysiology Class 04—Cancer epidemiology in Brazil and in the world Class 05—Public policies of relevance to the health of the woman related to breast cancer control
II	Class 01—Risk factors for breast cancer Class 02—Modification related to breast benign lesions Class 03—Main malignant changes in the female breast Class 04—Special situations for tracking the breast cancer Class 05—Degree of recommendation
III	Class 01—National strategies for tracking, early detection and diagnosis of breast cancer Class 02—Methods of treatment of breast cancer

cooperation and the construction of knowledge.

Other criteria included in the pedagogical didactic perspective, were also evaluated positively, more than 65%, by specialist judges, namely: participatory learning environment, cooperative and focused on interaction, promotes the exchange of experiences and the construction of knowledge, teaching is based on the interaction, cooperation and problematization and part of what students already know, the methodology is cooperative, interactive, problematizing and based on the identification and resolution of problems and the assessment is formative, continuous and allows the solution of problem situations, case studies emerging in the interaction spaces favoring autonomous learning.

The communicational and social perspective and the items that obtained more than 65% of satisfactory assessment by specialist judges who fully or partially agreed were: information space and sources of trading of the learning environment, the discursive tools, interaction and interactivity of the course, student and teacher profiles.

The web design specialists judges mostly (65%) attributed concept, good, very good and excellent in the following aspects of the technical and administrative perspective, namely: technical support, management and environment management tools, management tools of communities, professor and user authoring tools, the individual and community area tools, service tools, synchronous and asynchronous tools and assessment tools.

On the foregoing facts it is considered that this educational technology successfully meets and may be available for the formation of the Family Health Strategy nurses regarding the theme in breast health, drawing on the pedagogical framework of Vygotsky social interactionist design and the Meaningful Learning Theory of David Ausubel [6].

5. Conclusions

The continuing health education has emerged as a theoretical and pedagogical model to generate changes in the qualification and performance of professional and in-service training for health workers whose needs are detected in their work processes of health professionals which are urged to reflect and rethink their practice by modifying its context and professional life.

It is noteworthy that the results achieved in the construction and validation of the distance course in breast health inserted in the virtual learning environment of breast—AVAPMAMA follows the calling of the National Curriculum Guidelines for Undergraduate Nursing Course and the National Policy on Continuing Education in Health, when it offers a new way of training the health professionals, specifically nurses, posing as active, critical and reflective subject in learning process and the educator/teacher as mediator/facilitator of this process.

References

[1] Aguiar, R.V. and Cassiani, S.H.B. (2007) Development and Evaluation of a Virtual Learning Environment in Professional Nursing Courses. *Revista Latino-Americana de Enfermagem*, **15**, 1086-1091. http://dx.doi.org/10.1590/S0104-11692007000600005

[2] Barbosa, S.F. and Sasso, G.T.M.D. (2007) Internet e saúde: Um guia para os profissionais. Nova Letra, Blumenau.

[3] Bergmann, A., Mattos, I.E. and Koifman, R.J. (2004) Diagnóstico do linfedema: Análise dos métodos empregados na

avaliação do membro superior após linfadenectomia axilar para tratamento do câncer de mama. *Revista Brasileira de Cancerologia*, **50**, 311-320.

[4] Bloom, B.S., Engelhart, M.D., Furst, E.J., Hill, W.H. and Krathwohl, D.R. (1972) Taxonomia de objetivos educacionais: Domínio cognitivo. Editora Globo, Porto Alegre.

[5] Falkembach, G.A.M. (2005) Concepção e desenvolvimento de material educativo digital. *Revista Novas Tecnologias na Educação*, **3**, 1-15.

[6] Levy,L.F. and Santo, A.O.E. (2006) A psicologia vygotskyana e uma alternativa transdisciplinar. *Acta Scientiae*, **8**, 5-24.

22

Effect of Work Environment on Level of Work Stress and Burnout among Nurses in a Teaching Hospital in Nigeria

Guobadia Pauline Ojekou[1], Odetola Titilayo Dorothy[2*]

[1]School of Occupational Health Nursing, University College Hospital, Ibadan, Nigeria
[2]Department of Nursing, University of Ibadan, Ibadan, Nigeria
Email: paulineguobadia@yahoo.com, *odetolatitilayo@yahoo.com

Abstract

Nurses' roles expose them to a lot of stress based upon the physical labour, exposure to human suffering, lengthy work hours, poor staffing, and interpersonal relationships that are central to the work they do. Nurses are expected to deliver humane, empathetic, culturally-sensitive and proficient care in working environments with limited resources and increasing responsibilities. Such imbalance between providing high quality care with limited resources leads to physical and mental stress. This stressful nature of nursing can ultimately lead to job dissatisfaction and burnout which among health care providers are important issues since they affect turnover rates, staff retention and ultimately the quality of patient care. A thoroughly validated self developed questionnaire with a reliability coefficient of 0.78 was used to explore the effect of work environment on the level of work stress and burnout among nurses. A purposive sampling technique was utilized to select 100 participants from the medical unit of the hospital. Three hypotheses were tested at a significant level of 0.05. Data were analyzed using ANOVA and Pearson's Correlation. The study revealed that level of stress was higher among the staff nurses who had worked for only between 0 and 3 years, with mean stress score 46.0000. Findings further revealed that as the cadre rose, the nurses assumed that managerial roles were accountable for increased subordinates and oversee health related and administrative responsibilities and they experienced more stress. Also there is a significant relationship among work environment, stress and burnout among the nurses in the selected unit. In conclusion, though work conditions and environment are not favourable, there are job security and good interpersonal relationship among the nurses which cushion the stressful situations. It is therefore recommended that the management of the hospitals should provide a conducive work environment, providing necessary resources and adequate break periods to ensure staff welfare.

*Corresponding author.

Keywords

Work Environment, Stress, Burnout, Nurses

1. Introduction

Every work environment especially within a hospital setup needs to be conducive, friendly and stress free to promote quality care and wellbeing of health care workers whose job demands are increasing day by day. This is as a result of advancement in technology and patient's demand for quality in response to increasing health care cost. Stress is considered a normal part of life which is necessary occasionally as a push to increasing functional capacity, but when it is experienced over a prolonged period it becomes detrimental to health leading to a decline in productivity [1].

Stress can be defined as a particular relationship between the person and the environment that is assessed by the person as taxing or exceeding his or her resources and endangering his or her well-being [2]. Stress on its own does not have any damaging effect on an individual; however individuals' assessment of an event, their perceptions and interpretations give meaning and their coping ability determines whether events are viewed as threatening or positive. Personality traits also influence individual reaction to stress because what may be strenuous to one person may be stimulating to another [3].

As far back as the mid-1950s, stress was regarded as an occupational hazard and occupational stress cited as a significant health problem [4] while in the 1960s, patient's care, decision making, taking responsibility, and change were identified as sources of anxiety among nurses which predisposed them to work stress [5]. Nurse's role has long been regarded as stress-filled based upon the physical labor, human suffering, work hours, staffing, and interpersonal relationships that are central to what the work nurses do [6]. This stressful nature of nursing can ultimately lead to job dissatisfaction and burnout [7]. This statement is in line with some studies which conclude that the provision of health care services is demanding both physically and psychologically [8]. Nursing occupies a conspicuous position among the professions that have been identified as the most stressful worldwide as nurses relate with humans mostly in times of pain, suffering and death [6]. Nurses work tirelessly rendering care to critically and chronically ill patients who are between life and death in an environment where there is lack of tolerance for error [9]; all these can exert intense psychological and physical pressures on the health care giver leading to stress or burnout syndrome.

Among health care professionals, nurses have been found to be most prone to burnout [10]. This is more so because nurses are expected to deliver humane, empathetic, culturally sensitive, proficient and moral care, in working environments with limited resources, reduced supply of nurses and increasing responsibilities. Such imbalance between providing high quality care within an environment of limited resources leads to stress [11].

Job satisfaction and burnout among health care providers are important issues since they affect turnover rates, staff retention and ultimately the quality of patient care [12]. Burnout has been defined as "a syndrome of physical and emotional exhaustion, involving the development of stress which can lead to the development of negative self-concept, negative job attitudes and loss of concern for clients". Burnout has also been associated with high employment turnover, excessive absenteeism, negative job attitudes, low morale and a reduction in willingness to help others [10].

The way that an individual views and processes stress determines how much stress is felt and how close the person is to burnout. Perceptions of job stress and burnout are not just a product of work conditions because not all workers, exposed to the same conditions, develop burnout or perceive stress [3]. An individual can be exposed to few stressors but be unable to process the stress well and thus experience burnout. Another person, however, can be exposed to a significant amount of stressors, but process each well, and avoid burnout. How close a person is to a state of burnout is greatly dependent on individual differences [13].

According to psychological theories, stress is determined by the balance between the perceived demands from the environment and the individual's resources to meet those demands [14].

The International Council of Nurses (ICN) (2008) [15] declares that nurses, doctors, and laboratory technicians experience the highest job related stress with 45 percent reporting that their jobs are quite or extremely stressful. Likewise, the International Labour Organization has identified nursing as an industry with relatively high level of stress and burnout [16]. Stress can contribute to human errors and accidents.

2. Methodology

The study utilized a descriptive design to explore the role of work environment and conditions on the level of work stress and burnout among nurses in medical unit of University College Hospital (UCH) The Medical Unit is made up of 7 wards, rendering nursing care to both male and female clients on admission in the hospital receiving medical and long term care for acute and mostly chronic illness that does not require surgical intervention. The wards under the medical unit include: West Three ward, South West Three, Central Ward 3rd, East Three, South East Three, East Two and Multi-Drug Resistant Ward.

2.1. Study Population

The study population consisted of all professional nurses who are directly involved in patient care in the Medical Unit of University College Hospital, Ibadan. The professional nurses ranged between the cadres of Staff Nurse to Chief Nursing Officer.

2.2. Study Design

It was a descriptive study which utilized a convenience sampling technique to select all available and willing Registered nurses from each ward in the unit, making a total of 100 registered nurses.

2.3. Sample Size Determination

The sample size for this study was determined using sample size formula below [17]:

$$n = \frac{t_2 \times P(1-P)}{m^2}$$

where

n = Required sample size;

t = confidence level at 95% = 1.96;

P = Estimated population of professional nurses carrying out direct patient care in the medical unit = 80 out of a total nursing population of 1080 = 0.07;

m = margin of error tolerance at 5% = 0.05.

Sample size $n = \frac{1.96^2 \times 0.07(1-0.07)}{m^2} = \frac{3.84 \times 0.07(1-0.07)}{0.05^2} = \frac{0.249984}{0.0025} = 99.99$.

Calculated sample size 100.

10% of calculated sample size = 10 added to make up for attrition.

Total number of respondents = 110.

2.4. Sampling Technique

A purposive sampling technique was adopted. This implies that all the nurses who are directly involved in nursing care of the patients on all the wards of the Medical Unit ranging between the cadres of Staff nurses and Chief Nursing Officers were included in the study.

The calculated sample size was 100. Since 100 was the minimum sample size that can be studied, the researcher decided to increase the power of significance by including all the nurses in the Medical Unit who are involved in direct nursing care of patients and are willing to participate in the study in the sample frame, they were 110.

According to Suresh and Chandrashekara (2012) [18], determining the optimal sample size for a study assures an adequate power to detect statistical significance and that power proportionately increases as the sample size for study increases.

2.5. Exclusion Criteria

Professional nurses who are at the managerial post of Assistant Directors of Nursing as they are mostly on administrative schedule and are not directly involved in nursing care of the patients on the ward.

2.6. Ethical Consideration

The need for the research and procedure for data collection was explained to the participants. Verbal consent was obtained from participant to participate in the study. They were informed that participation was entirely voluntary, confidential and anonymous.

2.7. Instrument for Data Collection

The self-developed questionnaire was used to cover demographic characteristics, factors relating to job related stress from the work environment, work conditions and effect of stress on health. The instrument was trial-tested on 20 nurses in the medical unit of the State Hospital in Ibadan and the results had a co-efficient of 0.78. Showing that among similar groups, the questionnaire will consistently test and answer what it is meant for. Necessary corrections were made and the questionnaire was administered without any bias among the study population.

The researcher visited the wards in the selected unit of the hospital to serve the questionnaire personally to nurses who are willing to participate in the study, 110 questionnaires were served as some of the nurses were not around. Only 104 questionnaires were retrieved out of which only 100 were well filled the remaining 4 questionnaire were not adequately filled and could not be analyzed therefore were discarded.

The quantitative data was analyzed through content analysis. The responses were sorted out and grouped into similar and non similar responses

Comments were categorized and presented in simple percentages.

Hypotheses were tested using Analysis of Variance (ANOVA) and Pearson Correlation to relate work condition and work environment to stress and burnout among the nurses.

3. Results

The results are presented based on the objectives and hypotheses

4. Discussion

This study has revealed an either way relationship between work environment level of work stress and burnout among nurses. This is shown in **Table 1** and **Table 2**. **Table 1** shows a significant relationship between work environment and incidence of stress among nurses while **Table 2** indicated that there is no significant relationship between work condition and stress among nurses. This is also supported by **Table 3** and **Table 4**. **Table 3** shows that work environment is not too conducive, leading to stress while **Table 4** presented 69% of the res-

Table 1. Showing relationship between work environment and incidence of stress among nurses. For hypotheses 2 Pearson Correlation was used to relate stress and burnout to work environment.

	Stress	Remark
Work environment: Pearson correlation	0.351	
Sig. (2-tailed)	0.000	Significant
No.	100	

The results showed a positive correlation 0.351, the significance (2-tailed) is 0.000 in total respondents numbering 100. Correlation is significant at the 0.01 level (2 tailed), 0.000 is <0.01, this means that there is a significant relationship between work environment and stress and burnout among the nurses.

Table 2. Showing relationship between work condition and stress among nurses. For hypotheses 3 pearson correlation was used to relate stress and burnout to work conditions.

Work condition: Pearson correlation	−0.033	Not
Sig. (2-tailed)	0.745	Significant
No.	100	

Looking at work conditions, there is a negative correlation −0.033, the significance (2-tailed) is 0.745 in a total respondents numbering 100. 0.745 is >0.01, this means that there is no relationship between work conditions and stress and burnout among the nurses.

Table 3. Showing factors relating to job related stress from work environment.

	Always present	Often present	Rarely present	Not present	Total
Excessive noise disturbing my work on the ward	69 (69%)	20 (20%)	9 (9%)	2 (2%)	100%
Movement and interruptions from medical, para-medical and visitors disturbing my work on the ward	58 (58%)	34 (34%)	6 (6%)	2 (2%)	100%
Adequate lighting both day and night on the ward to promote work	8 (8%)	85 (85%)	6 (6%)	2 (2%)	100%
Adequate provision of privacy for procedures on the ward	12 (12%)	81 (81%)	5 (5%)	2 (2%)	100%
Pest and rodent such as flies, mosquitoes and rats	62 (62%)	21 (21%)	11 (11%)	6 (6%)	100%

Table 4. Showing effect of work environment and conditions on level of stress and burnout among the nurses.

	Not at all	rarely	Sometimes	Often	Always	Total
Do you feel run down and drained off physically and emotionally?	1 (1%)	1 (1%)	48 (48%)	45 (45%)	5 (5%)	100 (100%)
Do you find that you are prone to negative thinking about your job?	8 (8%)	69 (69%)	19 (19%)	4 (4%)	0 (0%)	100 (100%)
Do you find that you are less sympathetic with people than perhaps they deserve?	7 (7%)	21 (21%)	67 (67%)	4 (4%)	1 (1%)	100 (100%)
Do you find yourself getting easily irritated by small problems or by your team or co-workers?	8 (8%)	3 (3%)	86 (86%)	3 (3%)	0 (0%)	100 (100%)
Do you feel misunderstood or unappreciated by your co-workers?	5 (5%)	11 (11%)	81 (81%)	3 (3%)	0 (0%)	100 (100%)
Do you feel you have no one to talk to?	12 (12%)	61 (61%)	25 (25%)	2 (2%)	0 (0%)	100 (100%)
Do you feel that you are achieving less than you should?	3 (3%)	11 (11%)	72 (72%)	13 (13%)	1 (1%)	100 (100%)
Do you feel an unpleasant level of pressure to succeed?	3 (3%)	3 (3%)	54 (54%)	38 (38%)	2 (2%)	100 (100%)
Do you feel you are not getting what you want out of your job?	5 (5%)	7 (7%)	56 (56%)	30 (30%)	2 (2%)	100 (100%)
Do you feel you are in a wrong ward?	15 (15%)	67 (67%)	15 (15%)	3 (3%)	0 (0%)	100 (100%)
Is your job becoming more demanding on you?	2 (2%)	3 (3%)	42 (42%)	46 (46%)	7 (7%)	100 (100%)
Do you feel the hospital politics and protocols are frustrating your ability to do a good job?	2 (2%)	2 (2%)	27 (27%)	41 (41%)	28 (28%)	100 (100%)
Do you feel there is more work to do than you practically have the ability to do?	1 (1%)	6 (6%)	43 (43%)	35 (35%)	15 (15%)	100 (100%)
Do you feel you do not have time to do many of the important things in doing a quality job?	2 (2%)	4 (4%)	54 (54%)	35 (35%)	5 (5%)	100 (100%)
Do you find that you do not have time to plan as much as you would like to?	2 (2%)	3 (3%)	58 (58%)	30 (30%)	7 (7%)	100 (100%)

pondents indicating that they are rarely prone to negative thinking about their job and 67% rarely feel they are in the wrong ward. This means that despite the unfavourable work environment, work conditions are motivating. The socio-demographic characteristics revealed workers within the productive age with the younger nurses who form a greater percentage of the respondents being at the lower level of the professional ladder as presented on **Table 5** where 64% of the nurse respondents fall between ages 25 and 40 years. Testing for relationship between nurses' cadre and stress and burnout was not significant, **Table 6** p-value 0.530 > 0.05, However there is an interesting discovery in that level of stress was higher among the Staff Nurses who have worked for only between 0 - 3 years, most of them are never married with no family social support, they recorded a mean score of 46.0000. This can be associated to the fact that they are new in the institution of care, in a new and strange environment especially when expectations are not met, stress increases. As they get older in the establishment they acclimatize, adjust to the rules and regulations of the institution and experience less stress. This is reflected in the level of stress among the Nursing Officers and Senior Nursing Officers who have a lesser mean stress score of 44.2222 and 45.0625 respectively. As the cadre rises, the nurses assume managerial roles, are accountable for a lot of subordinates and oversee both health related and administrative responsibilities, they experience more stress. Same is reflected in the stress mean score of Principal Nursing Officers and Chief Nursing Officers who recorded 46.7778 for PNO's and 47.2500 for CNO's as presented in **Table 6**, relationship between the nurses'

Table 5. Biodata of respondent.

	Frequency	Percent	Valid percent	Cumulative percent
Age range of respondents				
21 - 30 years	25	25.0	25.0	25.0
31 - 40 years	39	39.0	39.0	64.0
41 - 50 years	23	23.0	23.0	87.0
Above 50 years	13	13.0	13.0	100.0
Total	100	100.0	100.0	
Sex distribution of respondents				
Male	1	1.0	1.0	1.0
Female	99	99.0	99.0	100.0
Total	100	100.0	100.0	
Respondents' marital status				
Never married	40	40.0	40.0	40.0
Married	56	56.0	56.0	96.0
Divorced	3	3.0	3.0	99.0
Widow	1	1.0	1.0	100.0
Total	100	100.0	100.0	
Number of children of respondents				
0	42	42.0	42.0	42.0
1 - 2	36	36.0	36.0	78.0
3 - 4	21	21.0	21.0	99.0
5 and above	1	1.0	1.0	100.0
Total	100	100.0	100.0	
Level of education of respondents				
Diploma in nursing	49	49.0	49.0	49.0
BSc./Bed.	36	36.0	36.0	85.0
MSc./Med.	1	1.0	1.0	86.0
Specialty programme	14	14.0	14.0	100.0
Total	100	100.0	100.0	
Respondents currently pursuing an educational programme				
Yes	41.0	41.0	41	41
No	59.0	59.0	59.0	100
Respondent's years of work experience in UCH				
0 - 3	41	41.0	41.0	41.0
4 - 6	27	27.0	27.0	68.0
7 - 9	15	15.0	15.0	83.0
10 - 13	7	7.0	7.0	90.0
>13	10	10.0	10.0	100.0
Total	100	100.0	100.0	
Respondents' professional cadre				
SN	40	40.0	40.0	40.0
NO	27	27.0	27.0	67.0
SNO	16	16.0	16.0	83.0
PNO	9	9.0	9.0	92.0
CNO	8	8.0	8.0	100.0
Total	100	100.0	100.0	

Table 6. Relationship between the nurses' professional cadre and incidence of stress and burnout.

	No.	Mean	Std. deviation	F value	P value	Remark
SN	40	46.0000	4.70134			
NO	27	44.2222	5.22813			
SNO	16	45.0625	7.63735	0.796	0.530	Not Significant
PNO	9	46.7778	5.76146			
CNO	8	47.2500	4.71320			
Total	100	45.5400	5.47247			

Using one way ANOVA to test stress by cadre at Alpha level 0.05, $P = 0.530 > 0.05$ we fail to reject the hypothesis, which means there is no significant relationship between nurses' cadre and stress and burnout among them.

professional cadre and incidence of stress and burnout. These findings are in line with Wu *et al.* (2007) [19] who also found that the burnout scores of women generally and from all dimensions of the burnout syndrome were higher among single members of the hospital staff. They stated further that this may be possible as the social support unit in which an individual is most likely to find shelter from the conflicts and difficulties of daily life is the family. Therefore, it was expected that married individuals would report lower levels of burnout syndrome than singles. In addition to illustrating a likely connection between nurse managers and staff nurse stressors [4], in her studies also reflected the demanding role of today's nurse managers who are often responsible for multiple patient care areas. This is also shown in **Table 6**, respondents who are Chief Nursing Officers (CNO) had the highest mean stress score of 47,2500 for relationship between the nurses' professional cadre and incidence of stress and burnout.

In another study, a general construct labeled "organizational support" exhibited the expected negative relationship with work exhaustion [20]. Similarly, social support from supervisors or colleagues demonstrated a negative association with work stress [21], as nurses felt more stress, they relied more on social support [4]. This is in agreement with the findings of some researchers who discovered that in management styles, relationship between staff nurses and nurse managers are particularly important when examining stress and burnout [22]. **Table 7** shows these findings, where 75% of the nurses indicated that there is good human relation among every staff on their ward and 59% said they can always go to their boss for assistance anytime they have a job or personal problem. Finally, it was discovered that group cohesion was higher and job stress lower when nurse managers used a more participative management style [4]. This is shown in **Table 7** where 75% of the nurses indicated that there is good human relation among every staff on their ward which is indicative of group cohesion.

5. Implications for Nurses

The results of this study show that environmental factors have a significant effect on the level of stress of the nurses more than work conditions. This can be attributed to the fact that as the nurses indicate, there is good interpersonal relationship among them which may go a long way in reducing stress and burnout in relation to work conditions. The younger nurses who are new in the system and most of them never marry experience a higher level of stress and burnout.

When workers are happy, it is reflected in the quality of their work output. In order to promote quality nursing care in the University College Hospital, the Board of Management should look into the unconducive work environment as this may affect not only the nurses but also other workers and patients within the hospital who are not included in this study.

Based on the findings and the implication of the study for nursing, it is suggested that nurses should ensure that

Table 7. Showing factors relating to job related stress from work conditions.

	SA	A	UD	D	SD	Total
The roster is done to favour individual request	3 (3%)	9 (9%)	8 (8%)	76 (76%)	4 (4%)	100%
There is enough time to complete my work and report for the shift	2 (2%)	11 (11%)	4 (4%)	79 (79%)	4 (4%)	100%
I have enough time to go for my break on every shift	0 (0%)	1 (1%)	4 (4%)	71 (71%)	24 (24%)	100%
There is adequate provision of functioning equipment to aid smooth nursing care	2 (2%)	38 (38%)	42 (42%)	9 (9%)	9 (9%)	100%
I am confident that my job is secured	6 (6%)	87 (87%)	4 (4%)	2 (2%)	1 (1%)	100%
My salary and other incentives are up to standard	1 (1%)	6 (6%)	8 (8%)	74 (74%)	11 (11%)	100%
I am always promoted when due	0 (0%)	8 (8%)	29 (29%)	55 (55%)	8 (8%)	100%
There is enough opportunity and encouragement to further my education and for seminars	4 (4%)	79 (79%)	6 (6%)	6 (6%)	5 (5%)	100%
All amenities needed for my comfort at every shift are provided	0 (0%)	0 (0%)	2 (2%)	37 (37%)	61 (61%)	100%
There is adequate staff covering every shift	0 (0%)	2 (2%)	1 (1%)	30 (30%)	67 (67%)	100%
There is good human relation among every staff on the ward	11 (11%)	75 (75%)	7 (7%)	4 (4%)	3 (3%)	100%
I can always go to my boss for assistance anytime I have a job or personal problem	8 (8%)	59 (59%)	23 (23%)	7 (7%)	3 (3%)	100%

the board of management of UCH provides means of promoting a conducive work environment by looking into the factors identified.

This study should be replicated in other units with less chronically ill patients who do not stay long in the hospital. It can also be replicated in other states in Nigeria, with a larger population.

References

[1] Salleh, M.R. (2008) Life Event, Stress and Illness. *Malays Journal of Medical Sciences*, **4**, 9-18.

[2] Irving, J.A., Dobkin, P.L. and Park, J. (2009) Cultivating Mindfulness in Healthcare Professionals: A Review of Empirical Studies of Mindfulness-Based Stress Reduction (MBSR). *Complementary Therapies in Clinical Practice*, **15**, 61-66. http://dx.doi.org/10.1016/j.ctcp.2009.01.002

[3] Robinson, M.D., Ode, S. and Hilmert, C. (2011) Regulated and Unregulated Forms of Cortisol Reactivity: A Dual Vulnerability Model. *Psychosomatic Medicine*, **73**, 250-256. http://dx.doi.org/10.1097/PSY.0b013e3182099deb

[4] Jennings, B.M. (2009) Work Stress and Burnout among Nurses: Role of the Work Environment and Working Conditions, Health Care Consultant. In: Hughes, R.G., Ed., *Patient Safety and Quality: An Evidence-Based Handbook for Nurses*. Agency for Healthcare Research and Quality, Rockville. bmjennings@cox.net

[5] Menzies, I.E.P. (1960) Nurses under Stress. *International Nursing Review*, **7**, 9-16.

[6] Lukpata, F.E., Lukpata, O.H., Ndiok, A. and Mgbekem, M.A. (2013) Nurses Workplace Stress and patient Safety in General Hospital Calabar, Cross River State, Nigeria. *International Professional Nursing Journal*, **11**, 87-92.

[7] Arafa, M.A. (2003) Predictors of Psychological Well-Being of Nurses in Alexandria, Egypt. *International Journal of Nursing Practice*, **9**, 313-320. http://dx.doi.org/10.1046/j.1440-172X.2003.00437.x

[8] Ilhan, M.N., Tuzun, H., Ceyhan, M.N. and Aygun, R. (2005) Turning the Mirror on Ourselves: The Association between Burnout Syndrome and Personal Characteristics and Working Conditions of the Research Assistants Working in a University Hospital. *Community and Physician*, **20**, 455-462.

[9] Rowe, J. (2003) The Suffering of the Healer. *Nursing Forum*, **38**, 16-20. http://dx.doi.org/10.1111/j.0029-6473.2003.00016.x

[10] Abushaikha, L. and Saca-Hazboun, H. (2009) Job Satisfaction and Burnout among Palestinian Nurses. *Eastern Mediterranean Health Journal*, **15**, 190-197.

[11] Khamisa, N., Oldenburg, B., Peltzer, K. and Ilic, D. (2015) Work Related Stress, Burnout, Job Satisfaction and General Health of Nurses. *International Journal of Environmental Research and Public Health*, **12**, 652-666.

[12] Atencio, B.L., Cohen, J. and Gorenberg, B. (2003) Nurse Retention: Is It Worth It? *Nursing Economics*, **21**, 262-268, 299, 259.

[13] Truby, B. (2009) Burnout Test. www.trubyachievements.com/..Stress_Management/Burnout.html

[14] Ursin, H. and Eriksen, H.R. (2004) The Cognitive Activation Theory of Stress. *Psychoneuroendocrinology*, **29**, 567-592. http://dx.doi.org/10.1016/S0306-4530(03)00091-X

[15] International Council of Nurses (ICN) (2008)

[16] International Labour Organization (n.d.) Occupational Safety and Health. http://www.ilo.org/public/english/protection/safework/stress/nursing.htm

[17] Smith, S. (2013) Determining Sample Size: How to Ensure You Get the Correct Sample Size. E-Book (c) Qualtrics Online Sample.

[18] Suresh, K.P. and Chandrashekara, S. (2012) Sample Size Estimation and Power Analysis for Clinical Research Studies. *Journal of Human Reproductive Science*, **5**, 7-13.

[19] Wu, S., Zhu, Z., Wang, Z., Wang, M. and Lan, Y. (2007) Relationship between Burnout and Occupational Stress among Nurses in China. *Journal of Advanced Nursing*, **59**, 233-239. http://dx.doi.org/10.1111/j.1365-2648.2007.04301.x

[20] Blau, G., Tatum, D.S. and Ward-Cook, K. (2003) Correlates of Work Exhaustion for Medical Technologists. *Journal Allied Health*, **32**, 148-157.

[21] Joiner, T.A. and Bartram, T. (2004) How Empowerment and Social Support Affect Australian Nurses' Work Stressors. *Australian Health Review*, **28**, 56-64. http://dx.doi.org/10.1071/AH040056

[22] Laschinger, H.K., Finegan, J. and Shamian J. (2001). Impact of Structural and Psychological Empowerment on Job Strain in Nursing Work Settings. Expanding Kanter's Model. *Journal of Nursing Administration*, **1**, 260-272. http://dx.doi.org/10.1097/00005110-200105000-00006

23

Structural Accessibility of Gynecological Nursing Clinics for Users with Motor Disabilities in Basic Health Units

Ana Talyne Pessoa[1], Beatriz da Silva Lima[1], Lorita Marlena Freitag Pagliuca[1*], Paula Marciana Pinheiro de Oliveira[2], Leilane Barbosa de Sousa[2], Paulo César de Almeida[1], Luciana Vieira de Carvalho[1], Aline Cruz Esmeraldo Áfio[1]

[1]Departamento de Enfermagem, Universidade Federal do Ceará, Fortaleza, Brasil
[2]Universidade Internacional da Integração da Lusofonia Afro-Brasileira, Fortaleza, Brasil
Email: *pagliuca@ufc.br

Abstract

A quantitative descriptive study aimed to evaluate the physical structure accessibility of gynecological nursing clinics and their bathrooms in basic health units for users with motor disabilities. A *checklist* tool/instrument was applied for analyzing 16 items in the bathroom and four in the nursing clinic. 157 basic health units were evaluated. In the nursing clinic, counters and tables (79.6%) were accessible, but stretchers (93%), seats (93.6%) and doors (87.3%) were inaccessible; moreover, 17.8% of the units examined proved totally inaccessible. In the bathroom, the items with the best evaluation were the height of the toilet flusher (47%) with operation by slight pressure (44.6%) and the wall-mounted sink (42.7%). Bathroom doors and turning area/space for wheelchairs were inaccessible. No bathroom reached full accessibility, and 31.2% were entirely inaccessible. Non-compliance was evident of the standard 9050:2004 of the Brazilian Association of Technical Standards. Raising the awareness of health and engineering professionals is recommended to learn technical accessibility standards and implement them.

Keywords

Nursing, Health Services Accessibility, Disabled Persons

1. Introduction

People with disabilities (PD) are those that have long-term impairments, whether being physical, mental, intel-

*Corresponding author.

lectual or sensory impairments. Full and effective activities of these people in society on a full and equal basis with others may be blocked because of the characteristics and environmental difficulties they may encounter that can prevent their social interaction [1].

In 2010, Brazil had 45,606,048 (23.9%) people who claimed having at least one disability, with the highest prevalence rate being in the Northeast with 26.63%, presenting an elevated position compared to the national average. As to gender, analyses had shown that 26.5% of the female population (25.8 million) had some disability compared with 21.2% of the male population (19.8 million). In this analysis, the female population had higher percentages of disability for all races or colors declared [2].

Physically disabled women report that they face distressing situations during consultations in health services. However, health professionals, especially nurses and the team leaders, responsible for gynecological care in the basic health units, must establish bonds of trust with users to promote quality care favoring sexual health promotion [3].

Primary health care is characterized as a set of actions that include health promotion and protection, disease prevention, diagnosis, treatment, rehabilitation, harm reduction and maintenance of health, individually and collectively. It should be a gateway for users. It follows the principles of universality, accessibility, connectivity, continuity of care, comprehensiveness of care, accountability, humanization, equity and social participation. Subjects are considered as an individual part of a socio-cultural environment, with the objective to develop comprehensive care [4].

Nurses are important members of the multidisciplinary team that is part of the Family Health Strategy (FHS) [5]. Among the actions carried out by primary care teams, those related to the control of cervical cancer (CC) can be highlighted. The following national goals have been established for CC control: expanding Pap test coverage in women between 25 and 64 years of age; treating 100% of women diagnosed with precursor cancer lesions; improving CC and breast cancer screening; universalizing these tests for all women, regardless of income, race, or color, thus reducing inequalities [6].

Among the main factors affecting the performing of Pap Smear examinations for wheelchair users, the design inadequacy of health services to this group of women can be emphasized, apart from the health team's unpreparedness in handling handling/treating these women with this particular condition [7]. The Ministry of Health's goals can only be achieved when all sexually active women have access to gynecological care. It appears that adult women with motor disabilities are culturally perceived as asexual and are excluded from the target audience for active CC control. Added to this scenario are physical barriers, which prevent these women from feeling empowered to seek gynecological care.

Women with disabilities are left on the fringes of the women's movement and the civil rights movement of this social group. It can be said that disability issues tend to be a considerable problem regarding public health and women's health. This share of the population has inexpressive actions addressed to their needs in primary health care services. Female clients in general have this care about their sexual and reproductive rights guarantee; on the other hand the disabled women are more vulnerable [8].

In Brazil, sexual and reproductive health interventions of women with disabilities were discussed and documented by the Ministry of Health for their promotion in the health network. However, public policies and care practices are still very incipient. Thus, women with disabilities do not receive adequate reproductive and sexual assistance. When they do exist, such assistance faces several barriers, especially when referring to physical disabilities [9].

In the face of the problems experienced by this population with regard to attending gynecological nursing consultations, this study aiming at evaluating the structural accessibility of gynecological nursing clinics for users with motor disabilities in basic health units (BHUs) has become relevant.

2. Method

A descriptive study using a quantitative approach composed of ordered and disciplined procedures used to acquire numeric information that resulted from formal measurement and analyzed in statistical procedures [10].

The study was carried out in BHUs of Maciço de Baturité's municipalities due to its geographic peculiarities and the lack of previous studies. Ceara state consists of 184 municipalities with 22 micro-regions and five macro-regions which make up the State Health System [11]. It was performed from August 2014 to January 2015. Access to the lists of health units was carried out through the National Registry of Health Facilities of the Ministry of Health. Exclusion criteria considered units that were leased in temporary spaces, were under construction or had access prevented due to hazard.

Data collection was conducted by applying a *check-list* instrument entitled Physical Accessibility Registry for Basic Health Units, which evaluated 16 items in the bathrooms and 4 items in the nursing clinics based on the Brazilian Standard (NBR) 9050:2004 of the Brazilian Association of Technical Standards (ABNT). This Standard sets criteria and technical parameters to be observed for when design, construction, installation and alteration of buildings, houses, urban spaces and equipment are done in order to obtain adequate conditions of accessibility [12].

The instrument offered information on unit identification, location (rural or urban) and municipality to which it belonged. For this study, the entry corresponding to Nursing Clinics was analyzed as described below.

Environmental evaluation was performed by analyzing the internal area of the clinics and their bathrooms. The evaluation of internal areas consisted of the nurse's clinic entrance door width that should be at least 80 cm wide; counters and work stations, which should be 75 to 85 cm from the floor (height); seats for the users/public, which should have a minimum of 45 cm depth, 46 cm from the floor (height), with grab bars or arm support; and a stretcher for clinical examination, which should be 49 to 53 cm from the floor (height) to facilitate user transfer.

In the private bathrooms the door was evaluated, which should also have a minimum width of 80 cm; maneuvering clearance area for a wheelchair, ensuring diagonal, lateral and perpendicular movement and 360˚ rotation, with the following dimensions being a reference: 1.20 m for straight movement; 1.20 m by 1.20 m for 90˚ rotation; 1.20 m by 1.50 m for 180˚ rotation and 1.50 m by 1.50 m for 360˚ rotation; clear sanitary and accessories that do not require transposition should be 1.20 m by 80 cm; presence of horizontal grab bars on the side and back walls with sanitary basin should be present, being at least 80 cm in length and 75 cm from the floor; the seat of the sanitary bowl should be 46 cm from the floor, presence of sanitary napkin disposal units 1.50 to 60 cm from the floor and 15 cm from the front edge of the sanitary bowl; flush control maximum height of 1m from the floor and working with light pressure; and a wall-mounted sink being a minimum height of 78 to 80 cm from the floor with a single lever faucet.

The instrument was filled out by the following possibilities: Accessible, if environment or object was suitable to the characteristics provided by item; Inaccessible when the features proposed in the item were not met; Non-existent if environment does not have object/device to be evaluated; Not Applicable when item addressed was not necessary in the assessed site; Not Collected, if the UBS or sector was not in use or closed at the time of data collection; Renovation, if the space provided the item is under renovation; Absent, if the UBS does not have the environment to be analyzed.

Data was processed by SPSS version 20.0 and later organized into tables. Mean and standard deviation were calculated. This study was approved by the Research Ethics Committee of the University of International Integration of African-Brazilian Lusophone No. 652.134/2014 and complies with the principles of Resolution 466/ 2012 of the National Health Council.

3. Results

The sample consisted of 157 public health units and the results were organized into four tables. **Table 1** and **Table 2** feature data analyzed from gynecological clinics, highlighting the analyzed variables and the frequency of accessible items, respectively. **Table 2** and **Table 3** present data from bathrooms and the frequency of accessible items.

Table 1 shows accessibility data referring to doors, counters and work stations, and seats and stretchers.

Regarding width of nursing clinic's entrance doors, most units were inaccessible (87.3%); counters and work stations were mostly accessible (79.6%); seats and stretchers were found to be considerably inaccessible (93.6%).

Table 2 shows distribution of the number of accessible items evaluated in nursing clinics' internal area.

In the internal area of nursing clinics, the following were evaluated: doors, counters/work stations, seats and stretchers. If these items are accessible in all units, there would be a total of 628 affirmative responses. However, no available items were observed in 28 (17.8%) units, 108 (68.8%) had one item and 21 (13.4%) had two items. In other words, no unit showed accessibility for three or four items analyzed.

Table 3 highlights accessibility conditions analyzed in the bathroom of nursing clinics, comprised of a door, maneuvering clearance area, grab bars, sanitary bowl, trash bin, flush control, sink and faucet.

Table 1. Distribution of the number of HBUs analyzed regarding accessibility of the gynecological nursing clinics.

Variables	Accessible	Inaccessible	Non-existent	Renovations	Not collected
	n (%)	n (%)	n (%)	n (%)	n (%)
Doors	19 (12.1)	137 (87.3)	-	1(0.6)	-
Counters and work stations	125 (79.6)	29 (18.5)	1 (0.6)	1 (0.6)	1 (0.6)
Seats	5 (3.2)	147 (93.6)	3 (1.9)	1 (0.6)	1 (0.6)
Stretchers	1 (0.6)	147 (93.6)	7 (4.5)	1 (0.6)	1 (0.6)

Table 2. Frequency of accessible items in internal areas of gynecological nursing clinics according to evaluated BHUs.

Accessible	N	%
0	28	17.8
1	108	68.8
2	21	13.4
Mean ± SD 0.96 ± 0.559		

Table 3. Distribution of the number of BHUs s analyzed regarding bathroom accessibility in gynecological nursing clinics.

Variables	Accessible	Inaccessible	Inexistent	Renovation	Not collected	Absent
	n (%)	n (%)	n (%)	n (%)	n (%)	n (%)
Bathrooms						
Door	7 (4.5)	102 (65.0)	-	1 (0.6)	9 (5.7)	38 (24.2)
Maneuvering clearance area						
1.20 straight movement	30 (19.1)	84 (53.5)	-	1 (0.6)	4 (2.5)	38 (24.2)
1.20 × 1.20 90° rotation	16 (10.2)	98 (62.4)	-	1 (0.6)	4 (2.5)	38 (24.2)
1.20 × 1.50 180° rotation	12 (7.6)	102 (65.0)	-	1 (0.6)	4 (2.5)	38 (24.2)
1.50 × 1.50 360° rotation	7 (4.5)	107 (68.2)	-	1 (0.6)	4 (2.5)	38 (24.2)
Transferring						
1.20 × 0.80 free space	6 (3.8)	108 (68.8)	-	1 (0.6)	4 (2.5)	38 (24.2)
Side and back grab bars	-	14 (8.9)	100 (63.7)	1 (0.6)	4 (2.5)	38 (24.2)
Horizontal grab bars	-	5 (3.2)	109 (69.4)	1 (0.6)	4 (2.5)	38 (24.2)
Lateral grab bars	-	6 (3.8)	108 (68.8)	1 (0.6)	4 (2.5)	38 (24.2)
Sanitary bowl	1 (0.6)	113 (72.0)	-	1 (0.6)	4 (2.5)	38 (24.2)
Napkin disposal units	1 (0.6)	73 (46.5)	40 (25.5)	1 (0.6)	4 (2.5)	38 (24.2)
Flush						
Maximum height	74 (47.1)	37 (23.6)	3 (1.9)	1 (0.6)	4 (2.5)	38 (24.2)
Light pressure	70 (44.6)	40 (25.5)	4 (2.5)	1 (0.6)	4 (2.5)	38 (24.2)
Wall-mounted						
Sink	67 (42.7)	42 (26.8)	5 (3.2)	1 (0.6)	4 (2.5)	38 (24.2)
78 to 80 cm from the floor	26 (16.6)	83 (52.9)	5 (3.2)	1 (0.6)	4 (2.5)	38 (24.2)
Single lever faucet	3 (1.9)	106 (67.5)	5 (3.2)	1 (0.6)	4 (2.5)	38 (24.2)

It is worth noting that of the 157 units evaluated, there were no bathrooms in 38 for the exclusive use by women; when present, they mostly had inaccessible doors and no maneuvering clearance area; lack of grab bars; mostly inaccessible paper towel disposal units and trash bins; flush control at appropriate height, but working with light pressure; wall-mounted sink but at inaccessible height and absence of single lever faucet.

Table 4 shows the distribution of the total number of accessible items in all bathrooms of nursing clinics evaluated.

Table 4. Frequency of accessible bathroom items in nursing clinics according to evaluated BHUs.

Accessible	N	%
0	49	31.2
1	14	8.9
2	31	19.7
3	33	21.0
4	18	11.5
5	4	2.5
6	4	2.5
7	3	1.9
8	1	0.6
Mean ± SD 2.04 ± 1.836.		

Most bathrooms had no accessible items (49% - 31.2%). Eight was the maximum accessible items found for the 16 items evaluated in bathrooms, and was in only one (0.6%) unit. If BHUs were all accessible, the total accessible items would be 2512.

4. Discussion

Ceará state corresponds to the third most populous state in the Northeast region, totaling at least 2.3 million people with disabilities. The percentage of the population with a disability living in the state (27.69%) exceeds the northeastern (26.63%) and the national (23.92%) rates. The most common disability is visual (22.15%), followed by motor-disability (8.08%) and hearing (6.23%) [2] [4].

The population of Maciço de Baturité consists of 625,524 inhabitants spread over 16 municipalities that are organized into two regions: Regional Coordination of Health 3 based in Maracanaú, including the municipalities of Maracanaú, Acarape, Barreira, Guaiuba, Maranguape, Pacatuba , Palmácia and Redenção; and Regional Coordination of Health 4 based in Baturité, and its other municipalities: Aracoiaba, Aratuba, Capistrano, Guaramiranga, Itapiúna, Mulungu and Pacoti [11].

Women with disabilities are prevalent in all municipalities in the Maciço de Baturité region, totaling 125,428 women, of which 92,926 live in the urban area and 32,502 live in rural areas [2]

The presented data indicate the importance of the creation and implementation of public policies being crucial to recognize and represent all the people with their diversity to effectively operate in the social control and guarantee rights of this significant portion of the population [13].

Most people face problems in access to health services, however disability people face the same obstacles and specific additional others [14]. The inclusion of people with disabilities in health services is achieved through architectural planning, which guarantees the right of access and mobility quickly and safely. A study [15] showed that inadequacies in the physical structure of health facilities hinder mobility on site, reducing the opportunity of equal service use. Investigating the difficulties encountered by disability people in accessing health services provides subsidies for properly planning health, thereby structuring and improving services that attend this population group.

The front door to the nurses' clinic serves as a basic means of access to the interior of this environment and ensures the user their right to come and go. However, as noted, the overwhelming majority was inaccessible. Therefore, the user who moves around with the aid of a wheelchair is prevented from entering the nursing office and will need help to enter the room, compromising their autonomy and independence.

Welcoming of gynecological consultations starts at the moment of service demand, but its significant value is in the moment patients enter the nursing clinic. Therefore, obstacles to privacy interfere with the quality of care [16].

Working stations were accessible, facilitating the communication between professionals and users, since it favors proper encounters and increased bonding. Unlike those, the seats were inaccessible (93.6%), thus hindering user mobility.

Health professionals are responsible for promoting an environment of trust and respect for patients to feel comfortable during consultation and thus experience this moment without fear to express difficulties and/or concerns [3]. The stretcher used for transferring patients with motor disabilities from their wheelchair to gynecological examinations was inaccessible in 93.6% of evaluated practices, augmenting this public's evasion to this kind of service, as the stretcher is an indispensable item for the user's comfort but was inaccessible.

The analysis of the gynecological nursing clinics' internal area showed that for the 628 items evaluated in the internal areas of 157 nursing clinics, a maximum of two positive responses was found in only 21 (13.4%) of them; and most units (68.8%) only had one accessible item. Women with motor disabilities avoiding consultations related to sexual and reproductive health is explained based on this finding. Inadequate physical infrastructure and furniture significantly contribute to public evasion of services provided by nursing in primary care, and especially in gynecological consultations, which require a comfortable and private environment for patients and professionals.

Preceding the performance of gynecological consultations and the collection of cervical examination materials, women must have an accessible bathroom adjacent to the gynecological nursing examination rooms available to them; in this way, users gain autonomy to prepare for the exam, and have their individuality and privacy respected. Again, 38 clinics had no bathrooms, and where available they (65.0%) were inaccessible, which prevents users with motor disabilities, particularly those who use wheelchairs, from entering this space.

The approaching area to the sanitary bowl must allow user transfer before and after use. But mostly, the space intended for transferring was inadequate. Grab bars help women with motor limitation to make the transfer from the wheelchair to the sanitary bowl; they should be placed in convenient locations and at heights which allow their use. Of the 157 units evaluated, 63.7% did not have this item, and no units had accessible grab bars, meaning that when present they were placed at inappropriate places and lost their functionality. Most toilets (72.0%) did not meet proper height, along with most paper towel disposal units (46.5%), and 25.5% did not even have any paper towels. Proper sanitary height requires less effort for transferring, as well as a flush control lower than a meter from the floor and working by light pressure; sanitary height was accessible in 47.1% of the units and 44.6% worked by light pressure flush.

Column sinks prevent wheelchair approximation, and also when height is over 80 cm above the floor they require additional effort for approaching and using the faucet; which should be of single lever type where a simple up and down lever movement with light pressure allows for proper hand hygiene/washing; the analysis showed that most sinks did not have columns, facilitating the approximation of wheelchair user to perform hand hygiene. However, most of these sinks (52.9%) had inadequate height, thereby hindering faucet reach by the user; faucets with rounded heads are difficult to use with wet hands, particularly for people with diminished strength. Faucets with movement sensors, which are hygienic because they do not require touch and are economical in rationing the use of water were not identified in any of the evaluated units.

These results corroborate another study [15] which revealed structural inadequacy of disability people toilets in health facilities, hampering access to these environments. This is partly due to a lack of knowledge of the legal system that protects disability people and partly because of the naturalization of actions of social actors; architectural and attitudinal barriers are imposed and represent symbolic violence against these people. It is unanimous that disability people face greater difficulties in access among users of the Unified Health System [17]. There are records showing that most health professionals do not receive specific training to attend to disability people during graduation, generating professionals who are unaware of the specific needs of this population segment [18].

Bathroom analysis revealed that the inaccessibility was predominant in the categories of door width and wheelchair maneuvering clearance area. Under these conditions, overweight or pregnant women also have compromised access and literally have to enter bathrooms backwards if they need to use the toilet. Tiny, low and uncomfortable toilets put at risk the safety of people with motor limitations and those who are overweight. Thus, the use of the sanitary bowl, flush control and paper towel disposals are impossible. Personal hygiene at the time of gynecological consultations is of utmost importance for enabling security and comfort to the patient.

To enable an overview of the accessibility assessment of gynecological nursing clinics' internal areas and their respective bathrooms, the area inside had four items evaluated in a sample composed of 157 clinics, so there should be 628 accessible items. As for bathrooms, 16 items of accessibility were evaluated totaling 1904 items that should be accessible, noting that 38 of the clinics did not have bathrooms. There were only two maximum accessible items of internal areas, with these being in only 21 of the analyzed clinics, and the most accessible item were the working stations (125). Doors were inaccessible in 137 clinics, so a wheelchair user could not go through the door, and at 125 units they could approach their wheelchair to the interview table, but in only one could they transfer to the examination table. A woman with a motor disability without a wheelchair does not even have a chair at her disposal in the clinic where she could sit comfortably and safely, considering they were only accessible in five BHUs.

So, a moment that is supposed to be enlightening and welcoming turns out to be an invasion of privacy and a major constraint which these users need to go through because of the inadequacy of physical infrastructure and lack of basic and necessary inputs to facilitate the service provided.

Low investment in professional training and health units being unable to absorb the demand and difficulties of municipal and state managers to define and establish flow in the various levels of care are aspects that can contribute to late diagnosis of CC and hinder its treatment [19]. A lack of available physical structure hinders and sometimes makes it impossible for users with physical disabilities to feel welcomed to participate in social life. They do not feel inclined to attend health services, since they are unable to offer minimum comfort and independence for moving around inside. Thus, a lack of adequate physical structure ends up excluding this population from gynecological nursing consultations.

Public policies and programs for women with disabilities exist, however their implementation is still inadequate and exclusionary. There is a considerable lack of knowledge on technical accessibility standards. The promotion of new ways of thinking, acting, building, communicating and using public resources is urgent in order to guarantee women with physical disabilities' their proper rights in health services. We express the need to disseminate such knowledge, essential for operationalizing health attention.

Society needs to be structured with inclusion and participation of all, by conducting quantitative research of this portion of the population to develop specific actions and professional training to attend them, considering that more than just technical standards is necessary; also awareness and sensitivity to the reality of this group in order to serve them in their basic and specific human needs.

5. Conclusions

The study results showed that BHUs had inaccessible physical structures, making the access of women with physical disabilities for gynecological consultations difficult and even impossible. Entrance doors, seats and stretchers in general were inaccessible in all clinics. Stretchers available to perform gynecological examinations were present in only one unit. In general, only working stations and counters were accessible.

With regard to the restrooms, we can mention the inadequate size, preventing freedom of movement and transferring to the sanitary bowl, so that users can get around with the aid of a wheelchair. Doors with tiny openings, and sanitary equipment such as a sanitary toilet and paper towel disposal units were mostly inaccessible; flushing and its operation by slight pressure were mostly accessible; grab bars were absent or often attached to inappropriate places, compromising their functionality; most of the sinks had no columns, facilitating approximation for their correct use, but most had inadequate height and the lack of single lever faucets was observed in most units. As a result, improperly distributed objects make it an uncomfortable and impossible environment to be used by a person in a wheelchair during preparation for gynecological consultations.

The exclusion of the female population with motor disabilities to such care exists because of prejudices linked to the myth that disabled people do not engage in sexual intercourse, and is exacerbated when the physical structure of gynecological clinics presents inaccessibility to women with physical disabilities.

It is urgent to clarify to administrators/managers and professionals who attend people with disabilities in health facilities about their proper care, thus guaranteeing them their right to access health care. This study can contribute to changes from its assessment of the reality and by arranging appropriate standards for structuring institutions. It also reinforces the need for deepening the theme because of the little amount of explored literature on the subject.

It is urgent to clarify managers and health professionals about the characteristics and needs of people with disabilities to access health facilities and their proper care, thus guaranteeing them their right to access health care. This study contributes to changes from assessing the reality and arrangement of appropriate standards for structuring institutions. It also reinforces the need for expanding the theme due to the low quantity of literature on the subject.

The study results will be presented and discussed with managers of health departments, health professionals and related fields that collaborate in the planning and implementation of the physical areas and equipment in health facilities. It is believed that this action will be a step to awaken an attentive eye to the physical accessibility issues of disabled people.

Among the limitations found in the study, we can mention the scarce amount of literature to discuss the data; the sample loss, although less than 10%, in this units was far from the municipal capital and restricted opening hours being incompatible with the data collection; and finally, professional resistance to allow the data collection.

Acknowledgements

To Fundação Cearense de Apoio ao Desenvolvimento Científico e Tecnológico and Conselho Nacional de Desenvolvimento Científico e Tecnológico, for the financial support and encouraging the development of this research.

References

[1] Secretaria de Direitos Humanos (2012) Convenção sobre os Direitos das Pessoas com Deficiência: Protocolo Facultativo à Convenção sobre os Direitos das Pessoas com Deficiência: Decreto Legislativo n° 186, de 09 de julho de 2008: Decreto n° 6.949, de 25 de agosto de 2009. Secretaria de Direitos, Brasília. http://www.pessoacomdeficiencia.gov.br/app/sites/default/files/publicacoes/convencaopessoascomdeficiencia.pdf

[2] Instituto Brasileiro de Geografia e Estatística (2010) Censo demográfico: Pessoas com Deficiência. Instituto Brasileiro de Geografia e Estatística, Rio de Janeiro. http://www.ibge.gov.br/home/estatistica/populacao/censo2010/caracteristicas_religiao_deficiencia/caracteristicas_religiao_deficiencia_tab_pdf.shtm

[3] Baptista, R.S., Pagliuca, L.M.F., Sampaio, A.F.A. and França, I.S.X. (2014) Sexuality: Experience of Women with Physical Disabilities. *Open Journal of Nursing*, **4**, 920-927. http://file.scirp.org/Html/3-1440383_52125.htm http://dx.doi.org/10.4236/ojn.2014.413098

[4] Brasil. Ministério da Saúde (2012) Política Nacional de Atenção Básica. Brasília: Ministério da Saúde. http://189.28.128.100/dab/docs/publicacoes/geral/pnab.pdf

[5] Melo, M.C.S.C., Vilela, F., Salimena, A.M.O. and Souza, I.E.O. (2012) O Enfermeiro na Prevenção do Câncer do Colo do Útero: O Cotidiano da Atenção Primária. *Revista Brasileira de Cancerologia*, **58**, 389-398. http://www1.inca.gov.br/rbc/n_58/v03/pdf/08_artigo_enfermeiro_prevencao_cancer_colo_utero_cotidiano_atencao_primaria.pdf

[6] Brasil. Secretaria de Atenção à Saúde. Departamento de Atenção Básica (2013) Controle dos cânceres do colo do útero e da mama. Ministério da Saúde, Brasília. http://bvsms.saude.gov.br/bvs/publicacoes/controle_canceres_colo_utero_2013.pdf

[7] Silva, M.G.O., Lopes, M.I. and Costa, P.V.L. (2014) Fatores que interferem na realização do exame papanicolau em mulheres cadeirantes. *Revista Interdisciplinar*, **7**, 99-105. http://revistainterdisciplinar.uninovafapi.edu.br/index.php/revinter/article/view/436/pdf_163

[8] Nicolau, S.M., Schraiber, L.B. and Ayres, J.R.C.M. (2013) Mulheres com deficiência e sua dupla vulnerabilidade: Contribuições para a construção da integralidade em saúde. *Ciência & Saúde Coletiva*, **18**, 863-872. http://www.scielo.br/scielo.php?script=sci_arttext&pid=S1413-81232013000300032 http://dx.doi.org/10.1590/s1413-81232013000300032

[9] Carvalho, C.F.S., Brito, R.S. and Medeiros, S.M. (2014) Contextual Analysis of Gynaecological Care Provided to Women with Physical Disability. *Revista Gaúcha Enfermagem*, **35**, 114-117. http://www.scielo.br/scielo.php?pid=S1983-14472014000400114&script=sci_arttext http://dx.doi.org/10.1590/1983-1447.2014.04.45335

[10] Polit, D.F., Beck, C.T. and Hungler, B.P. (2011) Fundamentos de pesquisa em enfermagem. 6th Edition, Artmed, Porto Alegre.

[11] Coordenadoria Regional de Saúde (2010) 3ª e 4° CRES compõe a Macrorregião de Fortaleza. http://www.saude.ce.gov.br/index.php/regionalizacao

[12] Associação Brasileira de Normas Técnicas (2004) NBR 9050: Acessibilidade a edificações, mobiliário, espaços e equipamentos urbanos. Associação Brasileira de Normas Técnicas, Rio de Janeiro.

[13] Conselho Nacional dos Direitos da Pessoa com Deficiência (2012) Cartilha Orientadora para Criação e Funcionamento dos Conselhos de Direito da Pessoa com Deficiência. Conselho Nacional dos Direitos da Pessoa com Deficiência.

Secretaria dos Direitos Humanos, Brasília; CONADE, Brasília.
http://www.pessoacomdeficiencia.gov.br/app/sites/default/files/arquivos/%5Bfield_generico_imagens-filefield-description%5D_145.pdf

[14] Eide, A.H., Mannan, H., Khogali, M., Van Rooy, G., Swartz, L., Munthali, A., Hem, K., MacLachlan, M. and Dyrstad, K. (2015) Perceived Barriers for Accessing Health Services among Individuals with Disability in Four African Countries. *PLoS ONE*, **10**. http://journals.plos.org/plosone/article?id=10.1371/journal.pone.0125915
http://dx.doi.org/10.1371/journal.pone.0125915

[15] Castro, S.S., Lefèvre, F., Lefèvre, A.M.C. and Cesar, C.L.G. (2011) Accessibility to Health Services by Persons with Disabilities. *Revista de Saúde Pública*, **45**, 99-105.
http://www.scielosp.org/scielo.php?script=sci_arttext&pid=S0034-89102011000100011&lng=en&nrm=iso
http://dx.doi.org/10.1590/S0034-89102010005000048

[16] Mendonça, F.A.C., Sampaio, L.R.L., Linard A.G., Silva R.M. and Sampaio L.L. (2011) Acolhimento e vínculo na consulta ginecológica: Concepção de enfermeiras. *Revista Rene*, **12**, 57-64.
http://www.revistarene.ufc.br/revista/index.php/revista/article/view/109

[17] França, I.S.X., Pagliuca, L.M.F., Baptista, R.S., França, E.G.F., Coura, A.S. and Souza, J.A. (2010) Violência simbólica no acesso das pessoas com deficiência às unidades básicas de saúde. *Revista Brasileira de Enfermagem*, **63**, 964-970.
http://www.scielo.br/scielo.php?pid=S0034-71672010000600015&script=sci_arttext
http://dx.doi.org/10.1590/S0034-71672010000600015

[18] Rebouças, C.B.A., Cezario, K.G., Oliveira, P.M.O. and Pagliuca, L.M.F. (2011) People with Physical and Sensory Deficits: Perceptions of Undergraduate Nursing Students. *Acta Paulista de Enfermagem*, **24**, 80-86.
http://www.scielo.br/pdf/ape/v24n1/en_v24n1a12.pdf
http://dx.doi.org/10.1590/S0103-21002011000100012

[19] Brito-Silva, K., bezerra, A.F.B., Chaves, L.D.P. and Tanaka, O.Y. (2014) Integrality in Cervical Cancer Care: Evaluation of Access. *Revista de Saúde Pública*, **48**, 240-248.
http://www.scielosp.org/pdf/rsp/v48n2/en_0034-8910-rsp-48-2-0240.pdf
http://dx.doi.org/10.1590/S0034-8910.2014048004852

24

Use of Religion: An Effective Method of Coping among Chinese Patients with Cancer

Huaxia Liu[1*], Hongwei Shi[1], Qianqian Yang[1], Aletha Rowlands[2], Minghua Han[3]

[1]School of Nursing, Taishan Medical University, Taian, China
[2]School of Nursing, West Virginia University, Morgantown, USA
[3]Taishan Vocational College of Nursing, Taian, China
Email: [*]huaxia66@163.com

Abstract

Religion and/or spirituality (R/S) plays a variety of important and inter-related roles for most advanced cancer patients. It has confirmed that religious involvement helps the patients to ease stress and provides individuals with positive coping strategies. However, much less attention has been given to how religion has been used to cope with cancer in China. The aim of this study was to explore the self-adjustment and experiences of religious coping among Chinese patients with cancer. A qualitative descriptive approach was chosen for this investigation. 16 Chinese patients with cancer were recruited from 4 hospitals in Tai'an, Shandong, China from April 2013 to October 2013 and completed 0.5 - 1 hour of in-depth interviews. Data were analyzed by modification of Colaizzi's phenomenological method. Three themes were derived from the experiences of the participants: 1) self-adjustment including cognitive adjustment, faith adjustment and behavior adjustment; 2) the experience of religion coping with the cancer patients including emotional, physical and social aspect; 3) hope and power including the hope to heal, to survive from cancer, and to live longer, the cure, the spiritual supporter and the helper. The use of religion is an effective method for patients coping with cancer. Cancer patients use religion to obtain physiological, psychological, and spiritual comfort. Such knowledge is imperative for evidence-based nursing practice. As point of care providers, staff nurses are well poised to design systems and processes to accomplish the goals of providing excellent nursing care, which is reflective of a holistic and multicultural environment.

Keywords

Cancer, Religious Belief, Coping, Qualitative Analysis, Phenomenological Method

[*]Corresponding author.

1. Introduction

Cancer has become a serious threat to public health. In China, cancer has become the leading cause of death in urban areas and the second most common form of death in rural areas [1]. Nearly all medical treatments for cancer such as chemotherapy and radiation have negative side effects that may threaten the lives of cancer patients [2]. In addition to the physical burden of cancer, psychological distress, including increased anxiety and depression and poor quality of life, seems to be greater in cancer patients than in the general population, particularly among patients with later stage cancers [3]-[5]. Religious coping refers to the use of religious beliefs or practices to cope with stressful life circumstance [6] [7]. Religion and/or spirituality(R/S) plays a variety of important and inter-related roles for most advanced cancer patients [8]-[10]. It has confirmed that religious involvement helps the patients to ease stress and provides individuals with positive coping strategies [11]. The study on the relationship between religion and cancer began in the 1990s which had gradually become a key topic in nursing, especially in the field of hospice care and palliative care [12]. Nowadays approximately 50% - 95% of cancer patients use religion to cope with disease, particularly among ethnic minorities, women, and older adults [13]. Although research has indicated that religious coping has a significant impact on patients' response to cancer, nothing is known about how Chinese cancer patients cope with cancer. This study employed a qualitative descriptive approach to examine how the patients used religion to cope with cancer, the function of religious coping, the factors influencing how cancer patients coped with religion and the experiences of individuals diagnosed with cancer in order to gain a more in-depth understanding of the religious coping in the context of Chinese culture. This study was based on two theoretical models within the spirituality literately: the general-attribution theory, behavioral-cognitive mechanisms and a meditational model [14] [15]. Results from this study may help health-care providers to facilitate their patients' spiritual journeys in dealing with their diagnoses and treatments.

2. Methods

A qualitative phenomenological approach was chosen to examine experiences of religious coping in patients with cancer. The purpose of phenomenological method is to uncover the genuine experience of the phenomenon under investigation [16] [17]. Modification of Colaizzi's phenomenological method was used to analyze data.

2.1. Sample

About 200 patients with cancer were approached from Taishan Medical University Affiliated Hospital, Tai'an Central Hospital, Tai'an Tumor Hospital and PLA 88th Hospital all in Tai'an, Shandong, China. But there were only 20 patients were eligible to the study (4 of them refused to attend the study). At last 16 participants were conducted by depth-interview from April 2013 to October 2013. Demographic data were collected from patients' charts to provide a context for understanding the experience of religious coping of cancer patients. The including criteria of participants were: 1) 18 years or older; 2) diagnosed cancer confirmed by a pathological exam; 3) conscious and able to express their own opinions; 4) believing in a religion. The criteria of exclusion for participants were: 1) having not any religion; 2) refusing to attend the study; 3) at termly-ill stage and unable to finish the interview. An oral informed consent was obtained from each participant.

2.2. Data Collection

Before each interview, the participant was informed of the purpose and the process of the study, the rights of the participants and the principle of confidentiality. The participant was assured that he/she could leave the research at any time without any obligation or penalty. Before the interview, the primary researcher entered the research environment as a trainee nurse in order to build a trust relationship with patients and created a harmonious, relaxed interview atmosphere. The first set of interviews was based on the following general questions: How are you feeling today? Did you attend church? The Interview Guideline begin with: "Do you have any religion?" If "yes", then to next: 1) What religion do you believe in? 2) How long have you believed in this religion? Did you start believing in this religion before or after getting cancer? 3) Why did you believe in religion? 4) What religious activities do you attend? 5) What changes have you had since you believed in religion? How do you think about diseases, health, death and meaning of life? 6) What influence does religion have on the treatment and rehabilitation of your disease? 7) What do you think about believing in religion generally? Each interview was conducted in patient's ward where no other individuals were present which lasted 30 to 60 minutes and was recorded using a digital recorder. At the end of each interview, the participant completed a "general situation questionnaire" and left his/her contact information in case the researchers needed clarification. Immediately after each interview, the researcher recorded the non-verbal behaviors of each participant. Each recorded interview was transcribed in a timely manner.

2.3. Data Analysis

Modification of Colaizzi's phenomenological method was used to analyze the transcripts of their interviews. The six steps are as follows:

1) All the descriptions are read in order to to acquire a sense of the whole.
2) From each transcript the significant statements and phrases were extracted.
3) Meanings were formulated from those significant statements and phrases.
4) Formulated meanings were organized into cluster themes.
5) Themes are integrated into an exhaustive description.
6) The validation of exhaustive description is sought by participants.

At Last, three themes and their sub-themes were discussed several times before the final decisions made among four researchers.

2.4. Ethical Considerations

The research was approved on May 16, 2012 by the ethics committee in the medical university where the researchers worked. After examining the clinical environment using a questionnaire, researchers requested nursing and medical staff to assist with participant recruitment. Through the word of mouth among the participants who were recruited early, additional patients who met the inclusion criteria were recruited. Verbal consent was obtained from all participants.

3. Results

3.1. Sample Description

The sample consisted of 10 females and 6 males with a mean age of 50.44 years (ranged between 26 and 63 years). Seven of them were diagnosed with lung cancer (n = 7, 43.75%), three were diagnosed with breast cancer (n = 3, 18.75%), two with gastrointestinal cancer, liver cancer, and ovarian cancer (n = 2, 12.5%, respectively). Six patients received primary school education, nine patients received secondary level education, and one patient received university education. More details are shown in **Table 1**.

3.2. Findings

Three themes about religious coping derived from the experiences of the participants include self-adjustment, dependence and support, and hope and power.

3.2.1. Theme I: Self-Adjustment

1) Cognitive Adjustment

Cognitive adjustment was the first step of self-adjustment among cancer patients. The participants expressed different perspectives of life, disease, and death, which helped them face the disease directly.

Some of the patients reconsidered the meaning of life. Different religions showed different explanations on the meaning of life. The meaning of life in Christianity is the glory of God and His forgiveness. On the other hand, the meaning of life in Buddhism is unremitting self-improvement.

For example, participant 7 stated: "I exhausted myself to make more money, which eventually dragged me down. Now I realized that the priority is to be healthy and have a happy family instead of money". Participant 13 said: "Instructed by God, I do my best to do everything well in life".

Some patients changed their perspective of sickness and death. Christian claims that anything in the universe was controlled by God. Disease is a test from God who offers patients hope and confidence to conquer the disease. For example, participant 12 noted: "Death is to go to the eternal life in heaven".

Participant 1 stated: "People believing in Buddhism will go to paradise after they die and death is the start of a new life".

Table 1. Characteristic of 16 participants.

No.	Gender	Age	Marital Status	Monthly Income (CHY)	Medical Diagnosis	Disease Duration (Months)	Religious Belief	Belief Duration (Months)
1	female	53	married	>2000	right lung cancer with thorax metastasis	16	Buddhism	16
2	female	49	divorced	>2000*	ovarian cancer	20	Buddhism	130
3	female	26	single	1000 - 2000	ovarian cancer	8	Buddhism	6
4	female	52	married	>2000	lung cancer with brain metastasis	16	Christianity	3
5	male	59	married	1000 - 2000	right lung cancer with thorax metastasis	20	Christianity	120
6	male	50	married	1000 - 2000	gastrointestinal cancer	15	Christianity	6
7	female	41	married	<1000	right breast cancer with post-operative metastasis	48	Christianity	160
8	male	53	married	>2000	liver cancer: terminal stage	60	Christianity	120
9	male	46	married	<1000	lung cancer with thorax metastasis	36	Christianity	24
10	female	38	married	1000 - 2000	right breast cancer: postoperative	10	Christianity	4
11	female	58	married	1000 - 2000	lung cancer	15	Christianity	10
12	female	59	married	>2000	Liver cancer: terminal stage	60	Christianity	56
13	male	50	married	<1000	lung cancer with general metastasis	18	Christianity	18
14	male	51	married	1000 - 2000	esophageal cancer	13	Christianity	13
15	female	63	married	<1000	lung cancer	20	Christianity	36
16	male	59	married	>2000	rectal cancer	24	Christianity	20

2) Faith Adjustment

Religion was found to have stimulated cancer patients' desire to live and their ability to accept being sick and to cope with their sickness optimistically. Participant 5 affirmed: "God cured my disease through the hands of doctors. The only thing I should do is to follow the will of God." Participant 4 stated: "I have to adjust myself to fight against disease. Whether it is good or bad, time goes away. Why don't I live happily?"

3) Behavior Adjustment

This study found that religion can enhance self-control, which enabled some participants to life a normal life. Participant 7 said: "Now I don't take myself as a patient. I do everything I can and never count on others. I try to keep a peaceful mind." "Now I will try to control my temper and put myself in other's position".

Most of the participants transferred their pressures from self to religion. Participant 16: "I have given myself to the hospital and God. Let them help me solve these problems".

3.2.2. Theme II: Experience of Religion Coping

The experience of religion coping can be summarized in three aspects: the emotional aspect, the physical aspect, and the social aspect.

1) The Emotional Aspect

The participants described that belief is the subject of their spirit. They believed that belief had the infinite power from God, could reduce the psychological distress. When they felt hopeless, God offered comfort and dependence, which encouraged them to live. For example, participant 4 noted: "In this group, people would offer help to me no matter what difficulties I have. This makes me feel loved beyond my family. Patients have a desire to receive more encouragement and support".

During the interview, some patients even had a positive change in personality. For example, participant 6 stated: "After I believed in religion, my personality has changed a lot. I was very bad-tempered, but now I am as mild as sheep". Participant 9 noted: "I go to religious activities every Thursday. I like these activities very much. People communicate with each other and I feel relaxed physically and mentally … throw away all the worries and stress".

Some reported an increased happiness while others demonstrated happiness. For example, participant 2 stated: "I am joyful and relaxed now". Participant 8 claimed: "I feel comfortable and happy everyday".

2) The Physical Aspect

Religion was found to have played an important role in health restoration and as a healer. Participants responded that religion could not only ease the emotional and psychological discomfort, but also improve the symptom management. Religious activities could reduce the side effects of chemotherapy. For instance, participant 1 believed: "Buddhism can cure cancer and free me from pains".

3) The Social Aspect

Participants responded that religion could promote interpersonal relationships and promote family harmony. Participant 7 explained: "After I believed in religion, I was much more open-minded, didn't care about what other people talk about me, and felt less anxious when communicating with others". Participant 12 said: "I have been a Christian for more than 10 years". "I have a harmonious family. Others might wonder how my family could be happy every day when it had a cancer patient at home". Participant 5 explained: "Since I believe in Christen, I reflect my fault first. I then talk about my husband's. We both changed and stopped gambling. Now we are getting along very well".

3.2.3. Theme III: Hope and Power

Based on their own experiences, participants claimed that religion had provided them with hope to heal, to survive from cancer, and live longer. They also believed that religion had provided a source of internal power to fight cancer. Words, such as "hope", "super power", "peaceful", "relax", "helpful", "comfortable", "stable and pure", "confident" and "no fear of death or cancer" were mentioned frequently by participants.

4. Discussion

The present study described self-adjustments and experiences of religion coping among Chinese patients with cancer. We found that religious coping is an effective way to cope with difficult situations. It has the effects of psychological treatment and affects patient's psychological, mental and physical health. It is estimated that over 100 million people in China believe in religion, and a majority of them suffer from major illnesses. It is of great significance to examine the relationship between the religious belief and health and disease. This study used qualitative methods to describe the cancer patients' experiences of using religion to cope with cancer religious. This study revealed that religion coping is an important coping mechanism used by patients with cancer.

4.1. General Condition of the Participants

We faced some difficulties to recruit the eligible participants because most of patients said that they had no religion. Another point as seen in **Table 1**, a majority of the participants are female farmers with low level of education and lower income. The result supported Pargament and Smith' study [14]. They found in their study that women, the elderly, and the poor are more likely to choose religion to cope with life events due to their lack of alternative means to solve problems. Religious coping refers to the use of religious beliefs or practices to cope with stressful life circumstance [6] [7]. It goes through a series of changes ranging from knowledge acquisition to behavior modification. In this process, many factors can affect the transformation including patients' cognitive level, cultural background, social view of religion, and others. Any of those factors may influence the effect of religious coping.

4.2. Self-Regulation

This study found that religious belief had led patients with cancer to have a new understanding of the meaning of life, disease, and death. For example, they believed "disease is a kind of test; death is not the end of the individual existence." Such finding is consistent with what Frankl reported. In 1958, Frankl established the link between spirituality and finding meaning. Frank felt that people who believed in God had an even stronger sense of meaning in life, even in the face of adversity and death. Spiritual people who believe in God have a constant "invisible witness present" who expects something of them in any given circumstance [18]-[20]. This view provides a good explanation of "Why me" for patients, which can quickly reduce the fear of cancer and death so that they can face the cancer and actively participate in cancer treatment.

Many factors affected the cancer patients' emotional adjustment such as spiritual support and the social support from religious groups. Such supports help patients with cancer to face the disease directly, adjust their attitude, and face life with an optimistic and positive attitude [17].

In the process of behavior modification, the participants mainly use some religious activities to relieve the pain of body and mind. For example, prayer has been used to enhance the confidence of patients and transfer the attention of somatic symptoms. Repentance has been used to reduce their mental stress which is conducive to treating the body and mind of patients. Twisting beads is used to adjust the state of mind so that the state of mind is peaceful.

4.3. Self Experience

During the Interview, almost all of the participants described that belief was their spiritual sustenance and reliance. Belief was one of the biggest psychological comfort factors for them, especially when they were in great distress. Faith had become the biggest spiritual pillar in their life. For example, some patients said "I feel there is a powerful force that supports me", and "I feel God always encourage me at any time". Regarding God as their listener, participants expressed their inner feelings through prayers to reduce psychological distress. Some studies have shown that cry and talk can release chemicals caused by fear, grievances, anger and other negative emotions, which is conducive to patient's physical and mental health [21]. Religion can help patients to eliminate pain and improve their immune function. It is reported that some patients refuse conventional medical treatment. Instead, they use religion to relieve symptoms and cure the disease [22]. Although the exact mechanism of how religion can produce such effects is unknown, the cognition of religious follower may play a key role. The present study confirmed that the use of religion is an effective method for patients to cope with cancer. Nurses could guide the patients to use religion to cope, enhance cognition. The study also has some limitations: such as a small sample since less people having a religion in China. And the study belongs to the qualitative research lacking of long-term follow-up across groups.

5. Conclusions

The study explained the phenomenon of religious coping among Chinese patients with cancer. In this study, we found that the use of religion was an effective method for patients to cope with cancer. Patients with cancer can obtain physiological, psychological, and spiritual comfort by use of religion. Current mental care for cancer patients is inadequate. Cancer patients have more psychological needs than physical needs. They need much more comfort and support from family, medical staff and community. The results of the study may improve health-care provider's understanding and recognition to the importance of religious coping among patients with cancer. And it may help health-care providers to facilitate their patients' spiritual journeys in dealing with cancer diagnoses and treatments. As point-of-care providers, staff nurses are well poised to design systems and processes to accomplish the goals of providing excellent nursing care in a holistic and multicultural environment.

The authors have no funding or conflicts of interest to disclose.

References

[1] Liu, J., Yang, X.L., Li, A., Chen, W.Q., Ji, L., Zhao, J., Yan, W., Chen, Y.Y. and Zhu, L.P. (2014) Epidemiological Patterns of Cancer Incidence in Southern China: Based on 6 Population-based Cancer Registries. *Asian Pacific Journal of Cancer*, **15**, 1471-1475. http://dx.doi.org/10.7314/APJCP.2014.15.3.1471

[2] Massie, M.J. and Holland, J.C. (1987) Consultation and Liaison Issues in Cancer Care. *Psychiatric Medicine*, **5**, 343-359.

[3] Derogatis, L.R. and Melisaratos, N. (1983) The Brief Symptom Inventory: An Introductory Report. *Psychological Medicine*, **13**, 596-605. http://dx.doi.org/10.1017/s0033291700048017

[4] Derogatis, L.R., Morrow, G.R., Fetting, J., Penman, D., Piasetsky, S., Schmale, A.M., Henrichs, M. and Carnicke, C.L. (1983) The Prevalence of Psychiatric Disorders among Cancer Patients. *Journal of the American Medical Association*, **249**, 751-757. http://dx.doi.org/10.1001/jama.1983.03330300035030

[5] Kimberly, K.L., Sandra, G.Z. and John, P.B. (2004) The Role of Spirituality in the Psychological Adjustment to Cancer: A Test of the Transactional Model of Stress and Coping. *International Journal of Behavioral Medicine*, **11**, 48-55. http://dx.doi.org/10.1207/s15327558ijbm1101_6

[6] Koening, H.G., Cohen, H.J., Blazer, D.G., Pieper, C., Meador, K.G., Shelp, F., Goli, V. and DiPasquale, B. (1992) Religious Coping and Depression among Elderly, Hospitalized Medically Ill Men. *Annals of General Psychiatry*, **149**, 1639-1770.

[7] Koenig, H.G., George, L.K. and Siegler, I.C. (1988) The Use of Religion and Other Emotion-Regulating Coping Strategies among Older Adults. *Gerontologist*, **28**, 303-310. http://dx.doi.org/10.1093/geront/28.3.303

[8] Sara, R., Michael, J., Holly, G., Amy, R., Andrea, C., Alexi, A., Susan, D., John, R., Lisa, A. and Tracy, A. (2010) "If God Wanted Me Yesterday, I Wouldn't Be Here Today": Religious and Spiritual Themes in Patients' Experience of Advanced Cancer. *Journal of Palliative Medicine*, **13**, 581-588. http://dx.doi.org/10.1089/jpm.2009.0343

[9] Astrow, A.B., Wexler, A., Texeira, K., He, M.K. and Sulmasy, D.P. (2007) Is Failure to Meet Spiritual Needs Associated with Cancer Patients' Perceptions of Quality of Care and Their Satisfaction with Care? *Journal of Clinical Oncology*, **25**, 5753-5757. http://dx.doi.org/10.1200/JCO.2007.12.4362

[10] Moadel, A., Morgan, C., Fatone, A., Grennan, J., Carter, J., Laruffa, G., Skummy, A. and Dutcher, J. (1998) Seeking Meaning and Hope: Self-Reported Spiritual and Existential Needs among an Ethnically-Diverse Cancer Patient Population. *Psychooncology*, **8**, 378-385. http://dx.doi.org/10.1002/(SICI)1099-1611(199909/10)8:5<378::AID-PON406>3.0.CO;2-A

[11] Holt, C.L., Qi, M. and Wang, L.C. (2011) Role of Religious Involvement and Spirituality in Functioning among African Americans with Cancer: Testing a Meditational Model. *Journal of Behavioral Medicine*, **34**, 437-448. http://dx.doi.org/10.1007/s10865-010-9310-8

[12] Kune, G.A., Kune, S. and Watson, L.F. (1992) The Effect of Family History of Cancer, Religion, Parity and Migrant Status on Survival in Colorectal Cancer: The Melbourne Colorectal Cancer Study. *European Journal of Cancer*, **28**, 1484-1487. http://dx.doi.org/10.1016/0959-8049(92)90549-H

[13] Abernethy, A.D., Chang, H.T., Seidlitz, L., Evinger, J.S. and Duberstein, P.R. (2002) Religious Coping and Depression among Spouses of People with Lung Cancer. *Psychosomatics*, **43**, 456-463. http://dx.doi.org/10.1176/appi.psy.43.6.456

[14] Pargament, K.I. and Smith, B.W. (1998) Patterns of Positive and Negative Religious Coping with Major Life Stressors. *Journal for the Scientific Study of Religion*, **37**, 710-724. http://dx.doi.org/10.2307/1388152

[15] Balboni, T.A., Vanderwerker, L.C. and Block, S.D. (2007) Religiousness and Spiritual Support among Advanced Cancer Patients and Associations with End of Life Treatment Preferences and Quality of Life. *Journal of Clinical Oncology*, **25**, 555-560. http://dx.doi.org/10.1200/JCO.2006.07.9046

[16] Turunen, H., Perälä, M.L. and Meriläinen, P. (1994) Modification of Colaizzi's Phenomenological Method: A Study Concerning Quality Care. *Hoitotiede*, **6**, 8-15.

[17] Moustakas, C. (1994) Phenomenological Research Method. Sage, London.

[18] Frankl, V.E. (1958) The Will to Meaning. *Journal of Pastoral Care*, **12**, 82-88.

[19] Frankl, V.E. (1966) What Is Meant by Meaning? *Journal of Existentialism*, **6**, 21-28.

[20] Albaugh, J.A. (2003) Spiritual and Life-Threatening Illness: A Phenomenologic Study. *Oncology Nursing Forum*, **30**, 593-598. http://dx.doi.org/10.1188/03.ONF.593-598

[21] Lin, B. (2002) On the Psychological Function of Religious Belief. *Journal of Fujian Teachers University*, **2**, 125-129. (In Chinese)

[22] Trevino, K.M., Balboni, M., Zollfrank, A., Balboni, T. and Prigerson, H.G. (2014) Negative Religious Coping as a Correlate of Suicidal Ideation in Patients with Advanced Cancer. *Psychooncology*, **23**, 936-945.

25

Correlation of Ceruloplasmin with Biomarkers of Cardiac Remodelling and Myofibrosis in Patients with Acute Decompensated Heart Failure Referred to a Tertiary Nurse Lead Heart Failure Clinic

Filip Málek[1,2*], Dagmar Vondráková[1,2], Oxana Komendová[1], Dana Říhová[1], Jana Vránová[2], Lenka Sedláčková[3], Táňa Andreasová[1], Petr Neužil[1]

[1]Department of Cardiology, Na Homolce Hospital, Prague, Czech Republic
[2]Third School of Medicine, Charles University, Prague, Czech Republic
[3]Department of Clinical Biochemistry, Haematology and Immunology, Na Homolce Hospital, Prague, Czech Republic
Email: *filip.malek@centrum.cz

Abstract

Background: Ceruloplasmin is an acute phase protein with plasma copper binding properties, and is a potent extracellular antioxidative enzyme. Inflammation and oxidative stress might explain the role of ceruloplasmin in the pathophysiology of heart failure. Study objective: The objective is to assess the correlation of ceruloplasmin levels with biomarkers of cardiac remodelling and myofibrosis in patients with acute decompensated heart failure. Patients and methods: Blood samples were taken and serum levels of soluble ST2, galectin-3, NT-proBNP and ceruloplasmin were analysed in 31 consecutive patients with systolic HF referred to tertiary care nurse lead heart failure clinic with acute decompensated CHF requiring i.v. diuretics. The mean patients' age was 68 years, mean left ventricular ejection fraction (LV EF) was 29%, 66% patients had ischemic aetilogy of CHF and 33% had atrial fibrillation. Results: The mean ceruloplasmin level was 0.243 g/l, mean galectin-3 level was 1.26 ng/ml, mean sST2 level was 38.15 ng/ml, and mean NT-proBNP was 1927 pg/ml. The ceruloplasmin level correlated with NT-proBNP ($r = 0.58$, $p < 0.05$) and with sST2 ($r = 0.77$, $p < 0.001$), sST2 levels correlated significantly with NT-proBNP ($r = 0.66$, $p < 0.01$). The ceruloplasmin level did not correlate with galectin-3 concentration. Conclusion: The ceruloplasmin level correlates with the biomarkers of cardiac remodelling (NT-proBNP, sST2), but not with the biomarker of myofibrosis (galectin-3). This finding supports the hypothesis of inflammatory re-

*Corresponding author.

sponse in acute decompensated heart failure.

Keywords

Acute Decompensated Heart Failure, Ceruloplasmin, NT-proBNP, sST2, Galectin-3

1. Introduction

Ceruloplasmin is an acute phase protein with plasma copper binding properties, and is considered to be one of the most potent extracellular antioxidative enzymes. Inflammation and oxidative stress might explain the role of ceruloplasmin in the pathophysiology of heart failure [1]. Historically, several epidemiologic studies showed the association of elevated ceruloplasmin levels with the risk of atherosclerosis, coronary heart disease, myocardial infarction and ischemic heart failure [2]-[5]. The Atherosclerosis Risk in Communities (ARIC) Study reveals the association of elevated ceruloplasmin levels with the risk of incident heart failure (HF), HF mortality and risk of cardiovascular disease (CVD) in healthy individuals [6]. In the patients with established chronic heart failure, ceruloplasmin levels correlated with the severity of heart and weakly with B-natriuretic peptide levels, but predicted all-cause mortality [7].

ST2 is a member of the interleukin-1 (IL-1) receptor family and consists of a trans-membrane ligand (STL2) and a soluble form (sST2). ST2 is released from cardiomyocytes and fibroblasts after mechanical strain. Soluble ST2 has been identified as a novel biomarker of cardiac stress and remodelling. In patients with acutely decompensated heart failure, the elevated sST2 concentrations predicted the risk of hospitalization and mortality, and this association was independent on natriuretic peptides levels and on other clinical variables [8] [9].

Galectin-3 is a protein secreted by activated macrophages and has a role in the development of fibrosis in injured tissues. Experimental studies showed increased galectin-3 secretion in the context of cardiac hypertrophy and heart failure models. Clinical studies identified galectin-3 to have additional prognostic information together with NT-proBNP in acute heart failure [10].

Relation of ceruloplasmin levels with the novel biomarkers of cardiac remodelling (sST2) and myofibrosis (galectin-3) has not been yet evaluated.

2. Study Objective

The aim of our study was to assess correlation of ceruloplasmin levels with biomarkers of cardiac remodelling (NT-proBNP, sST2) and biomarker of myofibrosis (Galectin-3) in patients with acute decompensated heart failure.

3. Patients Population and Methods

Blood samples were taken and serum levels of soluble ST2, galectin-3, NT-proBNP and ceruloplasmin were analysed in 31 consecutive patients, 22 men and eight women, with chronic systolic HF and left ventricular ejection fraction ≤35%, referred to tertiary care nurse lead heart failure clinic with acute decompensated CHF requiring diuretic dose adjustment between 1st January and 30th June 2015. Mean patients' age was 68 years (range 43 - 84 years), mean left ventricular ejection fraction (LV EF) was 29%, ischemic aetilogy of CHF had 20 (66%) patients and 10 (33%) had chronic atrial fibrillation. Patients were treated according to Guidelines for the diagnosis and treatment of chronic heart failure. Diagnosis of CHF decompensation was based of physical examination showing signs of fluid overload and/or worsening dyspnea. Patients with acute coronary syndrome, pulmonary emboly, acute infection, know malignancy and chronic inflammatory or autoimmune disease were not included in the study.

Blood samples were taken on the day of clinic visit.

Ceruloplasmin determination was performed with the use of immunoturbidimetric assay.

Normal value range is 0.220 - 0.440 g/l in healthy individuals.

The NT-proBNP analysis was performed with a commercially available chemiluminescence immunoassay for the determination of Human NT-proBNP: CLIA kit using Sandwich-CLIA as the method. The sST2 and galectin-3 was analyzed using a commercially available enzyme-linked immunosorbent assay kit. All biochemical analyses were realized on the analyser UnicelDxC 800 (Beckman Coulter Company, Germany) according to established methods.

An echocardiographic examination of the each patient was performed using a broadband transducer with a transmitting frequency from 1.7 to 4.0 MHz on commercially available equipment (Vivid 7, GE, USA). Left ventricular ejection fraction was calculated by Simpson's method.

All patients' data were collected and transcribed to statistical testing. Spearman's correlation coefficient *r* was used for statistical analysis. A *r* value > 0.6 and p value < 0.05 was considered significant.

The study was approved by Local Board Ethics Committee and conducted in accordance with the Declaration of Helsinki. All patients provided informed consent orally and in writing prior to enrollment.

4. Results

Results are shown in the table (**Table 1**). Mean ceruloplasmin level was 0.243 g/l, mean galectin-3 level was 1.26 ng/ml, mean sST2 level was 38.15 ng/ml, and mean NT-proBNP was 1927 pg/ml. As shown in the table, mean ceruloplasmin value in our study was 0.243 g/l and median 0.250 g/l was in range of normal healthy subjects (0.220 - 0.440 g/l).

Mean NT-proBNP level was 1927 pg/ml, and median value was 1103 pg/ml (range 465 - 7856 pg/ml), the values (mean and median) are above upper normal limit for acute heart failure (300 pg/ml).

Correlation of ceruloplasmin with biomarkers of cardiac remodelling and myofibrosis is shown in the table (**Table 2**). Ceruloplasmin level correlated with NT-proBNP ($p < 0.05$) and with sST2 ($p < 0.001$), sST2 levels corrrelated significantly with NT-proBNP ($p < 0.01$). Ceruloplasmin level did not correlate with galectin-3 concentration.

5. Discussion

Ceruloplasmin is a glycoprotein synthetized in the liver and transports copper. Ceruloplasmin decreases nitric oxide (NO) bioavailibility through NO oxidase activity. Ceruloplasmin also enhances low-density lipoprotein (LDL) oxidation. Oxidized LDL has proatherogenic role and decreased NO availability contributes to endothelial dysfunction [11] [12]. Based on this information, several studies suggested association of elevated ceuroplasmin levels with CVD and HF [13] [14]. Ceruloplasmin is an acute phase protein too and its levels correlate with

Table 1. Results—echocardiography and laboratory parameters.

Parameter	Mean	Median	Minimum	Maximum
LV EF %	28.89	30	16	35
EDD LV mm	63.39	62.50	53	80
LA mm	50.56	51	36	64
BMI kg/m^2	29.62	29.20	21.10	45.70
Potassium mmol/l	4.27	4.20	3.60	5.10
Sodium mmol/l	137.28	137.0	131.0	143.0
Urea mmol/l	9.46	8.0	3.30	27.80
Creatinine µmol/l	136.78	132.78	108.0	167.0
eGFR ml/sec	0.78	0.82	0.42	1.80
Cp g/l	0.243	0.250	0.140	0.320
NT-proBNP pg/ml	1927.25	1103.64	465.14	7856.53
sST2 ng/ml	38.15	31.50	14.60	112.00
Gal-3 ng/ml	1.266	1.021	0.212	3.220

Table legend: LV EF—left ventricular ejection fraction, EDD-LV—left ventricular end diastolic diameter, LA—left atrial diameter, BMI—body mass index, eGFR—estimated glomerular filtration rate (MDRD formula), Cp—ceruloplasmin, NT-proBNP—N-terminal B-natriuretic peptide, Gal-3—galectin-3.

Table 2. Correlation of ceruloplasmin with other heart failure biomarkers.

Parameter	Parameter	Corellation coefficient	Level of significance
sST2	NT-proBNP	$r = 0.66$	$p < 0.01$
Cp	sST2	$r = 0.77$	$p < 0.001$
Cp	NT-proBNP	$r = 0.58$	$p < 0.05$
Cp	Gal-3	$r = 0.24$	$p = 0.345$
Gal -3	NT-proBNP	$r = 0.41$	$p = 0.087$

Table legend: Cp—ceruloplasmin, NT-proBNP—N-terminal B-natriuretic peptide, Gal-3—galectin-3.

other inflammatory markers associated with CVD, e.g.: high-sensitivity C-reactive protein (hs-CRP) [13]. In the contrary with previous observations, ceruloplasmin levels were weakly associated with CVD in the ARIC study [6]. In the ARIC study, ceruloplasmin levels were associated with incident HF after adjusting for hs-CRP, N-terminal B-natriuretic peptide (NT-proBNP) and high-sensitivity cardiac troponin T. The genetic part of the study brought significant result showing that ceruloplasmin gene on chromosome 3 was not associated with incident HF but the ceruloplasmin level was.

In the patients with established chronic HF, ceruloplasmin levels correlated with CRP levels and showed independent association with the severity of heart failure as assessed by New York Heart Association class in non-ischemic cardiomyopathy [15].

Association of ceruloplasmin with other heart failure biomarkers was analyzed in several studies. In a study of patients with stable chronic HF, ceruloplasmin levels weakly correlated with B-type natriuretic peptide (r = 0.187, $p < 0.001$) [7].

In the patients with acute decompensated heart failure, ceruloplasmin correlated with NT-proBNP levels in a small study evaluated association of heart failure severity with the level of metabolic liver function [16].

Correlation of ceruloplasmin levels with the novel heart failure biomarkers, e.g.: marker of remodelling sST2 and marker of myofibrosis galectin-3 in the patients with decompensated heart failure has not been systematicaly yet studied.

In our study, ceruloplasmin level correlates with biomarkes of cardiac remodelling:

In our study, ceruloplasmin level in the patients with acute decompensated heart failure with fluid overload correlates with biomarkers of cardiac remodelling: NT-proBNP and sST2. On the other hand, ceruloplasmin levels did not correlate with the biomarker of myofibrosis (galectin-3).

6. Conclusion

Our findings support the inflammatory response and oxidative stress hypothesis in acute decompensated heart failure. It is possible that ceruloplasmin decreases the availability of NO and enhances the reactive oxidant species formation and oxidative cell injury. The cell injury might be associated with the increased wall stress leading to increased myocyte production of biomarkers of remodelling: NT-proBNP and sST2, but not with the increased expression of galectin-3. Galectin-3 is a protein secreted by activated macrophages and has a role in development of fibrosis in injured tissues [17].

Acknowledgements

Approval for the study was granted by Local Board Ethics Committee Na Homolce Hospital. Study was supported by institutional grant Na Homolce Hospital, Prague, Czech Republic IG 140505.

References

[1] Mak, S. and Newton, G.E. (2001) The Oxidative Stress Hypothesis of Congestive Heart Failure. *Chest*, **120**, 2035-2046.

[2] Reunanen, A., Knekt, P. and Aaran, P.K. (1992) Serum Ceruloplasmin Level and the Risk of Myocardial Infarction and Stroke. *American Journal of Epidemiology*, **136**, 1082-1090.

[3] Mänttäri, M., Manninen, V., Huttunen, V.K., *et al.* (1994) Serum Ferritin and Ceruloplasmin as Coronary Risk Factors

European Heart Journal, **15**, 1599-1603.

[4] Klipstein-Grobusch, K., Grobbee, D.E., Koster, F.E., *et al.* (1999) Serum Ceruloplasmin as a Coronary Risk Factor in the Elderly. *The Rotterdam Study British Journal of Nutrition*, **81**, 139-144.

[5] Ridker, P.M., Cushman, M., Stampfer, M.J., *et al.* (1997) Inflammation, Aspirin, and the Risk of Cardiovascular Disease in Apparently Healthy Men. *New England Journal of Medicine*, **336**, 973-979. http://dx.doi.org/10.1056/NEJM199704033361401

[6] Dadu, R.T., Dodge, R., Nambi, V., *et al.* (2013) Ceruloplasmin and Heart Failure in the Atherosclerosis Risk in Communities Study. *Circ Heart Fail*, **6**, 936-943. http://dx.doi.org/10.1161/CIRCHEARTFAILURE.113.000270

[7] Hammadah, M., Fan, Y., Wu, Y., *et al.* (2014) Prognostic Value of Elevated Serum Ceruloplasmin Levels in Patients with Heart Failure. *Journal of Cardiac Failure*, **20**, 946-952.

[8] Mueller, T., Dieplinger, B., Gegenhuber, A., *et al.* (2008) Increased Plasma Concentrations of Soluble ST2 Are Predictive for 1-Year Mortality in Patients with Acute Destabilized Heart Failure. *Clinical Chemistry*, **54**, 752-756. http://dx.doi.org/10.1373/clinchem.2007.096560

[9] Manzano-Fernández, S., Mueller, T., Pascual-Figal, D., *et al.* (2011) Usefulness of Soluble Concentrations of Interleukin family member ST2 as Predictor of Mortality in Patients with Acutely Decompensated Heart Failure Relative to Left Ventricular Ejection Fraction. *The American Journal of Cardiology*, **107**, 259-267. http://dx.doi.org/10.1016/j.amjcard.2010.09.011

[10] de Boer, R.A., Voors, A.A., Muntendam, P., *et al.* (2009) Galectin-3: A Novel Mediator of Heart Failure Development and Progression. *European Journal of Heart Failure*, **11**, 811-817.

[11] Shiva, S., Wang, X., Ringwood, L.A., *et al.* (2006) Ceruloplasmin Is a No Oxidase and Nitrite Synthase That Determines Endocrine No Homeostasis. *Nature Chemical Biology*, **2**, 486-493. http://dx.doi.org/10.1038/nchembio813

[12] Shukla, N., Maher, J., Masters, J., *et al.* (2006) Does Oxidative Stress Change Ceruloplasmin from a Protective to a Vasculopathic Factor? *Atherosclerosis*, **187**, 238-250. http://dx.doi.org/10.1016/j.atherosclerosis.2005.11.035

[13] Tang, W.H., Wu, Y., Hartiala, J., Hazen, S.L., *et al.* (2012) Clinical and Genetic Association of Serum Ceruloplasmin with Cardiovascular Risk. *Arteriosclerosis, Thrombosis, and Vascular Biology*, **32**, 516-522. http://dx.doi.org/10.1161/ATVBAHA.111.237040

[14] Engstrom, G., Hedblad, B., Tyden, P. and Lindgarde, F. (2009) Inflammation-Sensitive Plasma Proteins Are Associated with Increased Incidence of Heart Failure: A Population-Based Cohort Study. *Atherosclerosis*, **202**, 617-622. http://dx.doi.org/10.1016/j.atherosclerosis.2008.05.038

[15] Xu, Y., Lin, H., Zhou, Y., *et al.* (2013) Ceruloplasmin and the Extent of Heart Failure in Ischemic and Nonischemic Cardiomyopathy Patients. *Mediators of Inflammation*, **2013**, Article ID: 348145. http://dx.doi.org/10.1155/2013/348145

[16] Hendrichová, M., Málek, F., Kopřivová, H., *et al.* (2010) Correlation of NT-proBNP with Metabolic Liver Function as Assessed with ^{13}C-Methacetin Breath Test in Patients with Acute Decompensated Heart Failure. *International Journal of Cardiology*, **144**, 321-322. http://dx.doi.org/10.1016/j.ijcard.2009.03.022

[17] Sharma, U.C., Pokharel, S., van Brakel, T.J., *et al.* (2004) Galectin-3 Marks Activated Macrophages in Failure-Pronehy Pertrophied Hearts and Contributes to Cardiac Dysfunction. *Circulation*, **110**, 3121-3128. http://dx.doi.org/10.1161/01.CIR.0000147181.65298.4D

26

Nurse Managers Stress and Coping

AChiharu Miyata[1*], Hidenori Arai[2], Sawako Suga[3]

[1]Department of Human Health Sciences, Kyoto University Graduate School of Medicine, Kyoto, Japan
[2]National Center for Geriatrics and Gerontology, Obu, Aichi, Japan
[3]Department of Health Sciences, Kyoto Tachibana University, Kyoto, Japan
Email: *miyata.chiharu.4m@kyoto-u.ac.jp

Abstract

Objective: The purpose of this study was to gain insight into nurse managers' stress experiences and coping strategies in order to better support them. Design: A qualitative exploratory descriptive research design was used in this study. Subject: Fifteen nurse managers participated in this study. Results: Three descriptive themes related to nurse managers' occupational stress were identified: role overload, loneliness, and role conflict. We also identified three descriptive themes that contributed to their stress management: sufficient support and advice, taking mental breaks while off duty, and individual coping strategies. Conclusions: Our study proposes two recommendations to reduce nurse managers' stress. First, for nurse managers who experience work overload, hospitals should support them in learning how to work efficiently and how to manage their response to work demands. Second, nurse managers' primary stressors were loneliness and role conflict. Nurse managers are known to juggle multiple demands from the hospital nursing director and staff nurses. Although it is difficult to eliminate the role conflict, nurse managers should be guided on how to manage conflicting demands, the hospital nursing director and staff nurses.

Keywords

Nurse Managers, Role Stressors, Role Conflict, Coping Strategy

1. Introduction

Over the last decade, management in nursing has become increasingly demanding [1]. Nurse managers' roles have undergone a significant change as they take on more administrative management, and they now have much broader responsibilities for direct patient care, managing staff nurses, leadership, and organizational resource management. Shirey [2] reviewed the expansion of the nurse manager role from 1980 to 2003 and found increased demands on nurse managers, which led to increased job stress. Since this review was published, many

*Corresponding author.

other studies had supported Shirey's assertion that the nurse manager's role tends to be inherently demanding and stressful. A recent review indicates that nurse managers' leadership styles are responsible for creating healthy workplaces that will attract and retain the best nurses [3]. In addition, another study found that nurse managers have a significant impact on the health of their staff [4], and nurse managers' stress has been shown to be related to staff nurses' decreased satisfaction [5]. Thus, the poor health of nurse managers indirectly and negatively affects their staff's health. Furthermore, a number of studies [6] [7] have shown that nurse managers can be vulnerable and therefore at the risk of ill health and decreased psychological well-being. Nurse managers cannot perform their duties at a high level of professionalism without good health, and therefore, their health is clearly important. However, most of the research has focused on the stress of novice nurses and staff nurses in Japan, whereas few researchers have studied nurse managers' stressors. Therefore, the aim of this study was to address nurse managers' stress and coping strategies, and two research questions were developed based on this aim.

The research questions were as follows:

1) What are nurse managers' occupational stressors?

2) How do nurse managers cope with their stress?

2. Aim

The aim of this study was to gain insight into nurse managers' perceptions of stress and to learn their coping strategies.

3. Review of the Literature

Work-related mental health results primarily from increased workplace satisfaction and from mitigating work-related stress. Among nurses, specific environmental stressors have been identified, including unpredictable staffing and scheduling, lack of role clarity, little involvement in decision-making, poor status, and poor support [8]. Studies on nursing that specifically focus on nurse managers have focused more on the negative organizational outcomes from ineffective nurse managers than on their personal stress. For example, the nurse manager role is critical for organizational success, patient outcomes, and staff job satisfaction and empowerment [9]-[11]. However, most of the studies have focused on the effects of nurse managers' stress and have shown that it is induced by role overload, role ambiguity, fiscal responsibilities, inadequate human resources, and intrapersonal distress [12] [13]. In addition, Lee and Cummigs [14] reported that workload is negatively related to nurse managers' job satisfaction. Shirey *et al.* [15] conducted a qualitative study that focused on a variety of negative outcomes related to the stress of being a nurse manager. These included emotions such as anger, guilt, frustration, aggravation, and worry, as well as health outcomes such as sleeplessness, irritability, restlessness, impatience, exhaustion, shortness of breath, and tense muscles. These results have been supported by recent quantitative research that links nurse managers' stress with lower job satisfaction, lower organizational commitment, higher turnover intentions, and increased physical and mental health symptoms [12]. Another study revealed that some nurse managers thrive on the complexity of the role and enjoy the opportunity to lead others to achieve their personal, professional, and organizational goals, but others reported negative physical and psychological effects of role stress [16].

4. Study Design

A qualitative exploratory descriptive research design was used to gain an in-depth understanding of nurse managers' stress and coping strategies using semi-structured interviews.

4.1. Method

Data were collected from July to August 2012. All face to face interviews were conducted by researcher. The study was completed when the data has been saturated. Interview topic guide designed by researchers and experts from the faculty of psychology. The questions on the interview guide focused on the views of the job-stress of nurses [17]. Six questions were addressed using a qualitative descriptive approach:

1) What are the major occupational stressors that you face as a nurse manager?

2) How do you deal with your concerns?

3) Does your hospital offer any support?
4) Can you cope with your stress positively?
5) What do you do when you feel tired or stressed?
6) What do you think is the effect of your mental health on your staff?
All interviews lasted for 30 to 60minutes and were audio recorded in a private room at each hospital.

4.1.1. Study Inclusion Criteria

Fifteen nurse managers participated in this study. They were selected from five hospitals with 200 beds or more in the Kanto, Kansai, and Kyushu regions of Japan. Criterion sampling was used for intentional sampling, and each person had at least one year of experience as a nurse

4.1.2. Ethical Consideration

The study was approved by the Ethics Committee of the Kyoto University Graduate School and the Faculty of Medicine. Additionally, research permission was given by the nursing department directors of all five hospitals. After receiving approval from each hospital, we explained the project and procedures to the nurse managers.

4.2. Data Analysis

Data analysis was done simultaneously with data collection. The authors independently reviewed the transcriptions and constructed tables of code categories based on actual words or phrases (meaning units). We independently identified themes that represented one or more code categories and specific quotations that represented each code category; this qualitative content analysis approach was adapted from Graneheim and Lundman [18]. The researchers discussed the coding and the major themes that emerged from the data to reach consensus. Rigor and trustworthiness were ensured by our following qualitative principles and ensuring that there was a clear audit trail of the descriptive exploratory findings. Data analysis encompassed description, interpretation, and thematic development. Themes were emergent based on the data. The patterns identified offered an account that related to and answered the research questions.

5. Findings

Participant Characteristics (**Table 1**).

Table 1. Demographic characteristics of the nurse managers.

Age Mean (SD): 46.8 (6.0)	Experience as a nurse manager (years): 5.1 (2.3)	Academic background	Work unit Subhead
44	2	Diploma in nursing	Education
47	5	Diploma in nursing	Outpatient
50	1	Diploma in nursing	Internal medicine ward
50	9	Graduate university	Surgery ward
44	8	Diploma in nursing	Intensive care unit
47	7	Junior college graduate	Internal medicine ward
45	6	Junior college graduate	Orthopedics ward
51	7	Diploma in nursing	Surgery ward
50	4	Diploma in nursing	Internal medicine ward
45	5	Junior college graduate	Stroke care unit
49	7	Junior college graduate	Dental oral surgery ward
46	3	Junior college graduate	Gastrointestinal and breast surgery ward
46	3	Junior college graduate	Cardiovascular ward
47	4	Junior college graduate	Respiratory, blood and oncology ward
42	5	Junior college graduate	High care unit

The nurse managers were all women. The mean age was 46.8 years (range: 42 - 50 years). Mean years of work experience as a nurse manager was 5.1 years (range: one to nine years).

5.1. Stress Source

Three descriptive themes related to nurse managers' stressors were identified: role overload, loneliness, and role conflict (**Table 2**).

5.1.1. Role Overload

Role overload consisted of four subcategories: juggling many business roles; scheduling and coordinating human relationships; working with patients and families; and receiving numerous off-duty phone calls. Numerous and complex demands from staff members, colleagues, and families and multiple administrative duties caused overload, and high expectations also challenged nurse managers, who were asked to do too much for too many people in too little time. The nurse manager role has expanded over the years, mostly reflected in their greater responsibility for their staffs. The interviewees reported feeling overwhelmed, as reflected in the following comments:

"There is not enough time during the day. There are high expectations from staff, other health care professionals, and patients. There is not enough time during the day to manage multiple meetings, deal with patients' and families' complaints, and respond to staff needs."

"I've often said, if there were no staff allocation problem, this job would be good to do. Yet indeed, staff allocation is a pain in the neck and gets me down day after day."

5.1.2. Loneliness

The second major stressor identified by the participants was the sense of loneliness or isolation. This theme encompassed two subcategories: being solely responsible for managing ward-related problems and being unable to express fatigue because of the influence on staff members. Nurse managers expressed that because they could not share management problems with their chiefs and staff members, they worried about and experienced their problems on their own; they could not express their worries because of the influence on others, and they felt lonely. "We are stressed… a nurse manager is really lonely. I can consult the chief or staff members in my ward, but there are many things I cannot talk to them about—so I am carrying around the worries on my own".

5.1.3. Role Conflict

Role conflict consisted of two subcategories. Participants described feeling squeezed between conflicting demands: organizational performance targets from above and staff expectations from below and additional expectations from physicians and other department leaders, as reflected in the following comments:

"I do many things to improve the quality of nursing care. But sometimes it does not match the hospital policy. I can understand the feeling of the staff, but…"

"I consult the other department leaders and the physician about patient care. Sometimes, I feel anger, but it is not possible to show the anger."

5.2. Nurse Managers' Coping Strategy

We also identified three descriptive themes related to their coping strategies: sufficient support and advice, taking

Table 2. Stress source.

Theme	Sub-Category
Role overload	multiple business roles scheduling, coordinating human relationships working with patients and families numerous off-duty phone calls
Loneliness	managing ward-related problems alone inability to show fatigue because of the influence on staff members.
Role conflict	being caught between conflicting demands managing anger

mental breaks when off duty, and general coping (**Table 3**).

5.2.1. Sufficient Support and Advice

Regarding coping strategies, nearly half of the participants cited this theme as a significant stress mitigator. The theme consisted of three subcategories: advice from other administrators and nursing directors; sharing information with other nurse managers; and a hospital consulting system. Interviewee comments included:

"Fortunately, the senior nurse manager and vice nursing director listen to me. I receive advocating advice and criticism, too, but I feel happy that I can talk about my concerns to somebody else."

"I would be very happy if there were an opportunity to share all my concerns with other nurse managers after work and receive appropriate advice from senior nurses."

5.2.2. Taking Mental Breaks When off Duty

Another factor that decreased participants' stress was taking mental breaks while they were off duty. This theme consisted of two subcategories: awareness of the importance of taking time off and recognizing physical symptoms such as fatigue. Participants were aware of the need to take time off in order to reduce their stress and expand their chief nurses' training. Participants' comments included:

"I think we need to take some rest. Some nurse managers work all the time without taking rest, so I believe we need rest."

"In the past, even if I took rest, I received many phone calls, so I couldn't take sufficient rest. Today, I transferred my responsibility to the chief nurse so I can take rest. I think it improves the chief's motivation as well."

5.2.3. Individual Coping Strategies

This theme encompassed four subcategories: thinking positively; enhancing one's private life; separating private life from work; and identifying individual effective strategies. Stress-related emotions differed between the novice and experienced nurse managers, and coping strategies differed depending on the nurse manager's experience.

One novice nurse manager (with less than four years of experience) consulted other nurse managers as her coping strategy. Another eleven participants (who had more than four years of experience) spoke of coping strategies such as maintaining enriched relationships with their families, taking private time, and completely shifting from work to private life. Participants' comments included the following:

"I would say that the first thing to do for stress coping is to talk with other nurse managers." (a novice nurse manager)

"I have been in this position for seven years, and I have had a lot to learn. I am always trying not to think about my work when I am off duty and to give my attention to other areas such as my family." (an experienced nurse manager)

6. Discussion

Role overload and role conflict, which were extracted as stressors for nurse managers in this study, were consistent with the results obtained in other developed countries [13] [19]. Some researchers have suggested that nurse managers have the most demanding work schedules in the health care sector [20]. In addition, the scope of responsibilities, span of control, and work demands may be unrealistic for nurse managers [21] [22]. Role ambi-

Table 3. Nurse managers' coping strategy.

Theme	Sub-Category
Sufficient support and advice	advice from administrators and nursing directors sharing information with other nurse managers hospital consultation systems
Taking mental breaks when off duty	awareness of the importance of taking time off recognizing physical symptoms such as fatigue
Individual coping strategies	thinking positively enhancing private life keeping work and private life separate devising personal coping strategies

guity and diversity are considered to contribute to the excessive number of roles nurse managers must serve [12] [19], and the same situation is seen in Japan. Further, in Japan, there is little recognition of nurse managers' roles as nursing administrators among both the managers and staff nurses. As such, nurse managers tend to assume both administrative and staff management duties, which increase their workloads and complicate their work.

Next, the theme of coping strategies, such as seeking advice from superiors and coworkers and developing individual coping strategies, supported the results from previous studies. The increasing span of control is reported to cause effects such as lack of mentoring, increased stress, and decreased job satisfaction [23]. In this study, all participants mentioned the efficacy and importance of coping strategies, and when nurse managers did not have much experience, seeking advice from senior nurses and/or superiors and sharing their concerns with other nurse managers led to relaxation. In addition, in the past, nurse managers managed and monitored their wards on their own, and therefore, they had to remain at the hospital and never take a day off. However, they have recently become aware of the need to take time off in order to reduce their stress and expand their chief nurses' training.

By contrast, however, the sense of isolation that was extracted as a stressor in this study was not reported in other studies. Limited recognition of nurse managers' roles as administrators and their inability to manage stress are considered the background for the above. In particular, it was difficult for novice nurse managers to establish personal coping methods. Therefore, it is necessary to provide novice nurse managers with opportunities to seek advice from experienced managers so that they are not isolated on their wards and their stress does not increase. Further, nurses' need for continuing stress management education has been reported from clinical sites. Nurse managers are expected to achieve organizational objectives while establishing a healthy workplace for the staff in their units [24]. Therefore, we insist that the nurse managers who must care for their staff members' psychosomatic health must have sufficient stress management skills. Finally, lack of knowledge related to hospital operations, such as budgets and cost reduction, which was reported as a stressor in a number of previous studies, was not identified in this study [19]. However, in recent years, nursing directors in Japan have come to concurrently serve as hospital deputy directors, which require their greater knowledge of business and business administration. As a result, this new status may emerge as a new stressor in the future.

This study extracted general stress-related factors; "role conflict" and "sense of isolation" as stressors and "recognizing the need to rest" as a coping strategy were the primary factors extracted in this study, but the contents of specific stressors were not extracted. Therefore, in the future, it is necessary to collect quantitative data to supplement this study's results with specific individual stressors, using questionnaires. The study results suggest the need to establish a system in which nurse managers' duties are clearly defined and they can receive consultation and advice to reduce their stress.

7. Recommendations

In this study, we aimed to identify nurse managers' occupational stressors and coping strategies through interviews. The results can be utilized for future nurse manager stress management, including offering suggestions for reducing stress. In addition, for nurse managers who feel overloaded, hospitals should support them in learning how to work efficiently and how to manage their responses to their job demands. Nurse managers are known to juggle multiple demands from hospital nursing directors and staff nurses. Although it is difficult to eliminate role conflict, nurse managers should be given a safe place to discuss their concerns and receive advice on how to manage their conflicting demands.

8. Conclusion

We found that nurse managers' occupational stressors were role overload, loneliness, and role conflict, and their coping strategies included receiving sufficient support and advice from other administrators and nursing directors and taking mental breaks when they were off duty. However, individual coping strategies were very different. The nurse managers in this study appeared to recognize the impact of their stress on other staff members and also appeared to be aware of stress management strategies.

Acknowledgements

We thank all the nurses who took time from their busy schedules to participate in this study.

References

[1] Hyrkäs, K. (2005) Clinical Supervision, Burnout and Job Satisfaction among Mental Health and Psychiatric Nurses in Finland. *Issues in Mental Health Nursing*, **26**, 531-556. http://dx.doi.org/10.1080/01612840590931975

[2] Shirey, M.R. (2006) Stress and Coping in Nurse Manager: Two Decades of Research. *Nursing Economics*, **24**, 193-211.

[3] Cummings, G.G., MacGregor, T., Davey, M., Lee, H., Wong, C.A., Lo, E., Muise, M. and Stafford, E. (2010) Leadership Styles and Outcome Patterns for the Nursing Workforce and Work Environment: A Systematic Review. *International Journal of Nursing Studies*, **47**, 363-385. http://dx.doi.org/10.1016/j.ijnurstu.2009.08.006

[4] Nyberg, A., Bernin, P., Theorell, T., Westerlund, H., Vahtera, J. and Kivimäki, M. (2009) Managerial Leadership and Ischemic Heart Disease among Employees: The Swedish WOLF Study. *Occupational and Environmental Medicine*, **66**, 51-55. http://dx.doi.org/10.1136/oem.2008.039362

[5] Meyer, R.M., O'Brien-Pallas, L., Doran, D., Streiner, D., Ferguson-Pare, M. and Duffield, C.M. (2011) Front-Line Managers as Boundary Spanners: Effects of Span and Time on Nurse Supervision Satisfaction. *Journal of nursing management*, **19**, 611-622. http://dx.doi.org/10.1111/j.1365-2834.2011.01260.x

[6] Lindholm, M., Dejin-Karlsson, E., Ostergren, P.O. and Udén, G. (2003) Nurse Managers Professional Networks, Psychosocial Resources and Self-Rated Health. *Journal of Advanced Nursing*, **42**, 506-515. http://dx.doi.org/10.1046/j.1365-2648.2003.02650.x

[7] Luchinger, H.K.S., Almost, J., Purdy, N. and Kim, J. (2004) Predictors of Nurse Managers' Health in Canadian Restructured Healthcare Settings. *Nursing Leadership*, **17**, 88-105. http://dx.doi.org/10.12927/cjnl.2004.17020

[8] Williams, S., Michie, S. and Pattani, S. (1998) Improving the Health of the NHS Workforce. The Nuffield Trust, London.

[9] Duffield, C.M., Roche, M.A., Blay, N. and Stasa, H. (2011) Nursing Unit Managers, Staff Retention and the Work Environment. *Journal of Clinical Nursing*, **20**, 23-33. http://dx.doi.org/10.1111/j.1365-2702.2010.03478.x

[10] Lucas, V., Laschinger, H.K.S. and Wong, C.A. (2008) The Impact of Emotional Intelligent Leadership on Staff Nurse Empowerment: The Moderating Effect of Span of Control. *Journal of Nursing Management*, **16**, 964-973. http://dx.doi.org/10.1111/j.1365-2834.2008.00856.x

[11] Wong, C.A., Laschinger, H.K.S. and Cummings, G.G. (2010) Authentic Leadership and Nurses' Voice Behavior and Perceptions of care Quality. *Journal of Nursing Management*, **18**, 889-900. http://dx.doi.org/10.1111/j.1365-2834.2010.01113.x

[12] Kath, L.M., Stichler, J.F. and Ehrhart, M.G. (2012) Moderators of the Negative Outcomes of Nurse Manager Stress. *Journal of Nursing Administration*, **42**, 215-221. http://dx.doi.org/10.1097/NNA.0b013e31824ccd25

[13] Udod, S.A. and Care, W.D. (2011) Nurse Managers' Work Stressors and Coping Experiences: Unravelling the Evidence. *Canadian Journal of Nursing Leadership*, **24**, 57-72. http://dx.doi.org/10.12927/cjnl.2011.22601

[14] Lee, H. and Cummings, G.G. (2008) Factors Influencing Job Satisfaction of Front Line Nurse Managers: A Systematic Review. *Journal of Nursing Management*, **16**, 768-783. http://dx.doi.org/10.1111/j.1365-2834.2008.00879.x

[15] Shirey, M.R., Ebright, P.R. and McDaniel, A.M. (2008) Sleepless in America: Nurse Managers Cope with Stress and Complexity. *Journal of Nursing Administration*, **38**, 125-131. http://dx.doi.org/10.1097/01.NNA.0000310722.35666.73

[16] Paliadelis, P.S., Cruickshank, M. and Sheridan, A. (2007) Caring for Each Other: How Do Nurse Managers "Manage" Their Role? *Journal of Nursing Management*, **15**, 830-837. http://dx.doi.org/10.1111/j.1365-2934.2007.00754.x

[17] Kageyama, T., Nishikido, N., Kobayashi, T., Oga, J. and Kawashima, M. (2003) The Relationship of Work Stress to the Mental Health Status of Female Nurses in a Public Hospital. *Japanese Journal of Nursing and Health Sciences*, **4**, 1-10. (In Japanese)

[18] Graneheim, U. and Lundman, B. (2004) Qualitative Content Analysis in Nursing Research: Concepts, Procedures and Measures to Achieve Trustworthiness. *Nurse Education Today*, **24**, 105-112. http://dx.doi.org/10.1016/j.nedt.2003.10.001

[19] McCallin, A.M. (2010) The Role of the Charge Nurse Manager: A Descriptive Exploratory Study. *Journal of Nursing Management*, **18**, 319-325. http://dx.doi.org/10.1111/j.1365-2834.2010.01067.x

[20] Anthony, M.K., Standing, T.S. and Glick, J. (2005) Leadership and Retention: The Pivotal Role of Nurse Managers. *Journal of nursing Administration*, **35**, 146-155. http://dx.doi.org/10.1097/00005110-200503000-00008

[21] Judkins, S., Massey, C. and Huff, B. (2006) Hardiness, Stress, and Use of Ill-Time among Nurse Managers: Is There A Connection? *Nursing Economics*, **24**, 187.

[22] Shirey, M.R. (2007) AONE Leadership Perspectives: Competencies and Tips for Effective Leadership: From Novice to

Expert. *Journal of Nursing Administration*, **37**, 167-170. http://dx.doi.org/10.1097/01.NNA.0000266842.54308.38

[23] Silvetti, C., Rudan, V., Frederickson, K. and Sullivan, B. (2000) Where Will Tomorrow'S Nurse Managers Come From? *Journal of Nursing Administration*, **30**, 157-159. http://dx.doi.org/10.1097/00005110-200004000-00002

[24] Espinoza, D.C., Lopez-Saldana, A. and Stonestreet, J.S. (2009) The Pivotal Role of the Nurse Manager in Healthy Workplaces: İmplications for Training and Development. *Critical Care Nursing Quarterly*, **32**, 327-334. http://dx.doi.org/10.1097/CNQ.0b013e3181bad528

27

Life Adjustments of Elderly Hemodialysis Patients for Continuing to Attend Dialysis Facility

Utako Shimizu, Momoe Sakagami, Mieko Uchiyama, Hagiko Aoki

School of Sciences Faculty of Medicine, Niigata University, Niigata, Japan
Email: shirakaba@clg.niigata-u.ac.jp

Abstract

This study aimed to elucidate elderly patients' recognition of and life adjustment to attending dialysis facilities, and then to discuss factors for enabling such patients to continue attending dialysis facilities. Semi-structured interviews were conducted with 15 participants and interview data were analyzed using the modified grounded theory approach. The study was approved by the Ethical Review Board of Niigata University School of Medicine. The interview data yielded 21 concepts, comprising 2 categories and 7 subcategories. Patients who find themselves in a "Difficult Lifestyle" often try to maintain their health and lifestyle by using *required support for hemodialysis patients*. Factors for continuing to attend dialysis facilities were the ability to cope with the Difficult Lifestyle and to adjust to Hemodialysis as a Life Priority. It is thought that switching from a model of economic security to one of providing living support will be effective for maintaining elderly dialysis patients' life with only limited expenses. Additionally, it is necessary to consider the utilization of existing services.

Keywords

Elderly, Hemodialysis Patient, Living Support, Qualitative Research

1. Introduction

Hemodialysis is the main treatment for end-stage renal disease (ESRD) in Japan, where it accounts for 96.9% of chronic dialysis patients. In Japan, the mean age of dialysis patients has increased from 62.2 years in 2002 to 66.9 years in 2012 [1], compared with 62.1 years and 66.4 years [2] [3] in other developed countries such as the United States and the United Kingdom, respectively. In 4.2% of cases, hemodialysis initiation is due to kidney transplant (1601 of 38,055 cases in 2012) [1] [4].

Hemodialysis patients have to attend a dialysis facility three times a week, and hemodialysis greatly affects the lives of elderly patients. The burden of kidney disease in Japan, as measured by the Kidney Disease Quality of Life Short Form, is higher than in the US or Europe [5]. The percentage of Japanese dialysis patients who need assistance walking is 10.7% for individuals aged 45 - 74 years and 32.0% for those aged over 75 years [6], with the percentage increasing with age. Both in Japan and overseas, much remains unclear about the life condition of elderly hemodialysis patients. Therefore, it is important to elucidate elderly patients' recognition of attending dialysis facilities. Against this background, the present study aimed to elucidate elderly patients' recognition of and life adjustment to attending dialysis facilities, and then to discuss factors for continuing to attend dialysis facilities.

2. Methods

2.1. Research Design

A qualitative descriptive design was used to collect data through semi-structured interviews.

2.2. Participants

A total of 15 hemodialysis patients were selected by the head nurse of the hemodialysis unit of cooperating facilities. Hemodialysis complications often occur in patients who receive hemodialysis for more than 10 years. In addition, patients who are over 65 years old often experience decreases in their activities of daily living. Therefore, the eligibility criteria in this study were 1) receiving hemodialysis for more than 10 years and 2) over 65 years old.

2.3. Data Collection

Semi-structured interviews were conducted in Japanese at the participants' dialysis facilities by the first author, using a guide containing open-ended questions. Participants were asked to speak freely about their past experiences. Questions concerned patients' experiences feeling difficulty in attending dialysis facilities, utilization of services for attending dialysis facility, worry about continuing to attend dialysis facilities, and recognition of attending dialysis facilities. Data were collected in August to September of 2012. All interviews were audio recorded, and later transcribed verbatim in Japanese, and ideas and observations that arose during interviews were recorded.

2.4. Data Analysis

The modified grounded theory approach (M-GTA) [7] was used to analyze interview data. M-GTA is a qualitative analysis method derived from the original grounded theory approach [8]. The M-GTA focuses on organizing substantive theories for practical utilization, and is therefore more suited to our present purpose of conceptualizing a process from patients' recognition.

The verbatimtranscript was reread repeatedly for in-depth analysis of data. In M-GTA, the minimum analytical unit is the concept, and each concept is derived from several pieces of data (variations). Here, variations were extracted from the verbatimtranscript according to the analysis theme "What kinds of life management do elderly hemodialysis patients perform in order to continue to attend dialysis facilities?" Variations were collected after reading the verbatim transcriptrepeatedly until fully comprehending them. Variations with similar meanings were grouped to allow for the development of concepts. The M-GTA uses an analyzing worksheet to develop concepts, which also includes ideas for concept names and notes on interpreting variations. When a concept was created, similar or antithetical data related to the concept were examined to prevent arbitrary interpretation. Subcategories were created from the relationships between concepts, relationships between subcategories were examined, and the process of data comparison and analysis was repeated. The structure of the relationships between subcategories was clarified, identifying the categories. Data collection and data analysis were conducted until theoretical saturation was reached, as assessed by the absence of new concepts.

The research was supervised by one researcher specialized in chronic illness nursing and all results were considered by all authors to ensure accuracy and reliability. All categories, concepts, and variations were originally in Japanese and analyzed as such. The author translated these data into English, and a native English translator verified the translations.

2.5. Ethical Considerations

The study was approved by the Ethical Review Board of Niigata University School of Medicine (Approval No. 1443). Our study conformed to the principles set by the Declaration of Helsinki. Informed consent was obtained both verbally and in writing. All participants were informed that their participation was voluntary and that they could withdraw from the study at any time without penalty. The participants' physical condition was considered the first priority during the interview. The interview was suspended and rescheduled if so required by the participant required.

3. Results

A summary of the 15 participants (9 men, 6 women; 7 participants in their 60 s, 7 in their 70 s, 1 in her 80 s; duration of dialysis 12 - 28 years) is shown in **Table 1**. The interview data yielded 21 concepts, comprising 2 categories and 7 subcategories (**Table 2**). **Figure 1** shows the process of life adjustment for attending dialysis facility by elderly hemodialysis patients.

Hemodialysis patients had been conscious of the first category of "Hemodialysis as a Life Priority" from initiation of dialysis to the present. Hemodialysis as a Life Priority consisted of the subcategories *mental attitude of hemodialysis priority* and *life adjustment to hemodialysis priority. Mental attitude of hemodialysis priority* consisted of 4 concepts: living with goals, thinking of hemodialysis as a part of life, thinking about needing hemodialysis in order to live, and being determined to receive hemodialysis. Hemodialysis as a Life Priority was positively influenced by *feelings of support*. Dialysis patients who experience *living with poor physical condition*

Table 1. Summary of participants.

Participant	Gender	Age	Period of dialysis (years)	Primary disease	Job	Family	Access to dialysis facility	Family members in attendance	Commuting time, one way (min)
A	M	70 s	12	Nephrosclerosis	Unemployed	Wife	Private car	None	15
B	M	60 s	19	Glomerulonephritis	Independent business	Wife, Son	Private car	None	15
C	M	70 s	12	Glomerulonephritis	Independent business	Wife, Son	Private car	None	20
D	M	60 s	19	Nephrosclerosis	Temporary worker	Wife	Private car	None	40
E	M	70 s	26	Chronic nephritis	Unemployed	Alone	Private car	None	10
F	M	60 s	17	Glomerulonephritis	Temporary worker	Wife, Daughter	Private car	Wife	10
G	M	60 s	15	Pyelonephritis	Unemployed	Wife, Mother-in-law	Private car	None	25
H	F	60 s	28	Glomerulonephritis	Unemployed	Alone	Private car	None	1
I	F	70 s	18	Pyelonephritis	Unemployed	Husband	Private car	Husband, Son	10
J	M	60 s	28	Chronic nephritis	Unemployed	Alone	Private car	None	15
K	M	70 s	18	IgA nephropathy	Unemployed	Wife	Private car	None	30
L	F	70 s	25	Purpura nephritis	Agriculture	Husband, Son, Daughter-in-law, Grandchild	Private car	Husband, Wife	10
M	F	70 s	25	IgA nephropathy	Unemployed	Son, Daughter-in-law, Grandchild	Bus, Taxi	None	10
N	F	60 s	19	Pyelonephritis	Unemployed	Husband	Bus, Taxi	None	20
O	F	80 s	16	Glomerulonephritis	Unemployed	Husband	Bus	None	15

Table 2. List of categories extracted.

"Category", *sub-category*, concept
"Hemodialysis as a Life Priority"
Mental attitude of hemodialysis priority
Living with goals
Thinking of hemodialysis as a part of life
Thinking about needing hemodialysis in order to live
Being determined to receive hemodialysis
Life adjustment to hemodialysis priority
Not wanting to burden family
Scheduling around hemodialysis cycle
"Difficult Lifestyle"
Living with poor physical condition
Realizing a decline in health
Keeping a poor physical condition after hemodialysis
Forcing oneself to attend dialysis facilities
Difficulties of living with hemodialysis
Feeling time constraints
Feeling the inconvenience of transportation to dialysis facilities
Feeling inferior because of receiving social security for dialysis patients
Prospective worry about continuing to receive dialysis
Envisioning a decline in health
Worrying about future difficulty in attending dialysis facilities
Required support for hemodialysis patients
Requiring adaptable support for attending dialysis facilities
Not wanting to change hemodialysis cycle
Requiring financial support and car parking
Wanting to be able to freely contact sources of advice
Feelings of support
Feel be helped by security services for dialysis patients
Thought of being supported by medical professionals
Feeling grateful for the support of family

and *difficulties of living with hemodialysis* then begin to experience *prospective worry about continuing to receive hemodialysis*.

Elderly hemodialysis patients who realize this second category, Difficult Lifestyle, try to continue by taking advantage of the *required support for hemodialysis patients*, defined as requests for preferential treatment in attending dialysis facility. *Required support for hemodialysis patients* also consisted of 4 concepts: requiring adaptable support for attending dialysis facilities, not wanting to change hemodialysis cycle, requiring financial support and car parking, and wanting to be able to freely contact sources of advice. This addresses Difficult Lifestyle in accordance with patients' situations. *Required support for hemodialysis patients* was increased by patients' recognition of Difficult Lifestyle, and was decreased by recognition of Hemodialysis as a Life Priority.

4. Discussion

The lifestyle adjustments clarified in this study were largely divided into those where patients attempted to solve their problems themselves ("Hemodialysis as a Life Priority") and those where they would ask others for help (*required support for hemodialysis patients*). Hemodialysis as a Life Priority was disturbed by Difficult Life-

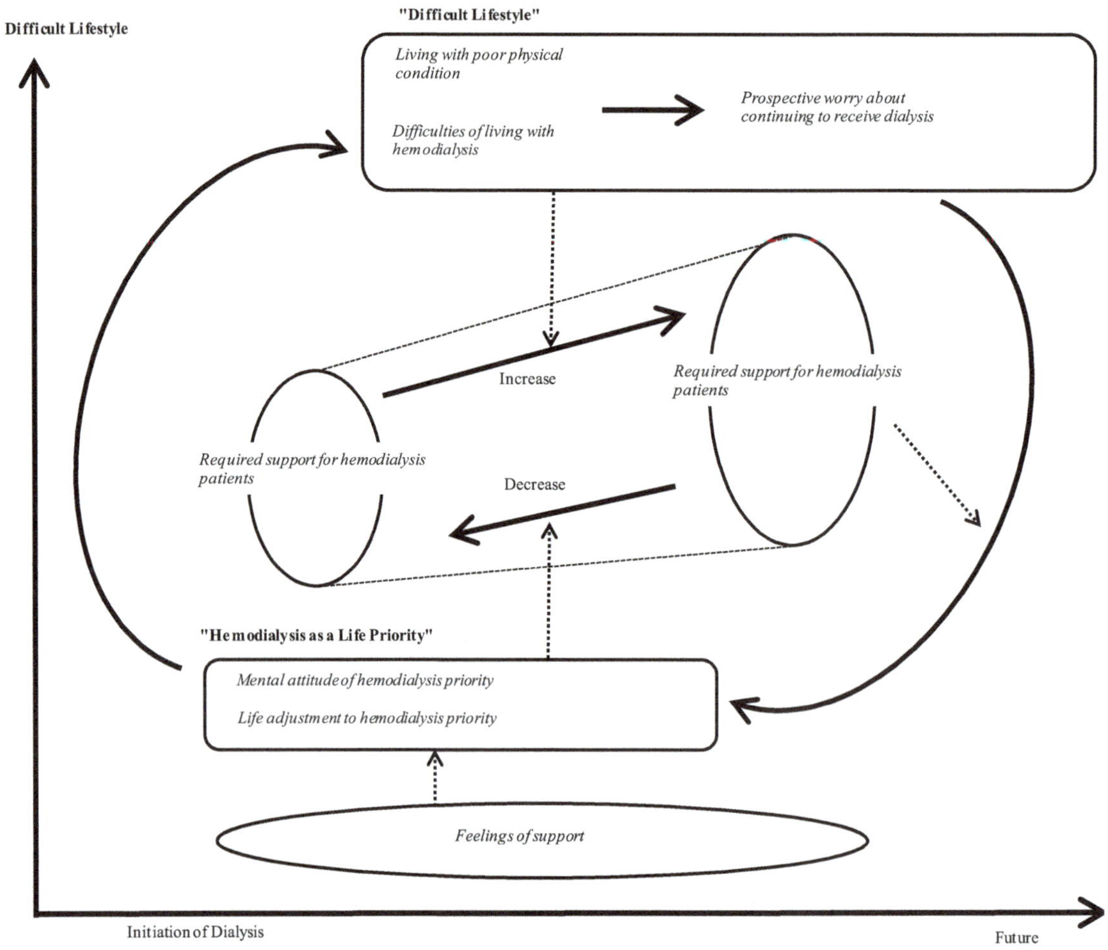

Figure 1. The process of life adjustment of elderly hemodialysis patients to attending dialysis facility.
Categories are indicated in rounded rectangular boxes and bold text. Subcategories are indicated in circles and italic text. Solid arrows indicate direction of change. Dashed arrows indicate direction of influence.

style. Because elderly hemodialysis patients could not avoid this Difficult Lifestyle, they tried to cope with it by strengthening their *required support for hemodialysis patients*. We consider that *required support for hemodialysis patients* played an important role in patients' continuing to attend dialysis facilities. *Required support for hemodialysis patients* differs from secondary gains [9] where patients take advantage of their kidney disease where possible, because patients in the present study made efforts concurrently under the category of Hemodialysis as a Life Priority. Thus, it is clear that in this study, elderly dialysis patients adjusted to life through their own efforts, not simply by receiving support, and that factors for continuing to attend dialysis facilities were able to cope with the Difficult Lifestyle and to adjust to Hemodialysis as a Life Priority. It is difficult to increase the number of transplants in Japan, as ethnographic research has shown that Japan departs radically from the traditional notion prevalent in Western Europe that organ donation is seen as the ultimate altruistic gift [10]. For this reason, ESRD patients often remain on hemodialysis throughout their life. Therefore, it is important to maintain hemodialysis patients' ability to cope with their hemodialysis.

Social security and welfare systems are available for dialysis patients in Japan. Although the individual medical expenses for dialysis total from 10,000 to 20,000 yen (US$ 94.5 - 190.0, 1 US$ = ¥105.848; OECD 2014) [11] a month [12], various forms of economic support for dialysis patients are provided, for example, tax reductions and discounted transportation fees. Therefore, all patients diagnosed with ESRD can initiate dialysis without anxiety about medical costs, unless they make a non-treatment decision [12]. However, because of rising healthcare costs, the remuneration for dialysis has decreased each year. Elderly dialysis patients have multiple disadvantages like declining activities of daily living, complications of dialysis, or solitary living/living in an aged household, which create difficulties for them to attend dialysis facility. In addition, elderly dialysis patients appear susceptible to social isolation, or difficulty in maintaining social relationships [13]. It is thought that switching from a model of economic security to a model of living support will be effective for maintaining elderly dialysis patients' lifestyle, because support for elderly dialysis patients must be provided with limited expenses. Furthermore, it is necessary to consider utilization of existing services. People over 65 years old who need long-term care may take advantage of the services provided by Long-Term Care Insurance, such as elder-care taxi, home repair, and lending/aid for purchasing welfare equipment will likely play an important role for the life adjustment of elderly dialysis patients, and provide an example of considerate support for life adjustment in Japan.

5. Limitations

Because there were participants from a limited residential area, it is possible that the study may reflect common local factors. Future studies should include more participants taken from a wider area.

6. Conclusion

Semi-structured interviews with 15 participants were conducted, and interview data yielded 21 concepts, divided into 2 categories and 7 subcategories. Elderly hemodialysis patients are conscious of Hemodialysis as a Life Priority. Patients who find themselves in a Difficult Lifestyle often try to maintain their health and lifestyle by using *required support for hemodialysis patients*. Factors for continuing to attend dialysis facilities were the ability to cope with the Difficult Lifestyle and to adjust to Hemodialysis as a Life Priority. It is thought that switching from a model of economic security to one of providing living support will be effective for maintaining elderly dialysis patients' life with only limited expenses. Additionally, it is necessary to consider the utilization of existing services.

Acknowledgements

This study was supported by a Grant-in-Aid for Young Scientists (B) from the Japanese Ministry of Education, Culture, Sports, Science and Technology.

References

[1] Nakai, S., Hanafusa, N., Masakane, I., Taniguchi, M., Hamano, T., Shoji, T., *et al.* (2014) An Overview of Regular Dialysis Treatment in Japan (as of 31 December 2012). *Therapeutic Apheresis and Dialysis*, **18**, 535-602. http://dx.doi.org/10.1111/1744-9987.12281

[2] United States Renal Data System (USRDS) (2014) USRDS Annual Data Report 2014. http://www.usrds.org/2014/view/Default.aspx

[3] Shaw, C., Pitcher, D., Pruthi, R. and Fogarty D. (2014) UK Renal Registry 16th Annual Report: Chapter 2 UK RRT Prevalence in 2012: National and Centre-specific Analyses. *Nephron Clinical Practice*, **125**, 29-53. http://dx.doi.org/10.1159/000360021

[4] The Japan Society for Transplantation, Japanese Society for Clinical Renal Transplantation (2014) Annual Progress Report from the Japanese Renal Transplant Registry: Number of Renal Transplantation in 2013 and Follow-up Survey. *Transplant*, **49**, 240-260. (In Japanese)

[5] Fukuhara, S., Lopes, A.A., Bragg-Gresham, J.L., Kurokawa, K., Mapes, D.L., Akizawa, T., *et al.* (2013) Health-Related Quality of Life among Dialysis Patients on Three Continents: The Dialysis Outcomes and Practice Patterns Study. *Kidney International*, **64**, 1903-1910. http://dx.doi.org/10.1046/j.1523-1755.2003.00289.x

[6] Canaud, B., Tong, L., Tentori, F., Akiba, T., Karaboyas, A., Gillespie, B., *et al.* (2011) Clinical Practices and Outcomes in Elderly Hemodialysis Patients: Results from the Dialysis Outcomes and Practice Patterns Study (DOPPS). *Clinical Journal of the American Society of Nephrology*, **6**, 1651-1662. http://dx.doi.org/10.2215/CJN.03530410

[7] Kinoshita, Y. (2003) Practice of Grounded Theory Approach. Koubundou, Tokyo, 35-46. (In Japanese)

[8] Glaser, B. and Strauss, A. (1967) The Discovery of Grounded Theory: Strategies for Qualitative Research. Transaction Publishers, Edison, 1-18.

[9] Larsen, P.D. (2009) Chronic Illness. 7th Edition, Jones & Bartlett Publishers, Burlington, 35-36.

[10] Crowley-Matoka, M. and Lock, M. (2006) Organ Transplantation in a Globalised World. *Mortality*, **11**, 166-181.

http://dx.doi.org/10.1080/13576270600615310

[11] OECD (2015) Economic Outlook No 97 - June 2015 - OLIS Version. http://stats.oecd.org/viewhtml.aspx?datasetcode=EO97_OUTLOOK97&lang=en

[12] Fukuhara, S., Yamazaki, C., Hayashino, Y., Higashi, T., Eichleay, M.A., Akiba, *et al.* (2007) The Organization and Financing of End-Stage Renal Disease Treatment in Japan. *International Journal of Health Care Finance & Economics*, **7**, 217-231. http://dx.doi.org/10.1007/s10754-007-9017-8

[13] Larsen, P.D. (2015) Labkin's Chronic Illness. 9th Edition, Jones & Bartlett Learning, Burlington, 101-125.

28

A Meaningful Life for Older Persons Receiving Municipal Care—Unit Leaders' Perspectives

Annica Kihlgren

School of Health and Medical Sciences, Örebro University, Örebro, Sweden
Email: annica.kihlgren@oru.se

Abstract

***Introduction*: In Sweden, new national guidelines for elderly care have been introduced containing core values and local guarantees of dignity that highlight the need for dignity, well-being and the organisation of the older person's daily life, so it is perceived as meaningful. Unit leaders play a crucial role in health care organisations when guidelines are to be implemented. *Aim*: The aim was therefore to describe unit leaders' experiences about what constituted a meaningful daily life for older persons receiving municipal care and the opportunities and obstacles that might exist. *Method*: Repeated interviews using reflective conversations with nine leaders were performed and analysed with qualitative content analysis. *Results*: Unit leaders felt a shared vision regarding a meaningful life was needed. Daily routines and habits that promoted independence, a feeling of community together with familiarity with the job, and got the little extra from knowledgeable staff were important. The historical collective paradigm in elderly care needed to be abandoned in favour of one promoting more individualism. Fundamental was the courage to ask the older person what was important and dared to follow through to "*Give power to the older person to decide what care to be given*". *Conclusion*: Organisational conditions affect unit leaders' ability to succeed in the implementation of the work. Further studies are required regarding the nature of the support that the unit leaders need to succeed in their work.**

Keywords

Action Research, Meaningful Daily Life, National Guidelines, Shared Vision

1. Introduction

This article focuses on unit leaders' perspectives on a meaningful daily life for older persons in need of municipal care and is part of a larger action research project [1] initiated as a result of reported shortcomings in Swedish elderly care. The government introduced new national guidelines for elderly care, which included core values and local guarantees of dignity that highlighted the need for dignity, well-being and the organisation of the older person's daily life, so it is perceived as meaningful to them [2]. Elderly care in Sweden is the responsibility of the municipalities and consists of home help service, nursing home care and home care in ordinary homes. The government gave each municipality the responsibility for the creation of its own guidelines, local guarantees and for the implementation of those guidelines.

Unit leaders play a crucial role in all health care organizations when guidelines are to be implemented. They affect both the quality of the care and the working environment [3]. The changes that have occurred and are taking place in elderly care have resulted in complex organisations, instability and uncertainty that must be addressed [4]. In addition, the number of leaders in elderly care has declined leaving fewer that are responsible for a larger number of staff. Staff education has also been questioned [5] and with inadequate skills, there is a risk that national and local targets for health care will not be met.

When introducing guidelines in elderly care, there is a need for shared visions among those working there. Hersey and Blanchard [6] state that once a leader has clarified and shared the vision, they can focus on serving and being responsive to the needs of the people with the understanding that the role of leadership is to remove barriers and help others achieve the vision. According to McCormack & McCance [7], the visions are the desired outcomes for person-centred practice stem from a therapeutic environment where the decision making is shared, staff members work collaboratively, leadership is transformational and there is support for innovative processes.

How leaders perceive relationships within the team and the impact of these relationships on practice is critical to the way that an effective practice context is created [8]. Leaders' attitudes influence how they administer, which will affect the staffs' possibility to implement the changes necessary to create meaningful daily lives for older persons.

There are few studies on perceived meaning-in-life among older persons receiving home care, but studies from those receiving nursing home care show that it is significantly associated with the physical, emotional, social, and functional well-being quality of life dimensions [9]. What constitutes a meaningful daily life for older persons, from the perspective of the older person, the relatives and the enrolled nurses, has been reported in the action research project [10]-[13]. However there is a lack of knowledge from the leaders perspective on what constitutes a meaningful life and how it can be created for older persons receiving municipal care. The aim of the present study was therefore to describe unit leaders' experiences about what constituted a meaningful daily life for older persons receiving municipal care and which opportunities and obstacles might exist.

2. Method

2.1. Design

The study was part of a larger action research project and combined the approach of Participatory Appreciative Action Reflection (PAAR) [14] and qualitative methods. The project aimed to seek opportunities and obstacles for the development of a meaningful daily life from the perspective of the older person by working together with them, their relatives, staff and leaders. Another aim was to use these data to formulate core values and local guarantees of dignity [1]. There were 20 repeated interviews in the form of reflective conversations with nine leaders. The leaders provided their analyses and reflections on what had been said regarding a meaningful daily life for older persons. Finally, an analysis of the data was performed by the researcher, based on a latent content analysis [15]. The regional Ethical Review Board in Uppsala approved the research project (Reg. No. 2011/009).

2.2. Participants

Recruited from one municipality in Sweden was the chief manager responsible for developing elderly care and leaders from five randomly selected nursing homes (n = 5) and three home care units (n = 3). A list of the nursing homes and home care groups based on the results of a user survey that rated the quality of the eldercare as favourable, average and low was used [16], to achieve variation [17]. The three home care units had received favourable, average, and low ratings in the user survey; among the nursing homes, two received favourable ratings, one had an average rating and two had low ratings. The leaders held leader positions at each unit and were responsible for the implementation of the guidelines as well as the core values and local guarantees at their units. There were seven women and two men with a mean age of 45 years (range 28 - 50) that had worked as units leaders between two and ten years.

2.3. Data Collection

The research was built on a co-creation of data and knowledge, focusing on the leaders' experiences of how meaningful daily life is envisioned by older persons. Seven leaders participated twice and two on three occasions in interviews conducted by the author. The leaders chose the time and location of the interviews, and all were carried out in their office.

The repeated interviews were conducted as reflective conversations on what factors could be important for a meaningful daily life thus leaving the direction of the conversation open [18]. The main questions were: *what is a meaningful daily life for an older person, and what can be the opportunities and obstacles to a meaningful daily life.* The interviews were digitally recorded and transcribed verbatim. The leaders read the transcriptions before the second and third interview; then together with the interviewer provided their analyses and reflections on the content of what had been said regarding a meaningful daily life. In the second and third interview, follow-up questions were asked such as: *what thoughts have you had about this since the last time we met, and do you remember what you mean by that.* These conversations were also recorded and transcribed verbatim.

2.4. Analysis

To analyse the data a qualitative content analysis was performed in steps [15]. The author first read the transcripts several times to acquire a general sense of the whole. Meaning units related to the same central meaning and relevant to the aim of the study were identified. The meaning units were then condensed into a description close to the text to grasp the manifest content. In the next step, the underlying meaning of the condensed meaning units was interpreted to determine the latent content, which was then coded. The codes were then compared and checked for differences and similarities; after which they were sorted into subthemes and five themes. The latent content in the themes was summarized and an overall theme emerged that described the leaders' experiences of what creates a meaningful daily life for older persons. The research group repeated the examination and discussion of the results during the analysis to ensure the trustworthiness of the data analysis and establish the best form for presentation.

3. Results

The leaders' experiences and reflections over what constitutes a meaningful daily life for older persons receiving municipal care were interpreted and five themes emerged: *Routines and habits are important for a meaningful daily life, Have the possibility to feel independent, Familiarity with the job and that little extra promotes meaningful daily lives, Community creates a meaningful daily life, and Understanding and accepting the history of elderly care.*

The themes constitute the unit leaders' perspectives of meaningful daily lives for older persons and the opportunities and obstacles that could exist. To give power to older persons over what care to be given was seen as a goal. The older person and the team around them working together would develop a care plan based on a shared vision on what a meaningful daily life was. Routines and habits were important as was the ability to feel as independent as possible. Knowledge and a good familiarity with the job, doing that little extra and a feeling of community were considered to be significant elements. The leaders felt elderly care should leave the collective thinking paradigm behind and strive for more individualised care. A place to start this process was to come to terms with the history of elderly care.

3.1. Routines and Habits Are Important for a Meaningful Daily Life

The leaders saw an opportunity for meaningfulness with routines that meshed with the habits and needs of the older person. For example: the importance of continued training to maintain or regain lost functions, being able to eat what the old person preferred, and having surroundings in a familiar manner. The leaders could see the necessity of good working routines but a degree of flexibility was important to ensure some individuality and opportunities for spontaneity.

"*We must have routines, but we can't create—your life should not be lived from our routines instead it's what's around your life that we set up our routines for, so that it will be safe and secure and function. You should be able to wake up in the morning and think; it would be really fun to go and take a look at the castle. But we can't have routines for that. But we can have routines for free time so that we can do it.*"

Knowledge of the older person's life story is an important key for shaping the routines around them. The leaders felt communication with older persons and their relatives would enhance their ability to individualise routines and create meaningfulness.

3.2. Have the Possibility to Feel Independent

A meaningful daily life from the leaders' perspectives was the ability of the older person to manage on their own and take care of themselves with as little help as possible. The leaders felt it was important if the older person was able to do things like: get out of bed, perform their own personal hygiene, dress and go to breakfast. The leaders also expressed that a meaningful life with dignity could be created by decreasing the staffs' physical presence as much as possible. With the use of security alarm systems, safety and security can be maintained without stifling older persons' freedom.

"*Meaningfulness and dignity can be created without our presence, take for example a security alarm, just by having it leads to an increased independence.*"

An opportunity for a meaningful life could be missed if the older person is prevented from living as they are accustomed because the staff considers the life style peculiar.

"*Sometimes we can wrinkle our nose when we meet people that have chosen to live a life we think is strange. We shouldn't sit ourselves in judgement over that. It is also dignified to let people live the life as they have lived, even if it doesn't conform to our model.*"

The leaders saw it as an opportunity for a meaningful life when their staff was able to interact with the older persons or their relatives and encourage them to do as much as possible for themselves. Obstacles occurred when the staff had difficulties communicating with the relatives and getting them to cooperate. There were also situations when the leaders felt their staff became locked in their routines and did not take advantage of the relatives' wishes to be involved in the care.

3.3. Familiarity with the Job and that Little Extra Promotes Meaningful Daily Lives

The leaders often reflected in the interviews on the importance of having staff that know what to do. To create meaningful daily lives it was important with both theoretical and clinical knowledge. It was also important that the knowledge was used effectively and in a dedicated manner. The leaders talked about a familiarity with the job among the staff, which can be very difficult to teach.

"*Some personnel just do it right and I don't think it's only something they have in them, rather it is an ability all people can cultivate in different ways, but can be difficult to teach. As such we can find ourselves in a situation where it is demanded that I appear, behave and relate in a certain way—that conveys a form of dignity, everyone can relearn.*"

All the leaders saw an opportunity for a meaningful daily life when the enrolled nurse felt a sense of responsibility for the older person and took pride in their work. Furthermore creating meaning in daily life is not only about what is done on a daily basis, but when something special is done. "To do that little extra."

"*Yes, a person thinks that all this is so special. A person thinks these small things aren't anything. To have the ability to eat and drink. That these basic things work. And if there is some problem with some of these basic things, that they be remedied.*"

Opportunities for a meaningful daily life could be found in the staffs' dedication to the older persons. They reflected over the importance of getting to know the individual staff members and the most effective way to work with and lead them on a more personal level.

"*A person that thinks it is fun to go to work. A person that thinks it is fun to meet the elderly in the morning: wonder what mood that pensioner is in today. What shape are they in today? What can we do? And that's in your genes in some way. I can't explain it. It is fantastic. And then there are those others that know they have to do certain things. But only because there are written routines.*"

According to one leader, when the staff use themselves as a tool in body and mind it could be an opportunity to create meaningfulness for older persons. But it could also turn into an obstacle if the staff member was having a bad day.

"*The body as a tool when I work. And if I should feel so bad that I can't manage that role, I need to stay home sick that day. If I am sad and depressed and can't leave it behind me when I walk in, it can't be allowed to spread, because if it does then the one laying in the bed will be infected.*"

The leaders also saw it as an obstacle when they as a leader did not dare to admit that some staff members were locked in the routines and were unable to remove their own values and expectations from the situation.

"*But if we don't dare to admit that rather many of the older staff especially, have worked a long time in elderly care, then our efforts will fail, how should we continue working to bring about meaningfulness?*"

3.4. Community Creates a Meaningful Daily Life

The feeling of community was considered important to create meaningful daily lives for older persons and the leaders reflected on staff that took time to for example sit down and drink coffee together with them.

"*At a doctor visit—accompanying with a doctor visit—that a person takes their time and sits down at the clinic and drinks a cup of coffee together. That's important.*"

Another opportunity for a meaningful daily life was when the staff creates alliances with older persons and relationships develop that lead to a feeling of community. The leaders also thought to achieve a meaningful daily life, the relatives should have increased involvement in the care of the older person. An obstacle arose when the staff had difficulties getting the relatives to cooperate.

"*It is difficult to accept. An example is that it is difficult to accept criticism. Eh-em... I have many co-workers and enrolled nurses that have a hard time listening to relatives.*"

One leader also pointed out that it was important not to pass judgement on the relationship between older persons and their relatives as there may be things in the family history they are not aware of. This leader also emphasized that the older persons were not complaining but instead felt sorry for the staff.

"*It is the relatives and the older persons that say to me sometimes; yea, it hasn't really been so good, I must talk to you about it. But, you can't blame the staff because they are so hard working and do the best they can. And you have to feel sorry for the personnel.*"

3.5. Understanding and Accepting the History of Elderly Care

According to the leaders one place to start with was to try to understand the history of elderly care and accept it. They described how important it was to remember how it was previously and which guidelines governed the care.

"*Our history influences us greatly. With the* 1992 *reform, long-term-care moved with all of its routines into another house that perhaps didn't look much like a hospital setting, but we took everything else with us. If we admit that, we can put our efforts into where it's seen the most.*"

With the acceptance of the history and changes within long-term-care the leaders felt they could understand why the staff sometimes acted as they did and could better initiate solutions and help support the staff to create meaningful daily lives for older persons.

"*And if we don't admit that it is so, then we continue without paying attention to the past into something new. To me that's dangerous. We must bring the history with us, we must dare to admit that that's how it was. It is first then we can identify: what's gone wrong. It has gone wrong for a person that shows clear tendencies of working undignified—as per definition dignity—however that should be. A person must look at that: why is it so?*"

The history is permeated by collectivism. Collective elderly care became an obstacle to individualised care. The leaders felt that with this history there was a risk that older persons could lose their dignity and the staff might interact accordingly. Another obstacle for a meaningful daily life was when the older person lost in the collective whole was a subject to depersonalized waiting.

"*There are nine people in a group, it's clear that of those nine there is someone that wants to sleep longer and another that likes to go up earlier. So there is a naturalness in it. But if you think about every morning here, Monday thru Friday there are three staff that should help nine people. And then some get help first and some get help last.*"

The question that needed to be reflected on as a team was: how to approach the concept of meaningfulness, dignity and individualised care. There is the experience of meaningfulness and dignity; there is no real recipe or measurement that will apply to everyone.

"*The knowledge part is the easiest part, to increase knowledge. The difficult part I think is to twist it and achieve individualisation. Nursing homes are per definition a collective solution for those that don't manage to live at home. It is a collective solution, but we must try to individualise the entire collective solution.*"

4. Discussion

This study highlights five areas that are important to create a meaningful daily life for older persons receiving municipal care. To start with the leaders felt it was important to be in agreement with what a meaningful daily life was for the older persons, and together with all the stakeholders find a common solution. A balance was needed in the daily routines that gave the older person the ability to feel as independent as possible. Familiarity with the job and the staff knowing what to do was important as was doing that little extra and creating a feeling of community for the older persons. Accepting the history of elderly care and abandoning the old doctrine of collectivism was considered necessary in order to develop care based on the new guidelines. The leaders felt that much is based on the vision for elderly care; to have the courage to ask the older person what is important and then dare to follow through to: "*Give power to the older person to decide what care is to be given*".

The leaders view on creating a meaningful daily life differs somewhat from the results of the larger project [1] as they were more focused on the staffs' involvement. The older persons living in nursing homes talk about having space to be themselves, a sense of belonging and a feeling of security. Obstacles to a meaningful day were the absence of space and feelings of insecurity. There was a longing for something to happen [10]. Older persons living at home with homecare actualise their own meaningful daily life by striving to maintain their routines and habits, and live their lives as normal as possible. They struggled between handling the increased demands and accomplishing everyday activities. The older persons created a reciprocity and collaboration with the staff to achieve a meaningful daily life. The ongoing dialogue between the older person and the staff becomes "the glue". Furthermore, for a meaningful daily life it was important to have a sense of belonging, a sense of closeness and togetherness, to retain previous relationships as well as establish new ones [11]. To maintain routines, habits and an everyday rhythm filled with meaning in a home like environment and in community with others, relatives felt a partnership was needed between the older person, their family members and the staff. [12]. Enrolled nurses create a meaningful daily life by being perceptive and responding accordingly to the older person. They read the older person in order to judge how the person is feeling, adapt to their daily life and share it with them [13]. The different stakeholders seem to share the same values regarding space to be yourself, habits and routines and a feeling of community to create a meaningful daily life for older persons. However the leaders differed somewhat with the other stakeholders in that they reflected over the importance of having a common vision, understanding and accepting the history and the individualisation of the collective solution in elderly care. This difference is understandable as they were the ones responsible for implementing the guidelines in their units and were more focused on how to lead to succeed with the work. However to succeed they might be more aware on their own role as leadership seems to be one of the key factors for implementation success. Their ability to create a culture receptive to evidence-based knowledge seems to be essential, together with their ability and willingness to provide feedback and to lead by own good example. A strong and clear leadership does not by it selves create changes. A supporting organization and a favorable culture also affect the process [19].

The results show that a common vision of a meaningful daily life is needed in order to shift the power regarding care to the older person, which is in line with person centred care that highlights a need for shared values [20]. Hersey and Blanchard [6] point out that when everyone supports the organizational vision it creates a deliberate focused culture that drives the desired outcomes. This is in accordance with McCormack & McCance [7] and their idea of the shared visions being the desired person-centred outcomes of: satisfaction with care, involvement with care, feeling of well-being and creating a therapeutic culture in which decision-making is shared, staff relationships are collaborative, leadership is transformational and innovative practices are supported.

The leaders in this study felt that understanding and accepting previous history, guidelines and practices was important. They saw the history permeated by collectivism that could become an obstacle to individualised care. The leaders felt that with this history there was a risk that older persons could lose their dignity and the staff might interact accordingly. Another obstacle was when the older person lost in the collective whole was a subject to depersonalized waiting. This can be seen as a collective memory existing among the stakeholders, one that is influenced by the history of elderly care, with a common knowledge [21] or shared experienced [22] within a group. The collective memory and the values it encompasses are shaped and reshaped by different processes and is influenced by various factors and actors [23]. In this dimension will it be important that the leaders choose the right tools for the implementation. Further investigation is needed on how to influence a new collective memory among all stakeholders where the older person has more power in their care.

Care for older persons in Sweden underwent significant changes during the 1990s when there was a reduction in the number of public nursing homes. Successive reductions in services for the majority of older persons and a pronounced trend to first help the oldest of older persons and those most in need of help was evident. This in turn has meant that persons who live in public nursing homes have become more dependent on health care efforts. Simultaneously, municipal problems with financing public care have increased. There seems to be a need to adopt a caring approach geared to meeting the needs that create meaningful spaces and places with person-centred care, and is something that requires further investigation. McCance *et al.* [24] show that patients and staff recognize moments of person-centeredness but there are long periods where person-centeredness is not the dominant focus in daily life.

The organizational conditions that these leaders have will affect their ability to succeed in the implementation of the work. There is a lack of knowledge on how managers can promote the implementation and probably not fruitful to study characteristics of the leader without taking into account the organization where the person works and its cultural climate. Success with implementation seems to be depended on the interaction between these three components [20]. There are often short-term solutions in the development of elderly care, therefore whatever resources the leaders have available must be used wisely. Despite hard savings in Swedish elderly care that have led to "slim downed" organizations, Larsson [25] explains in her thesis that there is room for development within the majority of the organizations. This requires however that the unit leaders prioritize the question of what is important, create space for creativity and flexibility, develop shared visions, and create time for learning and reflection.

5. Methodological Consideration

In action research it is important that the participants take part as co-researchers [26]. In the present study, the leaders can be seen as co-researchers in the collection of data. Thus, they were able to change, delete or advise shortcomings as well as add to the data. To achieve credibility in the study, in the repeated interviews the authors continually discussed and reflected together with the leaders. The results contain direct quotations, which give the reader an opportunity to judge the credibility. To strengthen credibility the same opening question was asked in each interview regarding what a meaningful daily life is for an older person [11]. The number of leaders who took part could be considered small. According to Sandelowski [27], the sample size in qualitative research should be large enough to achieve a variation of experiences and small enough to permit a deep analysis of the data. A strength, however, could be the repeated interviews, which totalled 20. The leaders considered participation in the research valuable and considered it to be a positive experience.

6. Conclusions

When implementing guidelines to create a meaningful daily life for older persons, the leaders in this study expressed that there was a need to start with a shared vision based on the guidelines. Understanding and accepting the history of elderly care are necessary if change is to occur. Routines and habits were important for the older persons as was the ability to feel as independent as possible. Knowledge and a good familiarity with the job, doing that little extra and a feeling of community were considered to be significant elements. The leaders felt that much was based on the vision for elderly care; to have the courage to ask the older person what was important for a meaningful daily life and then dared to follow through "*Give power to the older person to decide what care is to be given*".

The leaders felt elderly care should leave the collective paradigm behind and strive for more individualised care. The organizational conditions that these leaders will affect their ability to succeed in the implementation of the work. Further studies are required regarding the nature of the support that the unit leaders need to succeed in their work.

Conflict of Interest

The author declares no conflicts of interest.

Acknowledgements

The author is grateful for the participation of the leaders in the study. This study was supported by grants from Örebro University.

References

[1] James, I., Blomberg, K., Liljekvist, E. and Kihlgren, A. (2015) Working Together for a Meaningful Day for Older Persons: A Participatory and Appreciative Action and Reflection Project—The Lesson We Have Learned. *Action Research*, **2015**, 1-18.

[2] Swedish Ministry of Health and Social Affairs (2014) Government Office of Sweden. How It Works in Sweden. Stockholm, Sweden. http://www.government.se/government-of-sweden/ministry-of-health-and-social-affairs/

[3] McGuire, E. and Kennerly, S.M. (206) Nurse Managers as Transformational and Transactional Leaders. *Nursing Economics*, **24**, 179-185, 175.

[4] Anthony, A. and Milone-Nuzzo, P. (2005) Factors Attracting and Keeping Nurses in Home Care. *Home Healthcare Nurse*, **23**, 372-377. http://dx.doi.org/10.1097/00004045-200506000-00009

[5] National Board of Health and Welfare (2012) National Strategy for Approach to Eldercare Interim Report II. 2012 (In Swedish: Nationell tillsyn av vård och omsorg om äldre. Delrapport II. 2012). Stockholm, Sweden. http://www.ivo.se/globalassets/dokument/publicerat-material/rapporter/tillsynsrapporter/nationell-tillsyn-av-vard-och-omsorg-om-aldre-delrapport-2.pdf

[6] Hersey, P.K. and Blanchard, K. (1997) Management of Organizational Behavior: Utilizing Human Resources. Prentice Hall, Englewood Cliffs.

[7] McCormack, B. (2010) Person-Centred Nursing. Theory and Practice. John Wiley & Sons Ltd., Chichester. http://dx.doi.org/10.1002/9781444390506

[8] Rycroft-Malone, J., Harvey, J., Kitson, A., McCormack, B., Seers, K. and Titchen, A. (2002) Getting Evidence into Practice: Ingredients for Change. *Nursing Standard*, **16**, 38-43. http://dx.doi.org/10.7748/ns2002.05.16.37.38.c3201

[9] Haugan, G. (2013) Meaning-in-Life in Nursing-Home Patients: A Valuable Approach for Enhancing Psychological and Physical Well-Being? *Journal of Clinical Nursing*, **23**, 1830-1844. http://dx.doi.org/10.1111/jocn.12402

[10] James, I., Blomberg, K. and Kihlgren, A. (2014) A Meaningful Daily Life in Nursing Homes, a Place of Shelter and a Space of Freedom. A Participatory Appreciative Action Reflection Study. *BMC Nursing*, **13**, 19. http://dx.doi.org/10.1186/1472-6955-13-19

[11] Kihlgren, A., Blomberg, K. and James, I. (2014) A Reciprocal Relationship—An Opportunity and a Solution for a Meaningful Daily Life in Home Care—The Older Person's Perspective. *Clinical Nursing Studies*, **3**.

[12] Windahl, J., Kihlgren, A., Liedström, E. and James I. (2014) A Meaningful Daily Life in Nursing Homes and Home Care—The Relatives' Perspective. *Clinical Nursing Studies*, **2**. http://dx.doi.org/10.5430/cns.v2n4p129

[13] James, I., Fredriksson, C., Wahlström, C., Kihlgren, A. and Blomberg, K. (2014) To Have an Ordinary Day: Nurse Assistants' Experiences and Knowledge about How to Create a Meaningful Daily Life in Nursing Homes. *The Open Nursing Journal*, **8**, 34-42. http://dx.doi.org/10.2174/1874434601408010034

[14] Ghaye, T., Melander-Wikman, A., Kisare, M., Chambers, P., Bergmark, U., Kostenius, C. and Lillyman, S. (2008) Participatory and Appreciative Action and Reflection (PAAR): Democratizing Reflective Practices. *Reflective Practice*, **9**, 361-397. http://dx.doi.org/10.1080/14623940802475827

[15] Graneheim, U.H. and Lundman, B. (2004) Qualitative Content Analysis in Nursing Research: Concepts, Procedures and Measures to Achieve Trustworthiness. *Nurse Education Today*, **24**, 105-112. http://dx.doi.org/10.1016/j.nedt.2003.10.001

[16] Örebro Municipality (2010) Inflytande och delaktighet inom hemvården och särskilda boenden. Brukarundersökning särskilda boenden och hemvården 2010 (Influence and Participation in Nursing Homes and Home Care). Social Welfare Örebro Municipality, Örebro. http://www.orebro.se/download/18.47c6f44f12dd9e971378000211 5/S%C3%A4rskilda+boenden+f%C3%B6r+%C3%A4ldre%2C+deras+anh%C3%B6riga+och+hemv%C3%A5rden+hela+unders%C3%B6kningen+-+brukarunders%C3%B6kning+2010.pdf

[17] Patton, M.Q. (2002) Qualitative Research & Evaluation Methods. 3rd Edition, Sage, London.

[18] Gadamer, H.-G., Weinsheimer, J. and Marshall, D.G. (2004) Truth and Method. 2nd Edition, Continuum International Publishing Group, London.

[19] Sandström, B., Borglin, G., Nilsson, R. and Willman, A. (2011) Promoting the Implementation of Evidence-Based Practice: A Literature Review Focusing on the Role of Nursing Leadership. *World Views on Evidence-Based Nursing*,

8, 212-223. http://dx.doi.org/10.1111/j.1741-6787.2011.00216.x

[20] McCormack, B. (2004) Person-Centredness in Gerontological Nursing: An Overview of the Literature. *Journal of Clinical Nursing*, **13**, 31-38. http://dx.doi.org/10.1111/j.1365-2702.2004.00924.x

[21] Jimerson, R.C. (2009) Archives Power: Memory, Accountability, and Social Justice. Society of American Archivists, USA.

[22] Millar, L. (2006) Touchstones: Considering the Relationship between Memory and Archives. *Archivaria*, **61**, 105-126.

[23] Piggott, M. (2005) Archives and Memory. In: McKemmish, I.S., Piggott, M., Reed, B. and Upward, F., Eds., *Archives: Recordkeeping in Society*, Centre for Information Studies, Charles Sturt University, Wagga Wagga, 299-328. http://dx.doi.org/10.1016/b978-1-876938-84-0.50012-3

[24] McCance, T., Gribben, B., McCormack, B. and Laird, E.A. (2013) Promoting Person-Centred Practice within Acute Care: The Impact of Culture and Context on a Facilitated Practice Development Programme. *International Practice Development Journal*, **3**. http://www.fons.org/Resources/Documents/Journal/Vol3No1/IDPJ_0301_02.pdf

[25] Larsson, K. (2008) Mellanchefer som utvecklar: Om förutsättningar för hållbart arbete inom vård och omsorg (Unit Leaders Who Develop Conditions for Sustainable Work in Health Care). Doctoral Dissertation, Linkoping University, Linköping.

[26] Bradbury-Huang, H. (2010) What Is Good Action Research? Why the Resurgent Interest? *Action Research*, **8**, 93-109. http://dx.doi.org/10.1177/1476750310362435

[27] Sandelowski, M. (1995) Sample Size in Qualitative Research. *Research in Nursing & Health*, **18**, 179-183. http://dx.doi.org/10.1002/nur.4770180211

29

Quantitative Analysis of Pain during Mammography Using Electrical Stimulation

Mieko Uchiyama, Yongbum Lee, Utako Shimizu, Rika Saitoh

Graduate School of Health Sciences, Niigata University, Niigata, Japan
Email: Uchiyama@clg.niigata-u.ac.jp

Abstract

In order to quantitatively measure the degree of pain during mammography, we used a visual analog scale (VAS) and a device for quantitative analysis of perception and pain and performed regression analysis of the relationship between pain degree and VAS score. Twenty-four subjects underwent a typical mammogram and we found no correlation between pain degree using the device compared with VAS scoring. It is presumed that the system enables quantitative measurement and comparison more accurately than subjective markers such as VAS in quantitation of a pain produced in an examination with clearly defined physical size (such as mammography).

Keywords

Mammography, Pain Degree, Electrical Stimulation, Visual Analog Scale

1. Introduction

Mammography is widely performed as a standard breast cancer screening method in Japan and Western countries. In mammography, after the papillary glands are adequately stretched, the breast is compressed with a radiolucent paddle for fixation and a reduction in the breast thickness. In examinees undergoing mammography, not only breast compression but also fixation with the neck being rotated or the shoulder being flexed is necessary. These imaging techniques reduce X-ray exposure and ensure the image quality necessary for diagnosis [1].

Mammography screening, which is considered to be of the greatest benefit for early detection of breast cancer, is widely performed as a standardized procedure [2] [3]. Mammography is a radiological test during which the breast is compressed by parallel plates to make breast tissue as even and as thin as possible. Along with compression of the breast, positioning during mammography such as twisting the neck and keeping the arms up is burdensome. It is well known that mammography screening is physically hard on a woman. Many women feel the physical burden during mammography as pain [4]-[8].

The International Association for the Study of Pain (IASP) defined a pain as "an unpleasant sensory and emotional experience associated with actual or potential tissue damage, or described in terms of such damage" [9]. Therefore, when a pain is measured in humans, multiple areas including emotional and cognitive/evaluative aspects need to be taken into account comprehensively, in addition to the sensory aspects such as the intensity and location of a pain identified by the subject.

As for the physical and psychological burden experienced by the examinees at the time of mammography positioning, we have previously demonstrated empirically the relationship between muscle activity and pain based on the imaging method and the process of imaging [10]-[12]. Based on these results, we reported that patients experience more than moderate pain from the start of positioning through the entire course of breast compression and immobilization and that pain also occurs at sites other than the breast.

In the past, researchers have used subjective methods to assess pain in subjects undergoing mammography. Sharp *et al.* [13] used the visual analog scale (VAS) [14] [15] and Hafslund *et al.* [7] have used the McGill Pain Questionnaire [16]. Although subjective assessment of pain is widely used, it is regarded as inaccurate because it lacks objectivity and reproducibility. This has led to the invention of a method to quantitatively assess pain by applying electrical stimulation and comparing the pain sensation with the sensation of the stimulus [17]. They were those used to measure the pain during mammography. In this study, we quantitatively measured the degree of pain during mammography using this method.

2. Methods

The study included 24 healthy women. Their mean age was 24.0 ± 6.4 years, mean height was 159.5 ± 6.6 cm, and mean weight was 52.2 ± 5.6 kg. Of the 24 subjects, 2 had previously undergone mammography, and 22 had never had mammograms.

The subjects were given explanation on the study objectives, methods, and safety, and their informed consent was obtained. This study was conducted with the approval of the Research Ethics Committee of Niigata University School of Medicine (Approval Number 1946).

For this study, mammography was carried out only up to the completion of positioning, including compression of the breast, and the tissue was not x-rayed. Only positioning for the mediolateral oblique view of the right breast was performed. After the sham mammogram, a device for quantitative analysis of perception and pain (Pain Vision™ PS-2100; NIPRO Co. Ltd., Japan: Pain Vision™) was used to measure the degree of pain from mammography; at the same time, the subject assessments on the VAS were recorded. The criterion for judging pain measured was defined as maximum pain experienced upon compression of the breast during mammography. Typical thing in subjective pain measurement is VAS. This study is to compare the measured values of the quantitative pain and determination of subjective pain.

The sensory and pain analyzer Pain Vision™ emits a stimulatory electric current from an electrode attached to the skin; this pulsed electric current (50 - 3000 Hz; 0 - 150 μAms; pulse width, 0.03 mA) consists of not only single waves, but differential waves with a sharp tip. With electric stimulation, the pain threshold is measurable with the analyzer. The wave frequency emitted from the system stimulates Aβ fibers and some Aδ fibers of sensory nerves. A single wave with a sharp edge enables efficient stimulation of Aβ fibers and provides the subject with heteresthesia without pain [18].

The principle of measurement is based on the inability of humans to separately evaluate pain at more than one site simultaneously. At measurement, the minimum sensed electric current is measured three times, and the average electric current is defined as the minimum sensed threshold. Next, an electric current for electric stimulation is gradually increased and the subject is asked to push a button to indicate when he/she felt comparable pain intensity. That electric current level is defined as the pain-equivalent electric current. The reason why the minimum sensible electric current threshold is set up is to eliminate any inter-individual difference in recognizing relative positioning of electrodes and subcutaneous nerves and sensing it in the brain. With this system, "pain intensity" is calculated based on the pain equivalent electric current obtained in this manner and the minimum sensible electric current threshold according to the following formula (1).

$$\text{Pain degree} = \frac{(\text{a pain equivalent electric current} - \text{a minimum sensible threshold})}{\text{a minimum threshold}} \tag{1}$$

For measurement, a disposable distal electrode (EL-BAND, NIPRO) is attached on the medial side of the arm,

1 cm from the midpoint between the center of the bend of the elbow and the center of the wrist on the flexor side of the forearm (**Figure 1**). Pain degree of the measurement results are displayed in the bottom left of the screen (**Figure 2**).

The VAS is an assessment method of pain due to subjective factors. The subjects were asked to point to a position along a 100-mm line with 1-mm increments, its left end (0 points) representing "no pain" and right end (100 points) representing "worst pain imaginable," to indicate the level of pain they are experiencing as a score. **Figure 3** shows a diagram of the VAS. The participants were asked to point with their finger to the level of pain they were feeling during whole mammography.

Regression analysis was performed to define the relationship between degree of pain and VAS score. Statistical analyses were performed using SPSS 19J for Windows and the significance level was set at less than 0.05.

3. Results

For the 24 subjects studied, the mean VAS score (and standard deviation) during mammography was 51.0 ± 28.0, and the mean degree of pain value (and standard deviation) was 388.7 ± 355.0. A guideline for moderate to severe pain on the VAS is a score of ≥40, and the results of our study showed that the subjects had experienced at least moderate pain during mammography. Degree of pain can be said, in theory, to be "no pain" if the score is between 0 and 100, and a "perceivable quantity of stimulus" if the score is >100, suggesting that the subjects in our study experienced intense pain during mammography. However, there was a wide variation in values on the degree of pain measurement.

The relationship between VAS and degree of pain was $y = 68.10x + 23.766$, $r^2 = 0.289$ ($p < 0.01$), which showed no correlation (**Figure 4**). The values vary considerably, including cases where the VAS score was >60 although the degree of pain was <100, and cases where the degree of pain > 200 although the VAS score was <10.

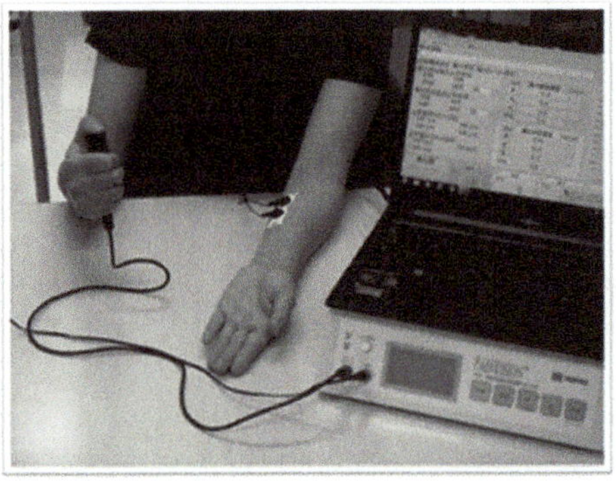

Figure 1. Measurements of pain degree that depends on the pain vision. For measurement, a disposable distal electrode (EL-BAND, NIPRO) is attached on the medial side of the arm, 1 cm from the midpoint between the center of the bend of the elbow and the center of the wrist on the flexor side of the forearm. An electric current for electric stimulation is gradually increased and the subject is asked to push a button.

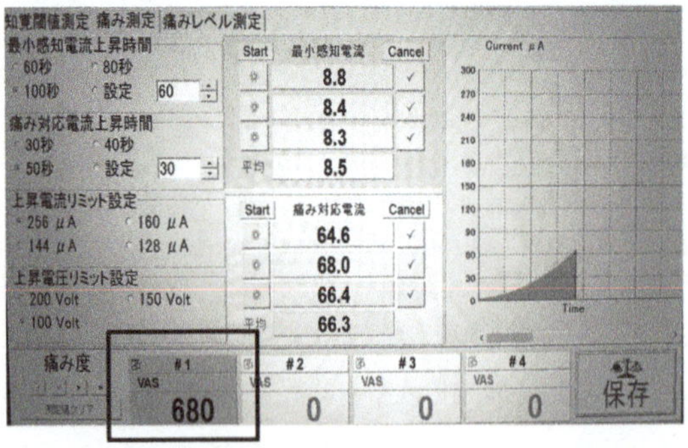

Figure 2. Computer display screen at the time of pain degree measurement. Displayed of minimum sensing current value (current perception threshold), pain corresponding current value and pain degree in Japanese version.

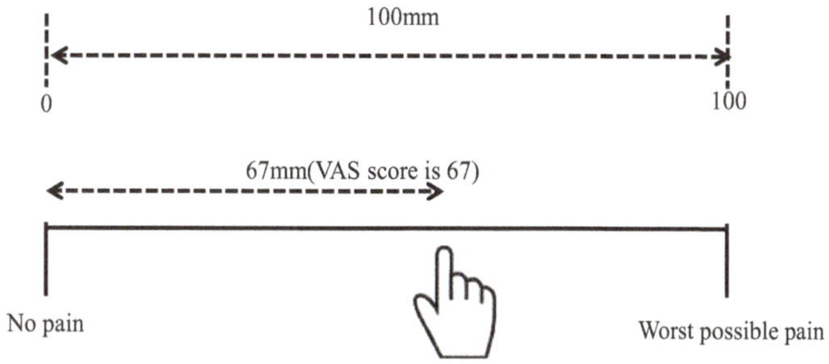

Figure 3. Visual analog scale for subjective pain assessment.

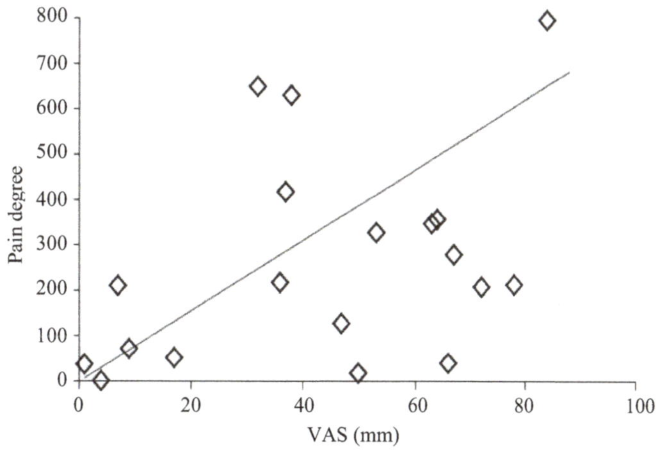

Figure 4. The correlation coefficient of the degree of pain during mammography assessed by degree of pain evaluation and VAS score.

4. Discussion

Whereas the VAS score is assessed within a range of 0 to 100, the degree of pain (without such range) can assess pain of a similar degree, as induced pain is converted to the pain one is actually experiencing. In situations where pain is largely affected by mental factors, VAS scores judge pain that has been subjectively overrated; however, the degree of pain score is considered to be less affected by psychological factors, because it can assess the degree of pain from a physical stimulus actually applied by the device.

A study on the effects of pain treatment using Pain Vision™ versus VAS scoring showed a strong correlation between the VAS score and degree of pain [19]. In our study, no significant correlation between the VAS score and degree of pain was found. This may have been due to psychological factors related to mammography and the temporal error caused by the delay between mammography and measurement of pain. However, one subject showed a moderate pain score of 40 on the VAS, whereas her pain degree score was high (approximately 700). Although the values vary between individuals, quantified measurements of pain or strain may allow for examination of various factors of pain during mammography. Further investigation of a greater number of subjects is needed.

This suggests that they influenced not only the pain and burden associated with breast compression directly involved in mammography but also a physical burden on the whole body and a psychological burden continuously present from the time before the screening, and were related to the results we had previously verified [20]-[23].

The results of this study suggested a few candidate situations for using the Pain Vision™ system. The first situation is in combination with a visual analog scale (VAS). As shown in the definition of pain by IASP, a pain is not measurable based solely on physical size. Since there is a difference in subjective sense of a pain, the threshold of a pain changes.

However, it is presumed that the system enables quantitative measurement and comparison more accurately than subjective markers such as VAS in quantitation of a pain produced in an examination with clearly defined physical size (such as mammography). It is thought that a combination with VAS is useful for elucidation of not only pain intensity but also the nature of a pain.

The other situation is evaluation of the benefit of care when intervention is considered for reduction of a pain. It is expected that the system will be used as a common tool in a large-scale survey for measurement of the effect because of the portability and potential availability of the equipment.

5. Conclusion

We quantitatively measured the degree of pain during mammography using Pain Vision™ and compared it to VAS scores. Twenty-four subjects underwent mammography and we found no correlation between degree of pain and VAS score. In the future, we believe that we should be verified in a larger number of samples.

Conflict of Interest

The authors declare that they have no conflict of interest.

Acknowledgements

This work was supported by JSPS KAKENHI Grant Numbers 26463372.

References

[1] Henrich, R.E., Baett, L., Botsco, M.A., Deibei, D., Feig, S. and Gray, J. (1999) Mammography Quality Control Manual: Patient Positioning and Compression. *American College of Radiology*, 30-75.

[2] Drukker, B.H. (1997) Breast Disease: A Primer on Diagnosis and Management. *International Journal of Fertility and Women's Medicine*, **42**, 278-287.

[3] Kerlikowske, K., Grady, D., Rubin, S.M., Sandrock, C. and Ernster, V.L. (1995) Efficacy of Screening Mammography. A Meta-Analysis. *Journal of the American Medical Association*, **273**, 149-154. http://dx.doi.org/10.1001/jama.1995.03520260071035

[4] Aro, A.R., Absetz-Ylöstalo, P., Eerola, T., Pamilo, M. and Lönnqvist, J. (1996) Pain and Discomfort during Mammography. *European Journal of Cancer*, **32A**, 1674-1679. http://dx.doi.org/10.1016/0959-8049(96)00140-2

[5] Kornguth, P.J., Keefe, F.J. and Conaway, M.R. (1996) Pain during Mammography: Characteristics and Relationship to Demographic and Medical Variables. *Pain*, **66**, 187-194. http://dx.doi.org/10.1016/0304-3959(96)03057-6

[6] Asghari, A. and Nicholas, M.K. (2004) Pain during Mammography: The Role of Coping Strategies. *Pain*, **108**, 170-179. http://dx.doi.org/10.1016/j.pain.2003.12.022

[7] Hafslund, B. (2000) Mammography and the Experience of Pain and Anxiety. *Radiography*, **6**, 269-272. http://dx.doi.org/10.1053/radi.2000.0281

[8] Sapir, R., Patlas, M., Strano, S.D., Hadas-Halpern, I. and Cherny, N.I. (2003) Does Mammography Hurt? *Journal of Pain and Symptom Management*, **25**, 53-63. http://dx.doi.org/10.1016/S0885-3924(02)00598-5

[9] Merskey, H and Bogduk, N. (1994) Classification of Chronic Pain: Descriptions of Chronic Pain Syndromes and Definitions of Pain Terms. IASP Press, 1-28.

[10] Uchiyama, M., Lee, Y., Kazama, K., Minagawa, Y., Tsai, D.Y., Sadakata, M. and Sayama, M. (2011) A Preliminary Study on Measurement of Muscle Activity during Mammography Positioning. *Japanese Journal of Radiological Technology*, **67**, 679-682. http://dx.doi.org/10.6009/jjrt.67.679

[11] Uchiyama, M., Lee, Y., Sadakata, M., Sayama, M. and Tsai, D.Y. (2012) Measurement of Muscle Activities for Evaluating Physical Burden and Pain during Mammography Positioning. *The Tohoku Journal of Experimental Medicine*, **228**, 53-58. http://dx.doi.org/10.1620/tjem.228.53

[12] Uchiyama, M., Lee, Y., Kazama, K., Minagawa, Y., Tsai, D.Y., Sadakata, M. and Sayama, M. (2012) Quantitative Assessment of Muscle Activity in Mammography Positioning. *20th IMEKO World Congress*, Busan, 9-14 September 2012, 9-14.

[13] Sharp, P.C., Michielutte, R., Freimanis, R., Cunningham, L., Spangler, J. and Burnette, V. (2003) Reported Pain Following Mammography Screening. *Archives of Internal Medicine*, **163**, 833-836. http://dx.doi.org/10.1001/archinte.163.7.833

[14] Keel, K.D. (1948) The Pain Chart. *Lancet*, **2**, 6-8. http://dx.doi.org/10.1016/S0140-6736(48)91787-5

[15] Turk, D.C. and Melzack, R. (2001) Handbook of Pain Assessment. 2nd Edition, The Guilford Press, New York.

[16] Merzack, R. (1975) The McGill Pain Questionnaire: Major Properties and Scoring Methods. *Pain*, **1**, 277-299. http://dx.doi.org/10.1016/0304-3959(75)90044-5

[17] Dinash, G., Daniel, K., Len, G. and John, G. (2001) Examining the Validity of Pressure Ulcer Risk Assessment Scales: Developing and Using Illustrated Patient Simulations to Collect The Data. *Journal of Clinical Nursing*, **10**, 697-706. http://dx.doi.org/10.1046/j.1365-2702.2001.00525.x

[18] Shimazu H., Seino, S.-I., Kato, S., Kobayashi, H. and Akimoto, M. (2005) Development of a Quantitative Measurement Method for the Magnitude of Pain Using Painless Electrical Stimulation and Its Evaluation Using Experimental Pain. *Transactions of Japanese Society for Medical and Biological Engineering*, **43**, 117-123.

[19] Hasegawa, J., Sugiyama, D., kumasaka, M., Hishinuma, M., Matsuo, K., Ide, S., Tanaka, S. and Kitoh, T. (2008) Evaluation of Pain Treatment by Pain Vision™. *Journal of Japan Society of Pain Clinicians*, **15**, 144-149.

[20] Uchiyama, M., Lee, Y., Sadakata, M., Tsai, D.Y. and Sayama, M. (2013) Effects of Mammography Positioning on the Autonomic Nervous Function. *Health*, **5**, 1335-1341. http://dx.doi.org/10.4236/health.2013.58181

[21] Lee, Y. and Uchiyama, M. (2014) Evaluation of Physical and Psychological Burden of Subjects in Mammography. *IWDM* 2014, *LNCS*, **8539**, 508-513. http://dx.doi.org/10.1007/978-3-319-07887-8_71

[22] Uchiyama, M. (2014) The Experience of Mammography Based on the Memoirs of Examinees. *Health*, **6**, 1310-1314. http://dx.doi.org/10.4236/health.2014.611160

[23] Lee, Y. and Uchiyama, M. (2015) The Effect of Humorous Stimuli on Alleviating Pain during Mammography: A Preliminary Study. *Health*, **7**, 659-664. http://dx.doi.org/10.4236/health.2015.76078

30

A Qualitative Study of Manager Experiences Using the RAFAELA System

Nina Berger Hustad[1*], Ragnhild Hellesø[2], Marit Helen Andersen[1,2]

[1]Division of Cancer Medicine, Surgery and Transplantation, Oslo University Hospital, Norway
[2]Faculty of Medicine, Institute of Health and Society, University of Oslo, Norway
Email: [*]nberger@ous-hf.no, ragnhild.helleso@medisin.uio.no, manderse@ous-hf.no

Abstract

Objective: The objective was to explore manager experiences using the RAFAELA system. Background: The RAFAELA system was developed in Finland during the 1990s to create a work situation where patients' care needs were balanced with personnel resources. The system is used in almost all hospitals in Finland and is implemented in several European countries. However, the system has never been evaluated outside Finland. This study, focusing on the managers' perspective, represents the second report from a larger Norwegian evaluation project of the RAFAELA system. Methods: An explorative qualitative design was chosen. Data were collected by individual in-depth interviews at a university hospital in Norway during 2012-2013. A total of 10 informants in various management positions were interviewed. The tape-recorded interviews were transcribed verbatim, and the transcripts were analysed using Kvale's method for content analysis. Results: Four main themes emerged from the qualitative data: making the invisible visible; a common language; a system for prospective planning; and a resource-demanding tool. Conclusions: The study indicated that the RAFAELA system provided useful information about the patients' care needs and nursing activities. Also the system provided a common reference frame for discussing nursing, staffing and allocation. Although the managers considered the RAFAELA to be time consuming in the implementation phase, they considered the system to be an important tool.

Keywords

the RAFAELA System, Patients' Care Needs, Nurse Staffing, Manager Experiences, In-Depth Interviews

1. Introduction

In an era of changes in health care settings and the need for quality care, documenting of health care delivery is

[*]Corresponding author.

essential for nursing care and for the managers. Advancements in medicine lead to increasingly complex patient needs and nursing tasks [1]-[3]. Research has shown that nurses' contribution to the care and treatment of patients has a positive impact on patient outcomes and that successful staffing positively affects the quality of patient care. Health personnel represents one of the largest expenses in hospitals, and a better hospital staff is associated with lower hospital costs over time [2] [4]-[7].

Instruments that provide readily available information about patient care quality, regarding the processes and outcomes of the delivery system, are essential aspects of the effective health care. Regular feedback between nurses and managers provides useful information and impacts patient safety and quality of care [3] [8]. In an integrative review study, the researchers attempted to identify the current practice of using patient classification systems [9]. The results confirmed that there was no "gold standard" for measuring the nursing workload. Hence, there is a need for additional measurement and valid systems that capture the complexity of these factors. Other studies also revealed the lack of valid systems that analysed patients' care needs, patient flow and the use of available resources in medical and surgical hospital wards.

A better understanding of patient classification systems is expected to make hospitals more prepared for monitoring the developments pertaining to analysing patients' care needs and determining how to use the available resources [4] [10]. According to the Norwegian Parliament's Coordination Reform of 2009, lack of appropriate systems for resource allocation may be one of the reasons why proper patient care is insufficient [11]. In 2011 a Norwegian regional project called "Better Resource Management" was established, demonstrating the need to improve the opportunities for managers to engage in purposeful resource planning [12]. This was also the background for performing a broad evaluation of the Finnish RAFAELA system at Oslo University Hospital. The RAFAELA system was designed during the 1990s to create a work situation in which patients' care needs were balanced with personnel resources [13]-[15].

The Norwegian evaluation project included 4 sub studies [16]. The objective of this paper, representing the second report from the project, was to explore manager experiences using the RAFAELA system.

2. Background

The RAFAELA system, based on thorough research and user experiences in hospital contexts, is currently being used by more than 90% of Finnish hospitals. Since 2010, Iceland, Norway, Sweden and the Netherlands also have become RAFAELA users [17].

The system is based on a three-part data collection system: i) daily patient classification as measured by the Oulu Patient Classification instrument (OPCq); ii) daily registration of nursing resources for direct care (N); and iii) professional assessment of optimal nursing care intensity level (PAONCIL). The workload is expressed in OPCq/N and is compared to the units' optimal standard for nursing intensity (NI) level defined by the nurses [13]-[15]. Hence, subjective perceptions are replaced by objective numbers. The OPCq instrument measures six sub-areas of patient needs and associated nursing interventions: 1) planning and coordination of care; 2) breathing, blood circulation and symptoms of disease; 3) nutrition and medication; 4) personal hygiene and excretion; 5) activity/movement, sleep and rest; and 6) teaching, guidance and follow-up in care, and emotional support. The nurses classify the patients once per day for the last 24-hour period. NI may vary for each sub-area between 1 - 4 points and are summed to a total score, ranging from 6 to 24 points per patient where 6 points indicate a patient with minimum needs and 24 points indicate a patient with intensive care needs. Total NI points at the unit were divided by the number of nurses, and the patient-related workload was obtained [13]-[15].

The assessment of optimal NI level per nurse is established by conducting a 4 - 6 weeks test using the PAONCIL instrument. On a scale from −3 to 3, where −3 indicate very low and +3 very high NI, the nurses assess to which extent they have had the possibility to meet the needs of their patient group during the shift. The idea of the RAFAELA system is that the daily NI is compared to the optimal NI level for the ward. When the actual NI is on the optimal level, a successful resource allocation is obtained [14] [15] [18].

3. Methods and Material

3.1. Design

An explorative qualitative design was chosen, and individual semi-structured interviews were conducted.

3.2. Participants

The participants were selected strategically to secure diversity and variation of the sample relevant to the aim of the study [19]-[20]. Eleven managers were asked to participate and a total of 10 informants (2 physicians and 8 nurses) agreed to participate. They represented all management levels of the division, being responsible for the treatment of patients, HR-planning, workload and budgeting. Background characteristics of the sample are demonstrated in **Table 1**.

3.3. Data Collection Procedure

The semi-structured interviews were performed in the period of September 2012 to April 2013. They lasted 40 - 60 minutes and took place in a suitable room with a relaxed atmosphere, starting with a briefing about the purpose of the study. One internal researcher and 1 external researcher attended the interviews to strengthen the scientific perspective and to ensure optimal ethical considerations. An interview guide consisting of open-ended questions was used to ensure that key aspects of the research question were covered. The guide was based on previous research within the field. It consisted of seven main questions covering the following areas: i) experiences with the daily use of the RAFAELA system, ii) the benefits and drawbacks of using the RAFAELA system, and iii) reflections and opinions about the future use of the RAFAELA system. At the end of the interviews, the participants were asked if there was anything they wished to add or comment on.

3.4. Data Analysis

The tape-recorded interviews where transcribed verbatim, and the transcripts were analysed using established methods for qualitative content analysis, containing five steps [21]. First, each interview was carefully read to obtain an overall impression of the data material. Then, the text was divided into meaning units, *i.e.*, meaningful parts to capture the most probable interpretation of parts of the text. Third, the statements were read, and the themes that dominated a meaning unit were identified. The fourth step consisted of analysing the meaning units in terms of the specific purpose of the study: to describe the managers' experience with using the RAFAELA system. In the fifth step, the essential themes of the entire interview were tied together in a descriptive statement [21]. The method thus involved a condensation of the expressed meanings into more essential meanings of the structure and style to identify the manifestation of the informants' experiences. Examples from the data analysis process are shown in **Table 2**.

To assure the validity of the data, a pilot interview was conducted before the start of the study to evaluate the interview guide and the interview setting. To secure trustworthiness, the interview data were coded and reflected within the research group until the themes that were suited to the aim of the study were achieved [19]. Further analysis was performed by a pair of researchers who verified each other's work. Conformability was established

Table 1. Background characteristics of the informants.

Informants	Managers	Number of nurses at the units	Years of experiences of mangers
Informant nr. 1	Unit manager	>50	<10
Informant nr. 2	Unit manager	=50	<10
Informant nr. 3	Division manager	>50	>10
Informant nr. 4	Section manager	>50	>10
Informant nr. 5	Section manager	>50	>10
Informant nr. 6	Division manager	>50	>10
Informant nr. 7	Unit manager	<50	>10
Informant nr. 8	Division manager	>50	>10
Informant nr. 9	Unit manager	<50	<10
Informant nr. 10	Unit manager	>50	>10

Table 2. Examples from the data analysis process.

Natural meaning units, statements	Meaning units	Sub themes	Theme
RAFAELA provides an increased awareness of what you spend time on during a day: those activities and all of the tasks a nurse performs in caring for patients. I do not think that you as a nurse is aware of all the tasks performed throughout the day. Hence, you are not aware of the value of the tasks.	RAFAELA provides increased awareness of what the nurses are spending their time on during the day and all the tasks they complete. The system provides awareness of the work and the value of nursing.	RAFAELA creates awareness within nursing. The system visualizes nursing and brings value to it.	*Making the invisible visible*
We think that we perform many coordination tasks in our unit. The RAFAELA reports support our assumptions. We almost perform more coordination tasks compared to direct nursing. However, we wish to perform more direct nursing work in the unit.	The RAFAELA system supports the fact that nurses perform numerous coordination tasks. The nurses wish they could provide more direct nursing tasks.	RAFAELA reports clearly demonstrate the different tasks and areas that nurses work in.	

by maintaining an audit trail. Steps were taken to enhance the credibility, including using Kvale's [21] framework for the analysis, supervision by experienced researchers, keeping a research diary and using the participants own words when reporting the results.

3.5. Ethical Considerations

The study was conducted in accordance with the Helsinki declaration and was approved by the Internal Study Board at the Oslo University Hospital (#2010/27572). Informed consent to participate was obtained from all the participants. In this study, the anonymity of the informants might be threatened because there were a few managers at each management level and thus the informants could be easily recognizable. Hence, we removed the recognizable statements to strengthen the anonymity and confidentiality of the data. The study was considered not to be a burden for the participants.

The RAFAELA system is owned by the Association of Finnish Local and Regional Authorities, and its use is managed by FCG—Finnish Consulting Group Ltd. The actual study was initiated by the university hospital. The license to use the system was acquired through a standard agreement between the actual hospital and FCG.

4. Results

The participants ranged in age from 35 to 61 years. Four main themes emerged from the data analysis: Making the invisible visible; A common language; A system for prospective planning, and A resource demanding tool.

Making the invisible visible

According to the informants, the RAFAELA system visualized nursing in several different ways that helped to make the nurses more aware of what they actually were doing during a day, referring to the RAFAELA sub-areas: planning and coordination of care; breathing, blood circulation and symptoms of disease; nutrition and medication; personal hygiene and excretion; activity/movement, sleep and rest; and teaching, guidance and follow-up in care/emotional support. Additionally, it was stated that the system defined each patient's needs for nursing care activities and helped the nurses assess their own work more thoroughly. The RAFAELA reports assisted the leaders by highlighting key nursing areas in the unit and thus contributed to make the nursing activities more visible. Data also showed that using the system provided increased awareness regarding nursing tasks performed during their shifts, and helped the nurses appreciate the value of their work:

"*The diffuse, but very important part of nursing care was made visible through the RAFAELA system.*"

"*It is important that the nurses can be aware of what they actually do. How do we use the nursing resources, what are the patient care needs, and what to do to meet them?*"

"*The RAFAELA system increases the awareness of what nurses spend time on. I think that the nurses are not fully aware of all tasks performed during a day and that they do not reflect on the value of their work.*"

Also the informants experienced RAFAELA reports to be useful for illustrating the resources used in each nursing area:

"I usually show the reports at monthly staff meetings. The nurses recognize the situations documented by the system, for instance, when it comes to those nursing areas that are the most challenging in our ward."

"The diffuse tasks being very important and very time consuming, these are made visible through the RAFAELA system."

A common language

The participants expressed that the RAFAELA system represented a common reference frame within nursing and across units. The system created a common understanding by encouraging nurses to discuss nursing and patient needs using terms, assessments and scales that were available from the system. Using a common model for resource-planning also made it easier to discuss and benchmark staffing across the wards:

"The system encourages discussions and contributes to a common understanding of what nursing is."

Several participants also mentioned that RAFAELA system supported them by providing arguments concerning the budgeting of nursing care. In their opinion, objective RAFAELA data provided credibility in discussions with nursing care executives confirming the reality at the wards:

"I just arrived from a meeting with experts from the economic department. I was told we are using too many temporary nurses from agencies. The RAFAELA system is a very effective tool for providing data relevant for such debates."

"There is something about being able to use graphs. The economists prefer tables and figures instead of assumptions, and in this way the RAFAELA system is a very useful tool."

A system for prospective planning

Another major theme dealt with the ability of the system to create a work situation where patients' care needs balanced with available personnel resources. This was related to daily resource planning, but also to revealing patterns of patient needs versus staffing over months and years:

"The managers get patient flow data that is very useful for the allocation of nurses. For instance, RAFAELA data documented less need for nurses on the Monday day-shift."

One of the informants also found the RAFAELA system to be a tool for knowledge development within decision making:

"Having this type of data in resource-planning is very important strategically for the future. It enables us to perform many analyses by ourselves without a lot of external consultants."

The informants expressed that system was useful for benchmarking and networking between different units, and enhanced the transparency in the organization:

"Then, examining the patients' composition according to their care needs and whether they should be in this unit or another unit... This is important information concerning the clinic's budget process, related to the assessment of how to allocate nursing resources."

Concerning need of skill mix within nursing, it was stated that the system contributed to illustrate the level of expertise needed in the units. However, the informants experienced that a weakness of the system was that the nurse competence variable not directly was registered by the system.

A resource-demanding tool

The informants stated that the implementation of the RAFAELA system required systematic education for a long period. They expressed the need of dedicated training personnel and the importance of being well prepared for the implementation process. The RAFAELA system was characterized as a complex system consisting of three different instruments entailing regular reliability and validity tests:

"Implementing RAFAELA was challenging, and we spent a lot of resources. Hence, it becomes important to experience the benefits and appreciate the value of it."

The mangers also expressed that one-to-one training for managers was needed to enable them to use the system in a comprehensive way. This included using the RAFAELA reports correctly, interpreting available information, and providing arguments for decision-makers in resource planning and allocating. In addition, it was stressed that it was important for managers to use the system actively and regularly.

5. Discussion

The findings of our study reflect two overall perspectives. The themes "Making the invisible visible" and "A common language" illustrate how RAFAELA contributed to awareness, and the visibility, of nursing care and thus provided the managers with an overall nursing perspective. The themes "A system for prospective planning" and "A resource-demanding tool" illustrate a management perspective.

The nursing perspective

Data indicated that through RAFAELA classifications, the nursing care activities were clearly defined based on the patients' care needs. Several factors may explain these findings.

First, RAFAELA allows each nurse in the unit to perform a patient classification based on a professional estimation of the patients' unique care needs and based on daily nursing resources spent on each patient. Second, the RAFAELA system is based on optimal nursing intensity levels at each unit, defined by the nurses over a period of 4 - 6 weeks every other year [13] [14]. This level seemed to be an important tool for the mangers in debating the situation of the unit, for instance, for the last month or the last week. The nurse mangers appreciated that the system allowed the manager and the staff to reflect on an increase or decrease in the nursing intensity level with reference to the optimal standard of the unit. In this way, the staff could actively participate in the allocation discussion together with their manager.

Another significant finding was that the RAFAELA system made nursing visible in the units. This, to a large extent, refers to invisible tasks essential for health service delivery [22]. An Italian study demonstrated that nurses described invisible care as reflexivity, review of care actions, collaborating with colleagues, being 'competent', and being aware of their clinical skills [23]. These phenomena were also mentioned by the participants when reflecting nursing activities being visible through the RAFAELA system. Our findings have been confirmed by other studies [24] [25], revealing the complex nature of nursing performance. Through descriptions of nursing and the use of patient classification systems, the profession's contribution to the patient's health was made visible. Some of the participants mentioned that one advantage of using RAFAELA data was that the system provided a reliable picture of the activities nurses perform during a shift. The importance of displaying the different areas of nursing activities, such as teaching, guidance or administration of medication also was stressed by the participants. Most likely, this is useful information for the nurse managers for recruiting purposes, staff education, and also for providing a profile of their unit. Previous studies have verified the importance of mapping nurse competency and established relevant nursing skills to deliver high-quality patient care [26] [27].

In a report by Fasoli & Haddock [9] the researchers argued that the lack of standardized language for communication and problems with describing what nurses do are obstacles for nursing workload measurement. However, one could present this argument in the opposite way. Using valid systems for workload measurement will contribute to common descriptions of what nurses do. Several studies have confirmed that measuring nursing care outcomes is important for nursing practice. Such information is crucial for increased quality within nursing [4] [24] [25].

In a review of conceptualization nursing workload, it was stated that the complexity of nursing makes it difficult to describe workload, and that there is no common definition of nursing workload in the literature [28]. Our findings indicated that the RAFAELA system contributed to a common language. The respondents in our study mentioned that the level of disagreement in the implementation process occurred when rating the six sub areas of the OPCq. The study of Andersen *et al.* supported this finding [16] and highlights the importance for nurses to be aware of their own work and participate in discussions about the nature of nursing. The participants stated that the system contributed to a professional understanding, not only for nurses, but also for the hospital managers because the same model and language were used in management discussions across units and clinics. In their report Brown et al stressed the importance of providing hospitals with common indicators describing nursing in addition to traditional medical outcomes [29]. This is in line with our findings demonstrating the managers' need of using feasible instruments providing professional understanding of patient needs and nursing workload.

The management perspective

According to the managers participating in the study the RAFAELA system was a useful tool for prospective planning. Among others the participants experienced the system to be an administrative tool for daily resource planning. Additionally, the system could support the managers in monitoring the sufficiency of available resources versus patient needs from day to day. A review study from 2011 supports our findings [30], revealing important factors that impact the nursing workload, such as nursing environment, nursing team, and the patient-nurse relationship. This finding is in line with the main idea of the RAFAELA system: to create a work situation in which patient care needs are balanced with personnel resources [13]-[15].

The participants experienced the RAFAELA system to be useful for revealing patient flow, allocation and benchmarking. Hence, in their opinion, the system was effective at addressing the increasing demands in the delivery of health care. In addition, they expressed that the reports could be used for discussions related to the quality of nursing care and how to meet individual care needs. The reports were also useful when debating staff planning at the level of administration managers and experts representing the finance department. In their review study Harper & McCully demonstrated the importance for nurse managers using patient classification systems to ensure quality care and predict staffing needs [31].

Our findings indicate that valid patient classifications system must be established to provide a basis for staff planning, estimating costs, and providing nurses reasonable time and the possibilities to provide high-quality care. This is supported by Baernholdt *et al.* recommending building in-hospital structures of information systems as useful management tools [32].

Some negative aspects using the RAFAELA system was mentioned. The participants agreed that implementing RAFAELA was a time-consuming process. Additionally, the implementation process was considered to be quite a challenging and complex process. The findings are supported by previous research of implementing patient classification systems [9] [10] [26] [29]. From a management perspective, this is easy to understand. Implementing a new patient classification system requires education of the entire staff, thorough discussions within the nursing group, including decision making, and quality assurance during the process. Our study provided new, detailed insight into the process of implementing new tools into a busy hospital setting. The RAFAELA system is based on three types of data collection and according to the manual, the system has to be tested for reliability and validity before implementing it into a hospital unit [13]-[15]. These tests are time consuming and complex and therefore implementing the system is scheduled to take approximately 3 - 6 months per unit [14]. To solve the aspects concerning implementing the system we propose individual web-based introduction programs. Further, interactive web-based training programs for managers of using and interpreting RAFAELA reports would be purposeful. To evaluate web-based introduction-and training programs new evaluation studies should be conducted.

The informants also stated that system revealed nurse competence to a very little extent. This is a well know weakness of the system as nurses' competence and skill mix play an important role when balancing patients' care needs with personnel resources. According to the inventors integrating nurse competence is considered central in further development of the system [17]. If nurse competency will be included to a certain extent for the future, we propose new investigations to study how this important factor interacts with the RAFAELA system.

Study Limitations

Some study limitations should be mentioned. Our sample was based on data derived from only one hospital setting. Hence, caution should be used when transferring information from this study to other contexts. On the other hand, our study represents the first study of manager experiences of the RAFAELA system as used outside Finland. Thus, our study adds scientific information to the existing knowledge concerning the RAFAELA system.

Ten managers participated in the study. It is possible that more informants would provide multiple nuances and variations to the results. We addressed this by including maximum variation sampling in the range of experience, management level, age and gender.

6. Conclusion

The study indicated that the RAFAELA system provided useful information about the patients' care needs and nursing activities. Also the system provided a common reference frame for discussing nursing, staffing and allocation. Although the managers considered the RAFAELA system to be time consuming during implementation, they considered it to be an important tool.

References

[1] Adams, A. and Bond, S. (2003) Staffing in Acute Hospital Wards: Part 1. The Relationship between Number of Nurses and Ward Organizational Environment. *Journal of Nursing Management*, **11**, 287-292. http://dx.doi.org/10.1046/j.1365-2834.2003.00361.x

[2] Lucero, R.J., Lake, E.T. and Aiken, L.H. (2009) Variations in Nursing Care Quality across Hospitals. *Journal of Advanced Nursing*, **65**, 2299-2310. http://dx.doi.org/10.1111/j.1365-2648.2009.05090.x

[3] McGillis Hall, L., Wodchis, W.P., Ma, X. and Johnson, S. (2013) Changes in Patient Health Outcomes from Admission to Discharge in Acute Care. *Journal of Nursing Care Quality*, **28**, 8-16. http://dx.doi.org/10.1097/NCQ.0b013e3182665dab

[4] Kane, R.L., Shamliyan, T.A., Mueller, C., Duval, S. and Wilt, T.J. (2007) The Association of Registered Nurse Staffing Levels and Patient Outcomes: Systematic Review and Meta-Analysis. *Medical Care*, **45**, 1195-1204. http://dx.doi.org/10.1097/MLR.0b013e3181468ca3

[5] Purcell, S.R., Kutash, M. and Cobb, S. (2011) The Relationship between Nurses' Stress and Nurse Staffing Factors in a Hospital Setting. *Journal of Nursing Management*, **19**, 714-720. http://dx.doi.org/10.1111/j.1365-2834.2011.01262.x

[6] Aiken, L.H., Cimiotti, J.P., Sloane, D.M., Smith, H.L., Flynn, L. and Neff, D.F. (2011) Effect of Nurse Staffing and Nurse Education On Patients' Death in Hospital with Different Nurse Work Environments. *Medical Care*, **49**, 1047-1053. http://dx.doi.org/10.1097/MLR.0b013e3182330b6e

[7] Aiken, L., Sloane, D.S., Bruyneel, L., Van den Heede, K., Griffiths, P., Busse, R., Diomidous, M., Kinnunen, J., Kózka, M., Lesaffre, E., McHugh, M.D., Moreno-Casbas, M.T., Rafferty, A.M., Schwendimann, R., Scott, A.P., Tishelman, C., Theo van Achterberg, T. and Sermeus, W. (2014) Nurse Staffing and Education and Hospital Morality in Nine European Countries: A Retrospective Observational Study. *The Lancet*, **383**, 1824-1830. http://dx.doi.org/10.1016/S0140-6736(13)62631-8

[8] Pastastavrou, E., Andreou, P. and Efstathiou, G. (2014) Rationing of Nursing Care and Nurse-Patient Outcomes: A Systematic Review of Quantitative Studies. *The International Journal of Health Planning and Management*, **29**, 3-25. http://dx.doi.org/10.1002/hpm.2160

[9] Fasoli, D.R. and Haddock, K.S. (2010) Results of an Integrative Review of Patient Classification Systems (Chap. 11). *Annual Review of Nursing Research*, **28**, 295-316. http://dx.doi.org/10.1891/0739-6686.28.295

[10] Perroca, M.G. and Ek, A-C. (2007) Utilization of Patient Classification System in Swedish Hospitals and Degree of Satisfaction among Nursing Staff. *Journal of Nursing Management*, **15**, 472-480. http://dx.doi.org/10.1111/j.1365-2834.2007.00732.x

[11] Report No. 47 to the Parliament 2009. The Coordination Reform 2008-2009.

[12] South-Eastern Norway Regional Health Authority (2012) Annual Report.

[13] Fagerström, L., Rainio, A.-K., Rauhala, A. and Nojonen, K. (2000) Validation of a New Method for Patient Classification, the Oulu Patient Classification. *Journal of Advanced Nursing*, **31**, 481-490. http://dx.doi.org/10.1046/j.1365-2648.2000.01277.x

[14] Fagerström, L., Rainio, A.-K., Rauhala, A. and Nojonen, K. (2000) Professional Assessment of Optimal Nursing Care Intensity Level—A New Method for Resource Allocation as an Alternative to Classical Time Studies. *Scandinavian Journal of Caring Sciences*, **14**, 97-104.

[15] Rauhala, A. and Fagerström, L. (2004) Determining Optimal Nursing Intensity: The RAFAELA Method. *Journal of Advanced in Nursing*, **45**, 351-359. http://dx.doi.org/10.1046/j.1365-2648.2003.02918.x

[16] Andersen, M.H., Lønning, K. and Fagerström, L. (2014) Testing Reliability and Validity of the Oulu Patient Classification Instrument—The First Step in Evaluating the RAFAELA System in Norway. *Open Journal of Nursing*, **4**, 303-311. http://dx.doi.org/10.4236/ojn.2014.44035

[17] Fagerström, L., Lønning, K. and Andersen, M.H. (2014) The RAFAELA System: A Workforce Planning Tool for Nurse Staffing and Human Resource Management. *Nursing Management*, **21**, 30-36. http://dx.doi.org/10.7748/nm2014.04.21.2.30.e1199

[18] Fagerström, L. and Rauhala, A. (2007) Benchmarking in Nursing Care by the RAFAELA Patient Classification System. *Journal of Nursing Management*, **15**, 683-692. http://dx.doi.org/10.1111/j.1365-2934.2006.00728.x

[19] Polit, C.F. and Beck, C.T. (2004) Nursing Research: Principles and Methods. 7th Edition, Lippincott Williams & Wilkins, Philadelphia.

[20] Patton, M.Q. (2002) Qualitative Research & Evaluation Methods. 3rd Edition, SAGE Publications, Thousand Oaks.

[21] Kvale, S. (2007) Det kvalitative forskningsintervju. Gyldendal Norsk forlag AS.

[22] Allen, D. (2007) What Do Nurses Do at Work? Profession Building and Doing Nursing. *International Council of Nurses*, **54**, 41-48. http://dx.doi.org/10.1111/j.1466-7657.2007.00496.x

[23] Canzan, F., Heilemann, M.V., Saiani, L., Mortari, L. and Ambrosi, E. (2014) Visible and Invisible Caring in Nursing from the Perspectives of Patients and Nurses in the Gerontological Context. *Scandinavian Journal of Caring Sciences*, **28**, 732-740. http://dx.doi.org/10.1111/scs.12105

[24] Hendrich, A., Chow, M., Skierczynski, B.A. and Lu, Z. (2008) A 36-Hospital Time and Motion Study: How Do Medical-Surgical Nurses Spend Their Time? *The Permanente Journal*, **12**, 25-34. http://dx.doi.org/10.7812/TPP/08-021

[25] Cornell, P., Riordan, M., Townsend-Gervis, M. and Mobley, R. (2011) Barriers to Critical Thinking Workflow Interruptions and Task Switching among Nurses. *The Journal of Nursing Administration*, **41**, 407-414. http://dx.doi.org/10.1097/NNA.0b013e31822edd42

[26] Harper, K. and McCully, C. (2007) Acuity System Dialog and Patient Classification System Essentials. *Nursing Administration Quarterly*, **31**, 284-299. http://dx.doi.org/10.1097/01.NAQ.0000290426.41690.cb

[27] Whelchel, C., Berg, L., Brown, A., Hurd, D., Koepping, D. and Stroud, S. (2013) What's the Impact of Quality Bundles at the Bedside? *Nursing*, **43**, 18-21. http://dx.doi.org/10.1097/01.NURSE.0000437481.30251.e1

[28] Morris, R., MacNeela, P., Scott, A., Treacy, P. and Hyde, A. (2007) Reconsidering the Conceptualization of Nursing Workload: Literature Review. *Journal of Advance Nursing*, **57**, 463-471. http://dx.doi.org/10.1111/j.1365-2648.2006.04134.x

[29] Brown, D.S., Donaldson, N., Burnes Bolton, L. and Aydin, C.E. (2010) Nursing-Sensitive Benchmarks for Hospital to Gauge High-Reliability Performance. *Journal of Health Quality*, **32**, 9-17. http://dx.doi.org/10.1111/j.1945-1474.2010.00083.x

[30] Myny, D., Van Gouberger, D., Gobert, M., Vanderwee, K., Van Hecke, A. and Defloor, T. (2011) Non-Direct Patient Care Factors Influencing Nursing Workload: A Review of the Literature. *Journal of Advanced Nursing*, **67**, 2109-2129.

[31] Harper, K. and McCully, C. (2007) Acuity Systems Dialogue and Patient Classification System Essentials. *Nursing Administration Quarterly*, **31**, 284-299. http://dx.doi.org/10.1097/01.NAQ.0000290426.41690.cb

[32] Baernholdt, M., Cox, K. and Scully, K. (2010) Using Clinical Data to Capture Nurse Workload. Implications for Staffing and Safety. *CIN: Computers, Informatics, Nursing*, **28**, 229-234.

31

The Agreement Rate about Unintended Pregnancy and Its Relationship with Postpartum Depression in Parents of Preterm and Term Infants

Maryam Ghorbani[1], Mahrokh Dolatian[2*], Jamal Shams[3], Hamid Alavi-Majd[4]

[1]Shahid Beheshti University of Medical Sciences, Tehran, Iran
[2]Department of Reproductive Health and Midwifery, School of Nursing and Midwifery, Shahid Beheshti University of Medical Sciences, Tehran, Iran
[3]Department of Psychiatry, Behavioral Research Center, Shahid Beheshti University of Medical Sciences, Tehran, Iran
[4]Department of Biostatistics, School of Paramedical Sciences, Shahid Beheshti University of Medical Sciences, Tehran, Iran
Email: [*]mhdolatian@gmail.com

Abstract

Introduction: Postpartum depression (PPD) affects women's health and self-confidence, and infant's social, emotional, cognitive and even physical development. Studies show that parents of preterm infants frequently experience symptoms of depression and anxiety. Women with unintended pregnancy are subjected to more risk of depression than women with planned pregnancy. Unintended pregnancy may lead to increased maternal exposure to psychosocial stressors, reduced social support by the spouse, increased levels of depressive symptoms and decreased life satisfaction. Findings: No significant difference was observed between term and preterm infants' mothers ($p = 0.85$) in terms of postpartum depression. However, two groups of fathers in terms of depression showed a significant difference ($p = 0.045$). McNemar's test showed that parents of term infants ($K = 0.322$, $p = 0.077$), and parents of preterm infants ($k = 0.17$, $p = 0.144$) agreed with each other on unintended pregnancy. Conclusion: Fathers of preterm infants are at higher risk for mental disorders than fathers of term infants and they need more attention in future studies.

[*]Corresponding author.

Keywords

Prematurity, Parents, Depression, Postpartum Depression, Unintended Pregnancy

1. Introduction

For most women, pregnancy is a time of positive changes, but it can also be a time of physical and psychological challenges, as pregnancy is associated with hormonal changes and can therefore increase susceptibility to incidence or recurrence of depression [1]. Postpartum depression is effective not only on women's health and self-confidence as a mother, but also on infant's social, emotional, cognitive and even physical development. Postpartum depression has been reported 10% - 15% in developed countries and 16% to 36% in developing countries. Numerous risk factors associated with postpartum depression have been recognized including mother's major depressive disorder, depression during pregnancy and family history of depression. Other important factors in some low-income countries include family fragmentation, lack of social support, dissatisfaction with having a baby girl, no breastfeeding, stressful life events, domestic violence, HIV/AIDS, infant diseases, infant prematurity and unintended pregnancy [1] [2].

Since changes occur in women's psychological and physiological function in the postpartum period, preterm delivery is likely to increase maternal distress and slow her physical recovery because of the special care required by a preterm infant [3]. The prevalence of preterm birth has been reported 5% in developed countries and 25% in developing countries. In Iran, the prevalence of preterm birth has been reported between 5.6% and 13.4% [4]. Although advances in technology result in more survival of preterm infants, mortality still remains high and imposes more emotional and financial burden to both family and the healthcare system [5].

Potentially stressful factors that can affect parents of preterm infants include problems related to the infant's health at the hospital and after discharge from the hospital, reduction in accountability, and concerns about the infant's mental development. Postpartum depression is a common experience in preterm infants' mothers [6]. According to several studies, experiencing emotional distress in parents of preterm infants is high and high levels of depression and anxiety symptoms appear during their baby's stay in the NICU [5].

Few studies have also investigated the effects of unintended pregnancy and have shown that women with an unintended pregnancy are at increased risk for depression compared to women with planned pregnancy. Unintended pregnancy may lead to increased maternal exposure to psychosocial stressors, reduced social support by the spouse, increased levels of depressive symptoms and decreased life satisfaction [1].

The aim of this study was to compare postpartum depression in parents of preterm and term infants, and review their agreement rate about unwanted pregnancy and its relationship with postpartum depression.

2. Patients and Methods

The current study used a descriptive-comparative, analytical design. The study population comprised parents of all preterm and term infants who presented at health centers in Qom, Iran to receive postpartum cares or to have their infants vaccinated. According to statistical analyses, the sample size was calculated as 82 couples and the subjects were selected using multistage stratified sampling during December 2012 to March 2013. Therefore, Because of existing different economic statue in Qom, the city was first divided into four economic classes. (The first stage of sampling was cluster sampling). All available health centers in the city were then listed and the sample size was distributed among the centers proportional to the number of their patients. (The second stage of sampling was quota sampling) Finally, centers from each class were randomly selected. Individuals were only recruited if they did not have any mental illnesses or a history of such diseases, were not on antipsychotic medicines such as antidepressants, and had no history of narcotic or psychoactive drug abuse. Parents of infants with any congenital or neurological defects were not included.

The present study used the following questionnaires:

Part one:

A questionnaire for the fathers:

The questionnaire consisted of two parts. The first part covered questions on demographic characteristics, having the intention to have a baby, the desired infant gender, and the history of mental illnesses of the first-degree relatives (6 items). The second part involved the adverse events which occurred to the father during his wife's pregnancy (27 items).

A questionnaire for the mothers:

The questionnaire included four parts. The first 12 items dealt with demographic characteristics of the mother, socioeconomic status of the family. The second part covered information on previous and current pregnancy (38 items). The third part of the questionnaire involved infant gender and their information and problem occurred because of infants after birth (15 items). The last 27 items explored the adverse pregnancy-related events.

The validity of these two questionnaires (demographic and obstetric) was determined with content validity. Moreover, in order to confirm the test-retest reliability of the questionnaire, 10 eligible couples who visited the mentioned health centers were selected and asked to complete the questionnaire twice with a two-week interval. The internal consistency of the tool was then computed as 98%.

Part two:

Beck Depression Inventory: To measure fathers' depression in this study, the-second edition of depression inventory was used. This is a self-report questionnaire with 21 items, to assess depression in adults and adolescents over 13 years and is scored Likertstyle according to the severity of symptoms. Among these items, 2items are dedicated to emotion, 11 items to cognition, 2 items to apparent behaviors, 5 items to somatic symptoms, and 1 item to interpersonal semiotics. Thus this scale determines different degrees of depression from mild to very severe and the subjects were divided into four groups considering the sum of the scores obtained: minimal or no depression (0 - 13 score), indicates mild depression(14 - 19 score),moderate depression (20 - 28 score)and severe depression (29 - 63 score) [7].

Edinburgh Postpartum Depression Scale: To assess mothers' depression status in this study, the globally applied screening scale for postpartum depression, Edinburgh depression scale, was used. The questionnaire includes 10 items about the common symptoms of depression based on Likertstyle. Mothers select the responses which show how they felt more often in the last week. Each item has four options and a score of 0 - 3. The sum of total score is 0 - 30 [8]. A score above 13 in the postpartum period was considered as depressed and a score lower than 13 as non-depressed.

In several studies, Cronbach's alpha coefficient of the questionnaire was reported 0.83 to 0.9 with high content validity [5]. To determine the validity and reliability of the questionnaire in Iranian population, and to determine the depression degree and estimate the effects of clinical trial, Dobson *et al.* in their descriptive-applied study in 2007 titled "Psychometric characteristics of the Beck Depression Inventory-II in a large sample of patients with major depressive disorder" evaluated 354 individuals who were diagnosed with major depression and were relatively recovered during the study. Participants responded the Beck Depression Inventory-II and Brief Symptom Inventory. To determine the validity of the mean and standard deviation, item-total internal consistency and alpha coefficients were calculated for each item. Total reliability coefficient was obtained 0.913 [9]. To determine the validity of the questionnaire, factor analysis and construct validity were used. Cronbach's alpha coefficient for this questionnaire was 0.873. Tashakori and Mehryarin 1994 obtained reliability coefficient of this questionnaire as 0.78 in Iran [10].

Edinburgh inventory was designed by Cox *et al.* in 1987 and includes symptoms of anxiety and concern. This tool is a widely used screening tool and there are different versions of this questionnaire in several languages [8]. The validity of Edinburgh inventory has been also investigated for screening postnatal depression with different scores, in several studies. Numerous studies have confirmed the validity of the instrument including studies by Jamil *et al.* (2006) with a sensitivity of 90% and a specificity of 60%, and Tesfaye *et al.* (2010) with a sensitivity of 78.9% and a specificity of 75.3%. In Iran, a 2010 study by Kamranpour *et al.* revealed the Cronbach's alpha more than 0.7, which confirms the reliability of the questionnaire [10]-[12].

3. Findings

According to the results of this study, in terms of age, there were no significant statistical differences between parents of term and preterm babies. However, higher levels of education in fathers of term infants in comparison to preterm infants, was obtained with Mann-Whitney test (Because of four classes for education including primary, pre high school, high school, university). This was a significant difference ($p < 0.001$).

Most mothers of both term and preterm groups were housewives (Chi-Square test: 84.1%). The majority of fathers of both term (Chi-Square test: 69.5%) and preterm (Chi-Square test: 78%) groups were self-employed.

120 to 240 USD In 41.5% of term group, and 240 to 300 USD was the average monthly salary of 46.3% of preterm group. About housing, most of the participants (37.7%) were owner of their place of residence and others lived in rental housing, governmental housing or lived with their families. Chi-Square test in two groups of parents showed no significant difference in terms of housing type, income and jobs (**Table 1**).

Most study units in both groups experienced their first childbirth. Chi-Square test in terms of number of childbirths, number of live births, number of sons and daughters, and gender of infant, type of labor, history of abortion, stillbirth's history, differences between the two groups were not significant.

Need for hospitalization ($p < 0.001$) and admission to neonatal intensive care unit ($p < 0.001$) showed statistically significant difference between two groups of infants (**Table 2**).

According to the current study results, mothers in term-infant group (25.6%) and mothers in preterm-infant group (24.4%) suffered from postpartum depression and chi-square test result showed no significant difference between the two groups in this regard ($p = 0.85$). Also, the majority of fathers in term group (91.5%) and in preterm group (80.5%) were not depressed. According to the Mann-Whitney test, fathers showed significant difference ($p = 0.045$) in depression (**Table 3**).

Most fathers in the term group (78%) and in the preterm group (63.4%) claimed the pregnancies were planned. Chi-square test revealed a significant difference between the two groups in terms of planned or unintended pregnancy ($p < 0.001$). Likewise, most mothers in the term group (75.6%) and mothers in the preterm group (59.8%) had planned pregnancies. Chi-square test revealed a significant difference between the two groups in terms of planned or unintended pregnancy ($p = 0.004$) (**Table 4**).

McNemar test results showed that term infants' parents ($p = 0.077$, $K = 0.322$), and preterm infants' parents ($p = 0.144$, $k = 0.17$) agreed with each other on the unintended pregnancy.

Logistic regression model showed no significant relationship between mother's age, mother's occupation, father's occupation, mother's education level, economic status, the number of pregnancies, preterm infant, birth weight, gestational age, history of infant hospitalization, history of hospitalization in NICU, planned pregnancy according to mother, planned pregnancy according to father, planned infant's gender according to mother and planned infant's gender according to father and maternal postpartum depression (**Table 5**). But according to this model, a significant relationship was observed between housing status, mother's age at marriage, infant's gender and maternal postpartum depression (**Table 5**).

Logistic regression model showed no significant relationship between father's age, father's occupation, education level, economic status, preterm infant, birth weight, gestational age, history of infant hospitalization, history of hospitalization in NICU, planned pregnancy according to mother, planned pregnancy according to father, planned infant's gender according to mother and planned infant's gender according to father and paternal postpartum depression. But according to this model, a significant relationship was observed between housing status, mother's age at marriage, infant's gender and maternal postpartum depression (**Table 6**).

Table 1. Data collected from demographic characteristics of parents of preterm and term infants.

Birth type Demographic data	Term	Preterm	Result
Parental age:	**mean (SD)**	**mean (SD)**	
Mother	28.22 ± 4.54	27.6 ± 6.25	p = 0.53 (t-test)
Father	32.83 ± 4.83	31.78 ± 6.22	p = 0.23 (t-test)
Parental education:(High school)	**N/(%)**		
Mother	42 (51.2)	36 (43.9)	p = 0.88 **(Mann-Whitney U)**
Father	24 (29.3)	54 (65.9)	p < 0.001 **(Mann-Whitney U)**
Parental job:	**N/(%)**		
Mother(housewife)	69 (84.1)	69 (84.1)	p = 1 (Chi-Square test)
Father (self-employed)	57 (69.5)	64 (78)	p = 0.21 (Chi-Square test)
Family's income level (self-employed)/N/(%)	34 (41.5)	38 (46.3)	p = 0.056 (Mann-Whitney U)
Mother's marriage mean age (SD)	20.63 ± 3.4	20.23 ± 3.6	p = 0.46 (t-test)

Table 2. Obstetric characteristics of parents of preterm and term infants and characteristics of newborns.

Birth type Pregnancy information	Term N/(%)	Preterm N/(%)	Result
First pregnancy	37 (45.1)	40 (48.8)	p = 0.71 (Mann-Whitney U)
Live child	39 (47.6)	43 (52.4)	p = 0.87 (Mann-Whitney U)
Abortion	15 (81.7)	22 (62.8)	p = 0.19 (Chi-Square)
Stillbirth	6 (7.3)	11 (13.4)	p = 0.2 (Chi-Square)
Natural childbirth	38 (46.3)	47 (57.3)	p = 0.11 (Chi-Square)
Mother's point of view about wanting pregnancy	64 (78)	51 (61.2)	p = 0.01 (Chi-Square)
Father's point of view about wanting pregnancy	64 (78)	47 (57.3)	p = 0.03 (Chi-Square)
Failure of contraceptive methods	10 (12.2)	23 (28)	p = 0.01 (Chi-Square)
Baby sex (son)	50 (61)	45 (54.9)	p = 0.42 (Chi-Square)
hospitalization's need	9 (11)	48 (58.5)	p < 0.001 (Fisher-Exact test)
NICU hospitalization	3 (3.7)	43 (52.4)	p < 0.001 (Chi-Square)
paying costs ability	80 (97.6)	70 (85.4)	p = 0.01 (Fisher-Exact test)

Table 3. Data collected about frequency distribution (absolute and relative) of Depression in mothers of both groups.

Birth type Mother's Depression	Term N (%)	Preterm N (%)	χ^2
Yes	21 (25.6)	20 (24.4)	p = 0/85
N/A	61 (74.4)	62 (75.6)	

Table 4. Data collected about frequency distribution (absolute and relative) of Depression in fathers of both groups.

Birth type Father's Depression	Term N (%)	Preterm N (%)	χ^2
Non depressed	75 (91.5)	66 (80.5)	p = 0/045
Mild depression	4 (4.9)	10 (12.2)	
Moderate depression	3 (3/7)	5 (6/1)	
Severe depression	0	1 (1/2)	

4. Discussion and Conclusion

Mental disorders such as depression include a wide range of disorders that can have a profound impact on people lives and interactions. Therefore, early diagnosis of these disorders can lead to faster treatment and improved quality of life. Mental disorders have examined parents of preterm infants in few studies and in most of the studies, fathers' condition evaluation is neglected.

The results of the this study in terms of depression are not consistent with those of Gambina *et al.* in 2011, which was conducted to compare the levels of stress, anxiety, and depression in preterm and term infant's mothers. In their study, mothers of delayed preterm infants experienced more depression than term infants' mothers [13].

The results of this study in terms of maternal depression is consistent with the results of Gary *et al.* in 2012, in Australia ,which was conducted with the goal of determining the parental stress levels and mental health in very preterm infants' mothers compared to mothers of term infants. In their study, no differences were observed between mothers of term and preterm infants in the results of the Edinburgh Postpartum Depression Scale. The difference between the methodology used by Gary and ours is that, we issued the questionnaires to the participants two months after birth to assess parents' mental disorders, but they did so 4 months after delivery. Furthermore, Gary *et al.* examined only mothers' mental state and fathers' mental state was neglected. Participants

Table 5. Depression of mothers in Logistic regression model.

	B coefficient	Expected B (OR)	p-value	CI B coefficient
Mothers age	0.615	1.849	0.046	1.1012 - 3.379
Mother's job	−1.279	0.276	0.278	0.028 - 2.782
father's job	0.493	1.638	0.380	0.544 - 4/931
Mother's education	−0.406	0.666	0.096	0.413 - 1.075
Marriage age	−0.486	0.615	0.048	0.380 - 0.995
Economic statue	−0.228	0.796	0/419	0.457 - 1.385
House statue	1.469	4.347	0.016	1.310 - 14.430
Number of pregnancy	0.069	1.072	0.781	0.659 - 1.743
prematurity	−0.323	0.724	0.538	0.259 - 2.024
Sex of baby	1.122	3.071	0.023	1.168 - 8.075
Birth weight	0.252	1.286	0.428	0.690 - 2.396
Gestational age	−0.104	0.901	0.836	0.337 - 2.413
Baby hospitalization	−1.041	0.353	0.158	0.83 - 1.496
NICU hospitalization	1.865	6.455	0.053	0.978 - 42.598
Wanted pregnancy from mother's viewpoint	−0.150	0.861	0.787	0.290 - 2.554
Wanted pregnancy from father's viewpoint	0.605	1.831	0.308	0.573 - 5.850
Wanted baby gender from mother's view	−0.327	0.721	0.633	0.188 - 2.763
Wanted baby gender from father's view	−0.479	0.536	0.620	0.136 - 2.817

Table 6. Depression of fathers in Logistic regression model.

	B coefficient	Expected B (OR)	p-value	CI B coefficient
Father's age	0.174	1.190	0.430	0.772 - 1.835
Father's job	−0.378	0.685	0.545	0.202 - 2.326
Father's education	−0.630	0.532	0.008	0.335 - 0.847
House statue	0.302	1.353	0.596	0.443 - 4.132
prematurity	−0.964	0.381	0.372	0.046 - 3.164
Sex of baby	0.709	2.032	0.136	0.799 - 5.167
Birth weight	0.427	1.532	0.209	0.788 - 2.979
Gestational age	−0.87	0.917	0.863	0.343 - 2.450
Baby hospitalization	−0.14	0.986	0.988	0.158 - 6.171
NICU hospitalization	−1.332	0.264	0.210	0.033 - 2.123
Wanted pregnancy from father's viewpoint	0.932	2.540	0.106	0.821 - 7.855
Wanted pregnancy from mother's viewpoint	1.011	2.748	0.058	0.967 - 7.803
Wanted baby gender from father's viewpoint	−0.301	0.740	0.662	0.192 - 2.851
Wanted baby gender from mother's view	−0.103	0.903	0.883	0.229 - 3.558

in the study of Gary *et al.* included mothers of infants delivered at 24 - 30 weeks gestation and they have infants were hospitalized to the Neonatal Intensive Care Unit. In the present study, mothers of preterm infants have babies with gestational age of 32 - 36 weeks and only 52.4% of them hospitalized in NICU [14].

Findings of the current research in terms of depression are not consistent with the research findings of Yurdakul *et al.* in 2009, which was conducted to assess symptoms of depression and anxiety and attachment of mother to baby in NICU. They concluded that the number of mothers with higher scores of depression in NICU was significantly more than mothers in the control group, but no difference was observed between anxiety and the type of mother's relationship and attachment of mother with infant. Yurdakul *et al.* have some differences with the present study in terms of mothers of infants admitted to Neonatal Intensive Care Units. A mother with a healthy term baby, participated as a control group. in the study Furthermore, STAI scale was used to evaluate anxiety and the research data were collected from mothers whose babies were in NICU [15].

To the best of our knowledge, no study was found that examined parents' agreement on unintended pregnancy and only a few studies investigated the relationship between unintended pregnancy and postpartum depression.

Al-Dallal *et al.* conducted a cross-sectional descriptive study in 2012 on 250 Bahraini Arab women who attended primary health care centers 8 weeks after delivery to screen their newborn. In this study, participants were randomly selected. The Arabic Edinburgh Postnatal Depression Scale was used for screening symptoms of postpartum depression. A researcher-made questionnaire was used to reflect demographic, maternal, newborn and psychological risk factors for postpartum depression. The significance level was considered 5%. With regard to demographic data, no significant relationship was observed between depression score ≥ 12, and mother's age at marriage, education level, parents' occupation, mother's marital status or the presence of another woman for their husbands. No significant relationship was seen between postpartum depressive symptoms, newborn gender, type of delivery, multiparity, prematurity, infant health status, history of neonatal death, separation from the infant, breastfeeding or breastfeeding problem. No significant relationship was observed between the score of postpartum depression and planned pregnancy, the time of previous pregnancy and pregnancy during contraceptive use [2].

Abdulbari Bener conducted a hospital-based study in 2013 and 1659 Arab women in the postpartum period participated in the study. The study was conducted in the form of face-to-face interviews by a researcher-made questionnaire containing questions about demographic and personal data, anthropometric measurements, medical history, and maternal characteristics. Depression, anxiety and stress were examined by Depression Anxiety Stress Scale (DASS-21). Depression and anxiety were significantly higher among preterm infants' mothers compared to term infants' mothers. Risk of depression in mothers of preterm infants that had low birth weight was two times more than term infants' mothers. While the risk of anxiety in mothers of preterm infants with low birth was 2.7 times more than term infants' mothers. Young mothers with low education level and less family income were more depressed and anxious after preterm birth than term infants' mothers. Psychological distress was higher in preterm infants' mothers [3].

Diababa *et al.* conducted a cohort study in 2013 in Ethiopia to investigate the relationship of unintended pregnancy during pregnancy, with social support and symptoms of depression. A total of 627 women participated in this study and the Edinburgh Postpartum Depression Scale was used to assess depressive symptoms during pregnancy. The relationship between independent variables and depressive symptoms during pregnancy was examined by multivariate logistic regression. Prevalence of depression symptoms during pregnancy was 19.9% and score of 13 was taken as cut of point. Women who reported their pregnancies as unintended were likely to experience depression symptoms almost twice more than women with planned pregnancy. Women who reported moderate levels of social support were less likely to report depressive symptoms [1].

Acknowledgements

This research is derived from the master thesis in the Shahid Beheshti Medical University. We appreciate the cooperation by honorable research deputy of university and all participants in this study.

Authors' Contribution

None declared.

Financial Disclosure

None declared.

Funding Support

We kindly express our gratitude to Research Deputy of Shahid Beheshti Medical University for providing the financial support.

References

[1] Dibaba, Y., Fantahun, M. and Hindin, M.J. (2013) The Association of Unwanted Pregnancy and Social Support with Depressive Symptoms in Pregnancy: Evidence from Rural Southwestern Ethiopia. *BMC Pregnancy and Childbirth*, **13**, 2-8.

[2] Al Dallal, F.H. and Grant, I.N. (2012) Postnatal Depression among Bahraini Women: Prevalence of Symptoms and Psychosocial Risk Factors. *Eastern Mediterranean Health Journal*, **18**, 439-445.

[3] Bener, A. (2013) Psychological Distress among Postpartum Mothers of Preterm Infants and Associated Factors: A Neglected Public Health Problems. *Revista Brasileira de Psiquiatria*, **35**, 231-236. http://dx.doi.org/10.1590/1516-4446-2012-0821

[4] Dolatian, M., Mirabzadeh, A., Forouzan, A.S., Sajjadi, H., Majd, H.A. and Moafi, F. (2013) Preterm Delivery and Psycho-Social Determinants of Health Based on World Health Organization Model in Iran: A Narrative Review. *Global Journal of Health Science*, **5**, 52-64.

[5] Melnyk, B.M., Crean, H.F., Feinstein, N.F. and Fairbanks, E. (2007) Maternal Anxiety and Depression after a Premature Infant's Discharge from the Neonatal Intensive Care Unit: Explanatory Effects of the Creating Opportunities for Parent Empowerment Program. *Nursing Research*, **57**, 383-394. http://dx.doi.org/10.1097/NNR.0b013e3181906f59

[6] Gray, P.H., Edwards, D.M., O'Callaghan, M.J. and Cuskelly, M. (2012) Parenting Stress in Mothers of Preterm Infants during Early Infancy. *Early Human Development*, **88**, 45-49. http://dx.doi.org/10.1016/j.earlhumdev.2011.06.014

[7] Beck, A.T., Steer, R.A. and Garbin, M.G. (1988) Psychometric Properties of the Beck Depression Inventory: Twenty-Five Years of Evaluation. *Clinical Psychology Review*, **8**, 77-100. http://dx.doi.org/10.1016/0272-7358(88)90050-5

[8] Kheirabadi, G.R., Maracy Mohammad, R., Akbaripour, S. and Masaeli, N. (2012) Psychometric Properties and Diagnostic Accuracy of the Edinburgh Postnatal Depression Scale in a Sample of Iranian Women. *Iranian Journal of Medical Sciences* (*IJMS*), **37**, 32-38.

[9] Dobson, K.S. and Mohammad Khani, P. (2007) Psychometric Characteristics Beck Depression Inventory-2 in a Large Sample of Patients with Major Depressive Disorder. *Iranian Journal of Rehabilitation in Mental Disorders*, **8**, 80-86.

[10] Azkhosh, M. (2008) Use of Psychiatric Tests and Clinical Diagnosis. 3rd Edition, Ravan, Tehran, 224-226.

[11] Gemmill, A., Leigh, B., Ericksen, J. and Milgrom, J. (2006) A Survey of the Clinical Acceptability of Screening for Postnatal Depression in Depressed and Non-Depressed Women. *BMC Public Health*, **6**, 1-8.

[12] Tesfaye, M., Hanlon, C., Wondimageqn, D. and Alem, A. (2010) Detecting Postnatal Common Mental Disorders in Addis Ababa, Ethiopia: Validation of the Edinburgh Postnatal Depression Scale and Kessler Scales. *Journal of Affective Disorders*, **122**, 102-108. http://dx.doi.org/10.1016/j.jad.2009.06.020

[13] Kamranpour, S.B. and Shakiba, M. (2012) Cesarean Section and Post Partum Depression. *Iranian Journal of Obstetrics, Gyneocology and Infertility*, **15**, 56-62.

[14] Gambina, I., Soldera, G., Benevento, B., Trivellato, P., Visentin, S., Cavallin, F., *et al.* (2011) Postpartum Psychosocial Distress and Late Preterm Delivery. *Journal of Reproductive and Infant Psychology*, **29**, 472-479. http://dx.doi.org/10.1080/02646838.2011.653962

[15] Yurdakul, Z., Akman, I., Kuscu, M.K., Karabekiroglu, A., Yaylali, G., Demir, F., *et al.* (2009) Maternal Psychological Problems Associated with Neonatal Intensive Care Admission. *International Journal of Pediatrics*, **5**, 35-39.

Permissions

All chapters in this book were first published in OJN, by Scientific Research Publishing; hereby published with permission under the Creative Commons Attribution License or equivalent. Every chapter published in this book has been scrutinized by our experts. Their significance has been extensively debated. The topics covered herein carry significant findings which will fuel the growth of the discipline. They may even be implemented as practical applications or may be referred to as a beginning point for another development.

The contributors of this book come from diverse backgrounds, making this book a truly international effort. This book will bring forth new frontiers with its revolutionizing research information and detailed analysis of the nascent developments around the world.

We would like to thank all the contributing authors for lending their expertise to make the book truly unique. They have played a crucial role in the development of this book. Without their invaluable contributions this book wouldn't have been possible. They have made vital efforts to compile up to date information on the varied aspects of this subject to make this book a valuable addition to the collection of many professionals and students.

This book was conceptualized with the vision of imparting up-to-date information and advanced data in this field. To ensure the same, a matchless editorial board was set up. Every individual on the board went through rigorous rounds of assessment to prove their worth. After which they invested a large part of their time researching and compiling the most relevant data for our readers.

The editorial board has been involved in producing this book since its inception. They have spent rigorous hours researching and exploring the diverse topics which have resulted in the successful publishing of this book. They have passed on their knowledge of decades through this book. To expedite this challenging task, the publisher supported the team at every step. A small team of assistant editors was also appointed to further simplify the editing procedure and attain best results for the readers.

Apart from the editorial board, the designing team has also invested a significant amount of their time in understanding the subject and creating the most relevant covers. They scrutinized every image to scout for the most suitable representation of the subject and create an appropriate cover for the book.

The publishing team has been an ardent support to the editorial, designing and production team. Their endless efforts to recruit the best for this project, has resulted in the accomplishment of this book. They are a veteran in the field of academics and their pool of knowledge is as vast as their experience in printing. Their expertise and guidance has proved useful at every step. Their uncompromising quality standards have made this book an exceptional effort. Their encouragement from time to time has been an inspiration for everyone.

The publisher and the editorial board hope that this book will prove to be a valuable piece of knowledge for researchers, students, practitioners and scholars across the globe.

List of Contributors

Noel D. Mbirimtengerenji
Kamuzu College of Nursing, University of Malawi, Lilongwe, Malawi

Oluyinka Adejumo
University of Western Cape, Cape Town, South Africa

Naohiro Hohashi and Junko Honda
Division of Family Health Care Nursing, Department of Nursing, Graduate School of Health Sciences, Kobe University, Kobe, Japan

Stig Jarwson, Merete Berg Nesset, Tom Palmstierna, Jim Aage Nottestad and Erik Søndenaa
St. Olavs Hospital, Forensic Department Brøset, Norwegian University of Science and Technology, Norway

Noel D. Mbirimtengerenji
Kamuzu College of Nursing, University of Malawi, Lilongwe, Malawi

Felicity Daniels and Penelope Martin
University of Western Cape, Bellville, South Africa

Thokozani Bvumbwe, Atupele Malema and Mep Chipeta
Faculty of Health Sciences, Mzuzu University, Mzuzu, Malawi

Christopher C. Griffin and Jonathan M. Cayce
DeRoyal Industries, Powell, TN, USA

Tammy Dean and Mary Anne Modrcin
Caylor School of Nursing, Lincoln Memorial University, Harrogate, TN, USA

Ronald Lagoe and Shelly Littau
Hospital Executive Council, Syracuse, NY, USA

Louise Pernisi
Upstate University Hospital, Syracuse, NY, USA

Yanli Zhao
Shanxi Cancer Hospital, Taiyuan, China

Ruifang Zhu
The First Hospital of Shanxi Medical University, Taiyuan, China

Elaine Amella, Martina Mueller and Jeannette Andrews
Medical University of South Carolina, Charleston, USA

Joy Wachs and Kimberly Sell
East Tennessee State University, Johnson City, USA

Mitsumi Masuda
Department of Critical Care Nursing, Graduate School of Nursing, Kitasato University, Tokyo, Japan

Hidenori Ohishi
Department of Medical Science, Graduate School of Medicine, Juntendo University, Tokyo, Japan

Noriko Terunuma and Ikuko Tojima
Nursing Department, Juntento University Hospital, Tokyo, Japan

Aud Moe, Aud Evensen, Karin Torvik and Hildfrid V. Brataas
Faculty of Health Science, Nord-Trøndelag University College, Steinkjer, Norway

Geraldine Jody Macdonald
Associate Professor, Teaching Stream, Bloomberg Faculty of Nursing, University of Toronto, Toronto, Canada

Brima Osaio Kamara, Rachel Rodriguez, Genesis Chorwe-Sungani and Angela Chimwaza
Kamuzu College of Nursing, University of Malawi, Blantyre, Malawi

Yi-Li Ko
Department of Nursing, College of Medicine, Fu Jen Catholic University, Taiwan

Wei-En Chu
Nurse, Kaohsiung Veterans General Hospital, Taiwan

Pi-Chu Lin
School of Nursing and Master Program in Long-Term Care, College of Nursing, Taipei Medical University, Taiwan

Anneli Pitkänen
Tampere University Hospital, Tampere, Finland

Raija Kontio
Helsinki University, Helsinki, Finland
Department of Psychiatry, Helsinki University Hospital, Helsinki, Finland

Mari Lahti
Turku University of Applied Science, Turku, Finland
Department of Nursing Science, University of Turku, Turku, Finland

Jouko Katajisto
Department of Statistics, University of Turku, Turku, Finland

Maritta Välimäki
Turku University Hospital, Turku, Finland

Amanda Hellström
Department of Health and Caring Sciences, Linnæus University, Kalmar, Sweden

Anna Condelius
Department of Health Sciences, Lund University, Lund, Sweden

Ania Willman
Department of Health, Blekinge Institute of Technology, Karlskrona, Sweden
Department of Care Science, Malmö University, Malmö, Sweden

Cecilia Fagerström
Department of Health, Blekinge Institute of Technology, Karlskrona, Sweden
Blekinge Centre of Competence, Karlskrona, Sweden

Zohreh Teimouri
Department of Midwifery, International branch of ShahidBeheshti University of Medical Sciences, Tehran, Iran

Mahrokh Dolatian
Department of Midwifery, School of nursing and midwifery, Shahid Beheshti University of Medical Sciences, Tehran, Iran

Sara Shishehgar
Faculty of Health, University of Technology, Sydney, Australia

Marjan Ajami
Department of Nutrition Iran University of Medical Sciences, Tehran, Iran

Hamid Alavi Majd
Department of Biostatistics, School of Paramedical Sciences, Shahid Beheshti University of Medical Sciences, Tehran, Iran

Birgitta Fläckman
Department of Health Care Sciences, Ersta Sköndal University College, Stockholm, Sweden

Kirsti Skovdahl
Faculty for Health Sciences, Buskerud and Vestfold University College, Drammen, Norway

Ingegerd Fagerberg
Department of Health Care Sciences, Ersta Sköndal University College, Stockholm, Sweden
Department of Neurobiology, Care Sciences and Society, Karolinska Institute, Stockholm, Sweden

Mona Kihlgren
Centre for Caring Sciences, Örebro University Hospital, Örebro, Sweden

Annica Kihlgren
School of Health and Medical Sciences, Örebro University, Örebro, Sweden

Yi-Li Ko
Department of Nursing, College of Medicine, Fu-Jen Catholic University, Taiwan

Pi-Chu Lin
School of Nursing and Master Program in Long-Term Care, College of Nursing, Taipei Medical University, Taiwan

Chi-Li Yang
Department of Physical Education, Shih Chien University, Taiwan

Chie-Pein Chen
Department of Obstetrics and Gynecology, Mackay Memorial Hospital, Taiwan

Huai-Jung Shih
Department of Dentistry, University of Szeged, Szeged, Hungary

Insook Lee, Kyung-Sook Bang, Sungjae Kim and Heeseung Choi
College of Nursing, The Research Institute of Nursing Science, Seoul National University, Seoul, Korea

Inju Hwang
College of Nursing, Seoul National University, Seoul, Korea

Izabel Cristina Falcão Juvenal Barbosa, Ana Fátima Carvalho Fernandes, Camila Brasil Moreira, Míria Conceição Lavinas Santos, Altamira Mendonça Félix Gomes, Ivna Silva Andrade and Anna Paula Sousa da Silva
Department of Nursing, Federal University of Piauí, Floriano, Piauí, Brazil

Guobadia Pauline Ojekou
School of Occupational Health Nursing, University College Hospital, Ibadan, Nigeria

Odetola Titilayo Dorothy
Department of Nursing, University of Ibadan, Ibadan, Nigeria

Ana Talyne Pessoa, Beatriz da Silva Lima, Lorita Marlena Freitag Pagliuca, Paulo César de Almeida, Luciana Vieira de Carvalho and Aline Cruz Esmeraldo Áfio
Departamento de Enfermagem, Universidade Federal do Ceará, Fortaleza, Brasil

Paula Marciana Pinheiro de Oliveira and Leilane Barbosa de Sousa
Universidade Internacional da Integração da Lusofonia Afro-Brasileira, Fortaleza, Brasil

Huaxia Liu, Hongwei Shi and Qianqian Yang
School of Nursing, Taishan Medical University, Taian, China

Aletha Rowlands
School of Nursing, West Virginia University, Morgantown, USA

Minghua Han
Taishan Vocational College of Nursing, Taian, China

Filip Málek and Dagmar Vondráková
Department of Cardiology, Na Homolce Hospital, Prague, Czech Republic
Third School of Medicine, Charles University, Prague, Czech Republic

Oxana Komendová, Dana Říhová, Táňa Andreasová and Petr Neužil
Department of Cardiology, Na Homolce Hospital, Prague, Czech Republic

Jana Vránová
Third School of Medicine, Charles University, Prague, Czech Republic

Lenka Sedláčková
Department of Clinical Biochemistry, Haematology and Immunology, Na Homolce Hospital, Prague, Czech Republic

AChiharu Miyata
Department of Human Health Sciences, Kyoto University Graduate School of Medicine, Kyoto, Japan

Hidenori Arai
National Center for Geriatrics and Gerontology, Obu, Aichi, Japan

Sawako Suga
Department of Health Sciences, Kyoto Tachibana University, Kyoto, Japan

Utako Shimizu, Momoe Sakagami, Mieko Uchiyama and Hagiko Aoki
School of Sciences Faculty of Medicine, Niigata University, Niigata, Japan

Annica Kihlgren
School of Health and Medical Sciences, Örebro University, Örebro, Sweden

Mieko Uchiyama, Yongbum Lee, Utako Shimizu and Rika Saitoh
Graduate School of Health Sciences, Niigata University, Niigata, Japan

Nina Berger Hustad
Division of Cancer Medicine, Surgery and Transplantation, Oslo University Hospital, Norway

Ragnhild Hellesø
Faculty of Medicine, Institute of Health and Society, University of Oslo, Norway

Marit Helen Andersen
Division of Cancer Medicine, Surgery and Transplantation, Oslo University Hospital, Norway
Faculty of Medicine, Institute of Health and Society, University of Oslo, Norway

Maryam Ghorbani
Shahid Beheshti University of Medical Sciences, Tehran, Iran

Mahrokh Dolatian
Department of Reproductive Health and Midwifery, School of Nursing and Midwifery, Shahid Beheshti University of Medical Sciences, Tehran, Iran

Jamal Shams
Department of Psychiatry, Behavioral Research Center, Shahid Beheshti University of Medical Sciences, Tehran, Iran

Hamid Alavi-Majd
Department of Biostatistics, School of Paramedical Sciences, Shahid Beheshti University of Medical Sciences, Tehran, Iran